Speaking of Apraxia

Speaking of Apraxia

A Parents' Guide to Childhood Apraxia of Speech

Leslie A. Lindsay, R.N., B.S.N.

Woodbine House ■ 2012

Cataloging-in-Publication Data

Lindsay, Leslie A.
  Speaking of apraxia : a parents' guide to childhood apraxia of speech / Leslie A. Lindsay. -- 1st ed.
    p. cm.
  Includes bibliographical references and index.
  ISBN 978-1-60613-061-2
  1. Speech disorders in children. 2. Apraxia. I. Title.
  RJ496.S7L55 2012
  618.92'855--dc23

                                                                                    2012002581

Manufactured in the United States of America

10 9   8   7   6   5   4   3   2

To Kate Riley—
my sweet, smart, and incredibly creative daughter.
Without you, I wouldn't have found my writing voice as easily.
For you, I give you a voice so that you may accomplish
whatever *your* heart desires.

To all those sweet voices yet to be heard...
their loving parents, grandparents,
speech-language pathologists, and teachers.

Table of Contents

. . . .

Preface

. . . .

I am not an expert, but I am a mom and I am concerned. When my sweet, fun, and beautiful daughter was diagnosed with Childhood Apraxia of Speech (CAS) at the age of two and a half, I didn't even know what it was, let alone know what to do about it.

What is Childhood Apraxia of Speech (CAS)? What caused it? What can we do about it? Not only did I have these questions, but additional concerns as well. I wondered how this would affect her social life, and how it would affect mine. I feared that CAS would hold her back academically as well.

Once I got over my initial shock—after about six months or so—I hit the local library in search of resources. I'm old-school at heart, and searching the Internet (although a wonderful resource) just didn't appeal to me. The friendly, grandfatherly librarian found one measly resource for me—a chapter within a book which just barely touched on CAS. Instead of offering a hands-on, practical education approach, it was focused primarily on nutritional aspects of treatment. As a *nurse*, I wanted something more *scientific*. As a *child-adolescent psychiatric nurse*, I wanted something more *holistic*. As a *mom*, I wanted something more *sympathetic*.

When I asked my daughter's speech-language pathologist (SLP) for recommended reading, she scratched her head and said, "There's not a lot out there, but I'll look into it." Her search came up with next to nothing.

Determined, motivated, and always looking for an excuse to learn, I decided that if there was to be a book about CAS written for parents, it was to be written by me.

So, I got started—and here it is!

Acknowledgements

I cannot thank enough the individuals who have helped this book go from idea to bookshelf. Special thanks to our speech-language pathologists, Jennifer Usher-Carr and Sylvia Garland, for "planting the seed" and for taking such good care of my girls' speech disorder. Special thanks also to Karin Sudlow, CCC-SLP, of Suburban Pediatric Therapies in Aurora, Illinois, for believing in me and allowing me to design and facilitate "Small Talk: All About Apraxia" through your clinic. Many thanks to parents, grandparents, teachers, and music therapists who attended those groups and provided me with insights and challenged my knowledge on Childhood Apraxia of Speech (CAS)—you got me thinking, writing, and researching your questions!

My deepest gratitude goes to my review board: Diane (Di) Bahr, CCC-SLP, Rhonda Banford, CCC-SLP, Lisa Circelli, M.Ed., Morgan Holubetz, CCC-SLP, Teri Kaminski Peterson, CCC-SLP, and Amy Moll. Thank you to Diane Nancarrow, CCC-SLP, of the Kaufman Center for reading an early version of some chapters. I also am quite appreciative of Tony Ebel, D.C., who took the time to provide some direction on chiropractic care, Kimberly Sena-Moore, BC-MT, for providing some "rhythm" to the music therapy section, and Emily Sevcik, MT-BC, for her assistance and willingness to attend *Small Talk: All About Apraxia* and provide parents with hints and tips on the value of music therapy. Thanks to Dr. Larry Shriberg who took a peek at the genetics connection to CAS. My sincerest thanks goes to Lloyd Wells, M.D., Ph.D., of the Child/Adolescent Treatment Program at the Mayo Clinic—my former workplace—for his review of the co-morbid conditions presented in Appendix A.

Also, thanks to Ruth Stoeckel, Ph.D., CCC-SLP, for review of portions of this book and her willingness to respond to my many email questions, as well as to Margaret (Dee) Fish, CCC-SLP, and Kathy Jakielski, Ph.D., CCC-SLP, for their support and suggestions for additional resources in writing this book (so glad I was introduced to you both at the 2009 CASANA conference in St. Charles, Illinois).

My understanding of CAS has been strengthened by my involvement in the Apraxia-KIDS listserv and the Windy City Apraxia Network, as well as through the connections I have developed through those organizations—you all are amazing individuals who care so deeply for children with CAS.

To those folks at Woodbine House—especially Susan Stokes—for seeing a need for such a book; thank you for giving me a place to share my knowledge on Childhood Apraxia of Speech and my desire to help others. My appreciation also goes to the staff at Eola Family Chiropractic for helping to "work out the kinks," literally and figuratively.

Of course, I couldn't have written this book without my precious little girls, Kate and Kelly. Thank you both for the inspiration, love, and understanding when I "take too long, mommy" at the library or coffee shop (thank you, Caribou Coffee for keeping me "grounded" in more ways than one). And most of all to my loving husband, Jim, for his support and encouragement. Sorry I missed out on afternoon snacks of popcorn and doughnuts and hiking in the woods, but without my weekly dose of "mom time alone," this book would not have gotten this far.

—Leslie A. Lindsay
Chicago, Illinois

How This Book Is Organized

You're a parent. You're short on time. You want answers and encouragement. Yesterday. I know. I have been there.

The good news is, you will find some answers here. Maybe not all of them, but at least a good amount. And if you don't find the answers you thought you would, don't worry; there is a section at the end of every chapter that points you in the right direction for further study. I call it ***Read On! Recommended Resources.***

But let's start at the beginning. Most chapters start with an anecdote about one of my family experiences relevant to the chapter. The characters you will come across are real and important to me. There is Kate—redheaded and blue-eyed, spunky, and smart, and yes—she has Childhood Apraxia of Speech (CAS). Kelly is my little precocious one, also redheaded and blue-eyed and once did express some symptoms consistent with CAS. My husband, Jim—Kate and Kelly's dad—and my rock. You may read, laugh, and cry at these introductions and completely relate to them, or you may skip them. Hopefully, they will give you a sense that "I've been there, too" and help you feel a little less alone on your journey to come to grips with CAS.

The Nuts and Bolts of This Chapter sections break the chapter down into tangible bullet points. You can glance over the list and see if "your" topic will be covered.

You will find sections and text boxes called:

➤ **What's a Parent to Do?**—offering a step-by-step approach to dealing with particular concern
➤ **Parents Cope**—helping you reframe a troubling moment

➤ **What Can You Do at Home?**—giving you a quick and simple activity you can do at home to help your child with apraxia. In fact, there is an entire chapter devoted to this topic, but you will still find these suggestions popping up in most chapters.

➤ **Parents Share**—giving you some insight and quotes from parents who have been right where you are now

I have talked to parents. Lots of them. Most have a child with apraxia. Some have children with other special needs. All of them love their children more than anything else in the world. They want to help you. You will find quotes from them offering *real-world advice, tips, or ideas.* There are other sections sprinkled throughout the book in the form of "Parents ask." These are questions I have heard often in this apraxia journey. Some of them I have asked myself! Following each question is a quick-and-easy answer.

I have talked to speech-language pathologists, too. Lots of them. Some are in private practice, others work within school districts, and still others are in research at universities. They know what they are talking about. Their advice and studies are peppered throughout the book.

Finally, I facilitated a support and education group in the Chicagoland area called Small Talk: All About Apraxia. Parents and grandparents came. They asked questions. I learned a lot about what is on your mind related to Childhood Apraxia of Speech. Parents from the group were kind enough to let me use some of the information they shared in the hopes that it may help another—you!

What Should You Do with This Book?

➤ Skim the book, decide where you want to start.
➤ You don't have to start at the beginning. Feel free to pick the chapters that you feel you need most.
➤ Come back to the ones you don't need just yet. Someday you may.
➤ If you have questions, ask your SLP or pediatrician or email me at: leslie_lindsay@hotmail.com.
➤ What are you waiting for? Turn the page... .

Tell Me More

The Straight Scoop On Speech Basics

Chapter One

Does My Child Have Childhood Apraxia of Speech?

At two years old, Kate was a beautiful, energetic, and happy toddler. But with the exception of one word—hi—Kate was as quiet as a mouse. We wondered if something was wrong. Even as a baby, Kate rarely babbled and cried; she was beautiful and unique with red hair and bright blue eyes. She was, in a word, "perfect." So why were we worried? After all, she could understand everything we said, even the big words.

"Play classical music. Dance with her. Babies need that so their brains can develop," others told us. And so we did. We talked to her as if she was a little adult, making conversations even though we didn't expect answers.

"She'll talk when she's ready," my mom-friends assured me. Only their toddlers were saying words like "elephant," and when we met at the park, I cringed and rolled my lips into a tight line, sucking in a deep breath.

Was Kate stressed because of her new sibling or our impending move? No, that wasn't it. We were providing her with a loving, stable environment. So, what was it? I was confused and frustrated.

*Sarah, age 2, was a puzzle to her parents. She was obviously quite bright and alert. She knew the names of all the birds in her **Big Book of Birds** and would point to the cardinal, chickadee, etc. when asked. But she struggled to say even the simplest words.*

Jake was an active three-year-old who loved cause and effect toys, an engineer in the making. He appeared to be a typically-developing child, with one exception: he was not talking. His grandmother kept saying, "Boys are late to talk—don't worry." But his parents were concerned. Could something else be going on?

Do these stories sound familiar? Does your child remind you of Kate or Sarah or Jake? If so, your child could have Childhood Apraxia of Speech (CAS).

I'll admit, when I first heard of Childhood Apraxia of Speech, I was totally stumped. We hadn't covered *this* in nursing school! So what *is* CAS, anyway? Like you, I had a ton of questions and concerns and little time to learn about it. But most of all—my child needed help. You may be feeling the same way.

The Nuts and Bolts of This Chapter

➤ A discussion on what CAS is, as outlined by the American Speech and Hearing Association

➤ A list of symptoms and red-flags related to CAS

➤ Terminology concerns—why are there so many names to represent one phenomenon?!

➤ Discussions on prevalence, intelligence, boys vs. girls, the likelihood of having CAS, as well as your child's future as it relates to communication.

Perhaps you have already been given a diagnosis of Childhood Apraxia of Speech (CAS) but are still searching for information to help you and your child cope with the condition (if that's the case, feel free to skip this chapter). Or, perhaps you are struggling to figure out exactly why your child isn't speaking in the same manner as other children her age. Perhaps you are wondering if it could be CAS.

What Is Childhood Apraxia of Speech?

Childhood Speech Apraxia (CAS), as most pediatric speech-language pathologists (SLPs) in the U.S. call it*, is best defined by what it is not. Historically, it's been one of the most debated disorders in the field of speech-language pathology. It took practitioners quite some time to find an easy, agreed-upon definition, list of symptoms, cause, and treatment. But they did!

If we were to define CAS in a table format, it would look something like this:

---

* Elsewhere in the world, the disorder is often referred to as Verbal Dyspraxia.

CAS IS NOT:	CAS IS:
A muscular disorder	A neurologically-based motor speech *disorder*, not a delay
A cognitive disorder	A neurobehavioral disorder
A developmental delay	A *disruption* in spatio-temporal parameters of speech movement (difficulty moving articulators—lips, jaw, tongue— through space with correct timing for accurate sequencing of sounds)
	Dynamic, ever changing
	Multifaceted

It's not a black and white answer. If this is still a bit confusing, don't lose heart.

The American Speech-Language-Hearing Association (ASHA) offers the following 2007 definition of CAS:

> *"A neurological childhood (pediatric) speech sound disorder in which precision and consistency of movements underlying speech are impaired in the absence of neuromuscular deficits."*

Let's break this down even more:

➤ *Neurological*—refers to the nervous system (brain and spinal cord to start with).
➤ *Childhood/pediatric*—generally refers to the ages of birth to adolescence.
➤ *Precision and consistency*—refer to the accuracy of speech sounds each and every time they are spoken.
➤ *Movements underlying speech*—refers to the movements of the articulators (lips, jaw, tongue, soft palate, hard palate) in smooth, sequential, and overlapping gestures necessary for intelligible speech.
➤ The *oral structures of the mouth*—are tongue, lips, jaw, and palate.
➤ *Neuromuscular deficits*—are things like abnormal reflexes and weakness and difficulties coordinating the muscles that are controlled by the brain to produce speech movements.

In plain language, kids who have been diagnosed with "pure" CAS have completely normal facial tone and musculature. Their reflexes are *typically* normal, yet they still can't coordinate their internal thoughts, shape them into verbal communication, and produce it in a manner we can all understand. ("Pure" refers to the fact that these children have no other neuro-developmental conditions; they are struggling with only

CAS.) So, when my daughter Kate would attempt to answer a simple question of what she wanted to do for the day, she knew what *she wanted to say, she just couldn't get her mouth to cooperate with her ideas.* She would go to the back door, dangle her shoes, and point in the general direction of the park. "Eh-eh?" She would say. Our little girl couldn't say "park," even when we asked her to *and* modeled the correct word, "Oh, you want to go to the *park*. Can you say, '*park?*'" Yet, we knew what she wanted, and so did she. (Of course, every child with CAS says things uniquely. Another child might be able to say "-ark" for park, thus making it much easier to piece together what she wants.)

The folks who wrote the *ASHA Technical Report on CAS* would impress upon us parents that when SLPs give the diagnosis of CAS, they are ruling out any weakness, decreased range of motion, low muscle tone, and coordination difficulties as contributing factors to your child's CAS. These children can still possibly have co-occurring (in addition to; also having) speech and language conditions such as dysarthria, phonological errors, and low tone. Children with CAS may also have developmental disabilities such as autism or Down syndrome, among others.

The problem with CAS occurs when the brain tries to tell the muscles what to do and the message gets scrambled somehow. The child typically knows what she wants to say, but her brain is not sending the correct instructions to move the mouth the way it should move. Thus, motor execution is affected. Words may or may not come out… and if they do, they are often unintelligible.

Generally speaking, the more a child with CAS *wants* to communicate, either to meet a need or to express something creatively, the harder it is for her. Automatic speech is easier. That is, the child hasn't stopped to think, "I want to say 'hi' when I see Grandma." She *knows* the word and *knows* it's socially polite to say hello as a greeting. She hasn't mentally planned on saying the word; it just happens that she says it at the right time. Sometimes a word or a phrase will just "pop" out and it may never happen again. In fact, Judy Jelm, CCC-SLP, a clinician in private practice in Naperville, Illinois, has coined the term "phrases out-of-the-blue" to describe this phenomenon in children with CAS.

Phrase Popping

I remember this "phrase popping" happening only once with my daughter Kate (diagnosed with CAS at the age of two and a half). It occurred when I was changing her diaper one day when she was just under two years old. In a hopeful moment of trying to teach independence and responsibility, I handed her the diaper all rolled up and asked, "What should we do with this?" I wasn't *really* expecting an answer, but she surprised me.

"Put it in the trash!" I heard it clear as day, as did Papa, who was within earshot. Little Kate toddled off, diaper in hand to the trashcan. We never heard so much from her again until years down the road.

Frustrating and discouraging, yes? If *you* are feeling these emotions, then imagine how your child might be feeling.

According to Dr. Kathy Jakielski, associate professor of the Department of Communication Sciences Disorders and certified speech pathologist at Augustana College in Rock Island, Illinois: "Children with CAS live with having to think about, practice, and sequence their words. When they're speaking, they are thinking about coordinating all of those movements that require motor planning."

One mom I spoke with summed it up this way: "Having apraxia is like trying to learn a foreign language." You have an idea of how things *should* sound, but you can't carry on a conversation in that language until you first master the letter sounds and basic words and *then* string them into sentences, and then—maybe even at the same time—"get" the grammar and meaning of all of the words. Only then can you become fluent in that foreign language. Oh, and of course you need to be able to practice that language a lot with others who also speak it.

Symptoms of CAS

Children with CAS often have a history of delayed speech development. They often come from families who have a history of speech or learning problems, but they can also be the first member in their family with the disorder. CAS is slightly more likely to occur in boys than girls, but it is still plenty common in girls. Below are some other warning signs, or red-flags to be aware of. Note that the defining characteristics will depend on the child's developmental age. The range of problems often unfolds as the child progresses. Ages presented here are meant to be general guidelines.

Warning Signs of CAS

Warning Signs in Infancy (Birth to Age 1)

- [ ] There is decreased cooing or babbling. Others comment on what a "quiet baby" you have.
- [ ] May have feeding difficulties.
- [ ] Your baby's first words appear late (after 14 months) or not at all.
- [ ] If first words *do* appear, they are often "easy," sounds (phonemes) replaced with even *easier* ones. For example, "hi" might sound like "I," but is used in a greeting context.

Warning Signs in Early Childhood (Age 1 to 3)

- [ ] Understands most of what is said, but cannot verbalize well. Large gap between receptive and expressive language.
- [ ] Cannot correctly use sounds.
- [ ] Difficulty imitating words and phrases (please see Chapter 7 for more information on imitation).

❏ Messy and distractible eating. Requires prompts to take a bite, chew, swallow, and drink; may overstuff or "pocket" food in the cheeks. Hyper- or hyposensitivity to oral activities such as eating different textures of foods or brushing teeth; difficulty identifying an object in the mouth through touch.

❏ Prosody (melody) of speech is affected. Also may only be able to repeat a word/sound/phrase in the context of a practiced routine; may "lose" words, and may have inability to repeat words when asked.

❏ May have developed elaborate nonverbal or gestural communication.

❏ Struggles with speech; "searching" (groping) for the right word.

❏ Leaves sounds out of words (e.g., "cookie" becomes "coo-ie").

❏ The longer the phrase attempted, the less understandable the child becomes.

Warning Signs at Any Age

Neurological problems (problems that affect cognition, body mechanics, or the sensory system) may occur with a variety of childhood conditions. Those that may accompany CAS include:

❏ The child often gestures and grunts in lieu of oral communication.

❏ Gross motor skills (running, jumping, climbing) may also be slow in developing.

❏ The child appears clumsy or uncoordinated, has poor body awareness (proprioception), or difficulty with fine motor skills (holding a pencil, using scissors).

❏ IQ testing shows high performance IQ (doing tasks) and low verbal IQ (talking tasks).

❏ Poor sequencing (the child has difficulties putting a series of movements in order—e.g., figuring out how to get on an unfamiliar piece of playground equipment, or sequencing events to relate to others).

❏ The child has poor auditory processing (listening and reacting appropriately) and others must repeat themselves often.

❏ Greater difficulties in learning to read, spell, and write.

❏ Difficulty with a variety of components of speech (pitch, quality, rate, etc.).

❏ Correctly saying "difficult" words is, well…difficult (e.g., "butterfly," "rocking chair," "exercise").

❏ The child can make the sound(s) of many letters when the letter is alone, but when combined in a sentence, will not be able to say it.

❏ Limited (correct) use of vowels and consonants.

❏ May have developed elaborate nonverbal and gestural communication.

❏ Family history of delayed language development, as well as a family propensity to have other learning problems.

Different Names, Same Thing?

Childhood Apraxia of Speech (CAS) has many different names. Curious as to what they are? These historical terms are reported in Joseph Duffy's 1995 text, *Motor Speech Disorders:*

➤ Developmental Dyspraxia
➤ Developmental Verbal Dyspraxia
➤ Developmental Aphasia
➤ Developmental Apraxia of Speech
➤ Dyspraxic Dysarthria
➤ Verbal Apraxia
➤ Oral Verbal Apraxia
➤ Developmental Verbal Apraxia
➤ Childhood Aphasia
➤ Executive Aphasia
➤ Congenital Articulatory Aphasia
➤ Dilapidated Speech
➤ Articulatory Apraxia
➤ Articulatory Dyspraxia
➤ Phonetic Disintegration
➤ Afferent Motor Aphasia
➤ Efferent Motor Aphasia
➤ Little Broca's Aphasia
➤ Ataxic Aphasia
➤ Sensorimotor Impairment
➤ Minimal Brain Dysfunction/Disorder
➤ Pure Motor Aphasia
➤ Speech Sound Muteness

(Note that **Apraxia and Aphasia are NOT the same thing!** In the hundred or more years before the terminology was standardized, a variety of labels were used that have now taken on different meanings.)

Why are all of these terms important to know? Well, as a curious parent, a studious scholar, or treating clinician, you will likely do some literature searches on the condition. Your librarian, your brain, and your search engine will get quite the workout as you type in all of these terms to get the information you want. Why so many different terms to describe one phenomenon? What many of these terms have in common is the root word "praxis." **Praxis** can be defined as planned movement, and **apraxia** is the *lack* of planned movement. Need a little more?

Sally Goddard, author of *Reflexes, Learning and Behavior,* identifies praxis as: "The brain's ability to select responses, arrange them in an appropriate order and orient them for proper execution." Therefore, one can assume that **apraxia** ("without praxia") *is the inability to select and arrange responses for proper execution, even though no motor paralysis exists.*

Besides apraxia of speech, which affects planning responses for speech, there are also other types of apraxias. One is *limb apraxia,* which causes difficulty moving the arms and legs in meaningful and purposeful ways. For example, a child may *want* to catch a ball, but simply cannot because her body and brain aren't working together. *Oral apraxia* is when a child is capable of puckering, smiling, blowing bubbles, etc., but simply can't when asked to do so. A child with CAS may also have limb apraxia or oral apraxia, but she may not.

Praxis may also be referred to as "motor planning." In this case, a motor skill is a highly refined pattern of movement performed automatically, and no longer requiring constant attention or reminders. It just happens. Typing on a keyboard is one such example.

ASHA's Official Stand on Terminology

In 2007, the American Speech-Language-Hearing Association (ASHA) released its important position paper on the terminology of CAS. Every parent of a child with CAS should have a copy. You can get one here: www.asha.org/docs/html/ TR2007-00278.html. While there wasn't universal agreement on the terminology, the paper made an impact and now (in the U.S.) we have just one term (CAS) instead of multiple.

How Do I Know If My Child Has CAS?

Just because your child has *some* of the symptoms listed above does not necessarily mean that she has CAS. Many childhood conditions can cause symptoms similar to those in CAS. And there are children who have no speech or language disorder at all who may display some of the listed symptoms when they are young. Please, if you have any concerns, it is best to seek advice—and an evaluation—from a licensed speech-language pathologist.

All speech and language disorders and delays are not treated the same, which makes it essential to pinpoint what is causing your child's speech-language concerns. There are other motor-speech disorders that may look like CAS. They are:

> *Dysarthria*—Caused by central or peripheral nervous system damage resulting in weakness, paralysis, or incoordination of the speech muscles themselves. Looks like: slurred speech, soft/whispery speech, slowed speech, limited tongue/jaw movement, abnormal rhythm, nasal or stuffy sounding speech.

> *Stuttering*—An interruption in forward flow of speech production. Also called "dysfluency." A child may really struggle to get the words out, stopping the flow of speech and often appearing as though she has gotten "stuck."

Or, you may find that your child has:

> *(An) Expressive Language Delay*—A delay in what a child is able to say and how it is said. It may look like you have a "shy" child (rarely initiates conversation/gives short answers to questions). She may over-generalize names of objects (*every* furry animal is a dog; *every* drink is juice), or she may "talk in circles," (a simple retelling of a story/event is very complex), or may find it hard to put sentences together in the right order.

> *Phonological Disorder*—difficulty in understanding the sound system and speech rules that other children naturally pick up on. A child may mispronounce a certain sound/letter in one word, but not others, whole groups of sounds may be mispronounced (e.g., all *g,* and *k* sounds may be pronounced as *t*). She may leave out endings to words, yet can say that sound when it occurs in the middle of the word (e.g., *book* is *booh*, but she can say *locker* or *hiking* fine). **Often, kids with CAS can "graduate" into a form of phonological disorder.**

In the case of suspected CAS, the first step is to see a speech-language pathologist (SLP) for a thorough assessment, or you may even consider starting with your pediatrician. Chapter 3 explains how to get started on the road to diagnosis.

Depending on your child's age and the extent of her speech delay, you may want to seek out a professional evaluation sooner rather than later. Elaine Weitzman, SLP and Executive Director of The Hanen Center, says, "We know that the window of opportunity [for language development] is greatest when a child is very young. If a toddler is late in his or her language development, parents will never regret acting early. They might, however, regret acting too late."

The bottom line: it's best to get an assessment from a licensed SLP when you start noticing your child isn't reaching developmentally appropriate speech-language milestones.

Can CAS Occur with Other Conditions?

You may be wondering if CAS can occur with other conditions—and the answer is gray, at best. There are times where apraxia is the only concern a child has. This may be referred to as "pure" apraxia. There are also children who have CAS on top of another condition. They may have a condition that typically causes communication delays or problems, but the CAS means that they have *even more* trouble speaking than someone with that condition normally does. It can be especially difficult for these children to get a diagnosis of CAS without being told, "Oh, it's just the Down syndrome [for example]."

The most common of these other conditions are autism spectrum disorders, attention-deficit/hyperactivity disorder (ADHD), Down syndrome, and sensory processing disorders. Other, rarer genetic conditions that can include CAS symptoms are Cri du Chat and Prader-Willi syndrome. Please refer to Appendix A for more information.

Teresa of Chicagoland talks about her experience with dual diagnosis:

> *"My son Nick has Down syndrome, but he was also diagnosed with CAS at the age of five. His speech was quite delayed and often it seemed like he was grasping to try to say words, like the cat got his tongue. He was definitely more behind in his speech than his peers who had Down syndrome. Once we got the CAS diagnosis, the speech therapy became tailored to address this issue. He did a lot more repetitive work along with pairing speech with motor play. So many of these disorders and their symptoms overlap and there are certainly a lot of gray areas when deciding why a child's speech is delayed."*
> (Refer to Chapter 6 for more information on the CAS and Down syndrome connection).

If your child has apraxia, recognize it early, get the appropriate help, look for ways to cope, and find resources to help your child. These topics are all covered in this book. I know you are thinking, "Easy for you to say!" Don't forget—I was once where you are, too. It's anything *but* easy. **You will get through this; your child will get through it, too.**

Parents Ask...

Can a smart child have apraxia?

Yes! **CAS has nothing to do with intelligence.** If you are dealing mostly with CAS, then your child probably does not have cognitive delays. In fact, many of these kiddos are quite intelligent—gifted and talented in many ways! *Just because you are pursuing a speech-language evaluation, it does not mean you are questioning your child's intelligence.*

Sometimes CAS occurs with another condition that is associated with cognitive delays. For example, children with Down syndrome frequently have both muscle function and motor planning concerns and may be diagnosed with CAS. In this case, the CAS doesn't mean the child's intelligence will be *more* affected than is usual for someone with Down syndrome.

"But isn't apraxia a 'special need'?" Well, yes. If your child is evaluated by the school district and it is determined that her delay in speech is significant enough to receive services (and you, the parent, consent) then your child will be labeled as having a 'special need.' I know—this isn't easy to hear. But remember that just because your child is receiving "special education" doesn't mean she is not bright. Nowadays, special education covers a wide range of services to meet a child's individual needs.

How Many Kids Have CAS?

The answer may surprise you for a variety of reasons. For one, just as with other neurobehavioral disorders (genetic/metabolic) such as autism spectrum disorders (ASD) and ADHD, CAS is also on the rise.

In the past decade, approximately 3.4 to 4.3 percent of all children in the United States with a speech delay of "unknown origin" were found to have suspected CAS. One preliminary population estimate, based on clinic referral data, is that CAS may occur in 1 to 2 children per 1,000. Yet another study indicates it could be as high as 1 to 10 children per 1,000. In other words, the incidence appears to be somewhere between 0.1 percent and 1 percent of all children.

How do you respond when someone asks you, *"How many kids have apraxia?"* A lot…some…it's rare. OK, this isn't a multiple choice exam, but almost all of those answers are right. Let me explain:

➤ It may seem like a lot because you deal with CAS every day. You likely will meet others who deal with it, too (other parents, SLPs, and teachers). Birds of a feather flock together, right?

➤ But when you first heard of it, you thought that maybe it was pretty rare. After all, *you* had never heard of CAS before.

➤ And once you started hearing a little more about it, you realized that it's not really rare, but it's also not very common.

Parents Ask…

Why doesn't anyone know the precise incidence?

For one, there are a good number of overlapping symptoms and co-occurring disorders (having more than one concern/disorder at the same time) that may blur even the best-trained diagnostician's eye. During an evaluation, most SLPs rely on behavioral checklists consistent with the symptoms of CAS, possible red-flags in the child's personal and family history, and observation of the child's speech. Keep in mind, too, that other speech-language issues (such as limited vocabulary or auditory processing disorders) may make for some gray areas, even for the SLP completing the evaluation.

Let's Talk about Sex: Are Boys or Girls More Likely to Have CAS?

Over the last 100-plus years, most research has found that boys are more likely to have CAS. The boy : girl ratio varies from study to study. According to Penny Hall's 1993 book, *Developmental Apraxia of Speech,* 74 percent of kids with CAS are boys.

"But, I have a daughter with CAS," you say.

Let me explain. Raise your hand if you have ever said, "I've had it up to here!" as you point to the top of your head to your kids? Think of that statement as your "threshold" for their poor behavior.

Well, imagine that there is a *threshold* for apraxia that your child has reached.

Keep this analogy in mind because we are now going to borrow a concept model from the study of genetics.

The prevalence rate of 74 percent is attained when a certain threshold is reached (or crossed). Somehow it's "easier" for boys to reach that point.

What that means for your daughter with CAS is that she has to have more symptoms, before it is recognized as CAS. In genetics speak, that is referred to as a **greater loading of factors.** Thus, the greater loading of factors = more severe form of CAS.

Penny Hall, Associate Professor Emeritus from the Department of Communication Sciences and Disorders at the University of Iowa, and her colleagues hypothesized that girls may actually have CAS just as often as boys, but when they do have it, it is more severe. That is, girls tend not to be diagnosed with CAS unless they have more severe symptoms.

Of course, some girls have just a mild version CAS. And some boys have severe CAS. Researchers haven't gotten to the bottom of why that is, though.

One mother of a daughter with CAS says this when speaking of gender differences: *"I always thought it was boys who were more likely to have a speech problem. Aren't boys kind of late in developing speech, anyway? I was so surprised when my daughter had apraxia and my son was a chatterbox!"*

What Does CAS Mean for Your Child's Future?

I wish I could take away all of the confusion you feel right now. I wish I could ease your fears. *If I could—believe me—I would.*

There is a light at the end of the tunnel. **Children with CAS do make progress; they do get better.** But it takes hard work on everyone's part. Every child with CAS will have different symptoms and her own pattern of strengths and challenges.

Keep in mind that CAS is a dynamic, ever-changing speech disorder. There are a lot of factors that go into making a prognosis:

➤ age at diagnosis,
➤ type and amount of therapy,
➤ at-home practice,
➤ involvement of family,
➤ school involvement,
➤ child's temperament and personality,
➤ child's motivation.

Of course, there's a genetic piece, too; especially if your child is struggling with additional diagnoses.

Improvements Over Time

You are probably wondering how other parents responded—and got through—the early years of CAS. You'll hear from three parents here.

Ally's mom, Susan, says: *"Her progress, when it started, was very fast and furious. She wanted to talk with an intensity that also took my breath away. Ally was diagnosed at 2 years, 10 months and her speech was age appropriate by age 5. Her speech at age 7 is perfect, only breaking down slightly when she is very tired."*

Tanner's mom, Brandy, shares this: *"It's a scary thing when your child isn't speaking [like other children his or her age]. But have faith. Our son Tanner has progressed so much over the last four years. At seven, he is—for the most part—understood by all of his friends and teachers."*

Diane relates these feelings regarding her son William's experience with CAS: *"As a parent, I asked myself how I was going to protect [my son], how could I make him speak better? My son worked extremely hard [in speech therapy], and I am happy to report that William was dismissed from speech therapy last year. The path has been bumpy at times, but we are making our way and are beginning to see the light."*

So, with that in mind, ***most children with "just" CAS will make wonderful progress in being able to express themselves verbally.*** Treatment must be completed by a trained SLP and be intense and frequent, and the child must have parent/home support.

Your child with CAS won't simply "grow out of it," as some may suggest. When a child is correctly diagnosed with the condition, CAS *tendencies* typically remain throughout one's life (this *does not* mean that the individual won't be able to talk). These tendencies may or may not be apparent to the person at the checkout stand or the soccer coach, but your child (and her close friends, family, or trained SLP) may notice that she avoids multisyllabic words or transposes words/sounds when she is especially tired or stressed.

Despite these continuing tendencies, most children who have pure CAS when young have as much chance as any other child of growing up to lead happy, successful adult lives. If given proper support and treatment, CAS will likely not affect a child's ability to succeed in school, to pursue her interests, and to excel in music, sports, academics, or wherever her talents lie. As adults, people with CAS may choose careers in which they don't have to do much public speaking, but other than that, the sky's the limit!

The prognosis for developing effective speech when a child has CAS along with another condition such as autism or Down syndrome is not as clear cut. Whether your child will be speaking effectively depends on the child as well as the specific characteristics of her other special need(s). Your child may need to use some kind of low-tech or high-tech communication system (sign language, electronic devices, communication books, etc.) to help get her message across. But with the right kinds of therapy and support, they can definitely make progress in understanding and using speech and language.

See Chapter 15 for more details on prognosis.

Whether you have a sneaking suspicion your child has CAS, or you know for a fact that she does, you are in good hands. This book will give you the inside scoop from how to find the right help to navigating the school system and coping with your feelings. Childhood Apraxia of Speech is quite treatable if you start the journey early and stay the course.

Say That Again?! Chapter Summary

We started the chapter with a basic definition of CAS, or so it seemed. But once we got into the nitty-gritty of it, we learned there really is more to the disorder than meets the eye. Even speech-language pathologists (SLPs) grapple with the terminology and diagnostic characteristics. Warning signs for parents to keep track of were outlined, as well as discussions on prevalence, intelligence, your child's future, and co-occurring conditions.

Read on! Recommended Resources

➤ Please take a look at the **American Speech-Language-Hearing Association's (ASHA)** webpage: www.asha.org. Pay particular attention to the 2007 Technical Document on CAS: www.asha.org/docs/html/TR2007-00278.html.

➤ **Apraxia-KIDS/CASANA** is the largest nonprofit U.S. organization on CAS. You'll find it's a nice online resource for parents and professionals. Here you can access articles and a "family start guide" to apraxia, as well as join a listserv: www.apraxia-kids.org.

➤ *Hope Speaks: An Introduction to Childhood Apraxia of Speech* (DVD) is a half-hour documentary that is both educational and inspirational. It is designed as an introduction to parents of children who have recently been diagnosed with CAS. You can order it through the Apraxia-KIDS store at www.apraxia-kids.org.

➤ You may also like *I Want to Be Your Friend,* an illustrated book designed for preschool through early elementary-aged children about young Emma, who has CAS. Told from Emma's point of view you learn that while she can't communicate as well as others, she is still just a "normal kid." Written by Emma's mother, Angela Baublitz, this is a great introduction to CAS for parents and children alike. Find your copy at Apraxia-KIDS: www.apraxia-kids.org.

➤ **The Hanen Center** is recognized as an international leader in early language development through parent- and educator-focused programs. For more information, visit www.hanen.org or call 877-426-3655.

➤ *It Takes Two to Talk,* by Jan Pepper and Elaine Weitzman (of the Hanen Center), gives parents simple and successful tips for working with their children on communication skills—whether it's "just" a speech delay, or something more. (Order at www.hanen.org.)

➤ *Play to Talk: A Practical Guide to Help Your Late-talking Child Join the Conversation,* by James MacDonald and Pam Stoika (Kiddo Publications, 2007), gives parents a step-by-step approach to helping their children with essential skills on conversation and socialization, all backed by 30 years of clinical research.

➤ For speech-language concerns in general, you may appreciate *Childhood Speech, Language, and Listening Problems: What Every Parent Should Know* by Patricia McAleer Hamaguchi (John Wiley and Sons, 2001).

➤ **The ChildTalk blog** by Becca Jarzynski, CCC-SLP, is a parent-friendly and very helpful resource if you are looking for strategies in working with your child and gaining valuable speech-language information: www.talkingkids.org

➤ Debbie Feit's book, *A Parent's Guide to Speech and Language Problems* (McGraw-Hill, 2007), is down-to-earth and easy to read.

➤ You may also want to look for *The Late Talker: What to Do if Your Child Isn't Talking Yet* by Marilyn Agin, Lisa Geng, and Malcolm Nicholl (St. Martin's Griffin, 2004).

➤ *Ready Bodies, Learning Minds,* by Athena Oden, a pediatric PT, gives lots of suggestions on expectations, goals, and how to help children with vestibular skills, motor planning (praxis), and visual and auditory skills (David Oden, 2004).

. . . .

Chapter Two

An Introduction to Speech, Language, and Listening

. . . .

"Imagine if you will, a little boy who has a dream, a dream to communicate. He wishes he could answer your question so that you understand his response. He wishes he could ask for clarification when he doesn't know exactly what you want him to say or do. He wishes to connect with his friends in their verbal play, or to raise his hand in eagerness to answer his teacher. Because in his mind, he knows what he wants to say, yet he just can't get it out. Imagine this little boy is yours."

Communication is part of our everyday life. It's in the news, the radio, on television. It's on the road, in the grocery store, at school, at work. It's everywhere. When you exchange a few words with your neighbor, you don't think much about the process of talking. In fact, it doesn't seem all *that* complicated. You have a thought, you open your mouth (insert foot—sometimes), and the thought comes out in the form of words others can usually understand. This chapter is all about talking. How it happens, why it happens, and what happens when there's a glitch in the process. Since talking also requires listening, we'll talk about that, too.

A recent conversation I had with my neighbor had to do with the weather, the past weekend, and what the kids were up to. Really, the context of what we were talking about was so simple, yet so complex to articulate, at least at a neuromuscular level.

> ### The Nuts and Bolts of This Chapter
>
> ➤ The "basics" of speech—definitions of common terms to get the ball rolling
>
> ➤ Typical childhood speech development (and a few tips on what you can do to help it along), including easy access charts
>
> ➤ The physiology of speech, language, and listening
>
> ➤ A little on the stigma and myths associated with late-talkers

When I mentioned my daughter's difficulty with speech, I joked and said something like, "I don't understand why she has such difficulty talking and eating...those happen to be two of my favorite things!" My neighbor nodded and smiled sympathetically. She knew I was concerned, she knew Kate was in speech therapy, and she could relate—her own child had received speech therapy at one time, too.

But really, talking *is* complicated. There is a high-order process going on, involving speech, language, listening, and comprehension. Is it all in your mind? Yes, in fact, one important language center *is* located in the front part of your brain, in an area called the premotor cortex. This region is responsible for the planning and coordination of speech. It is primarily the left side of the brain that is "in charge" of *understanding* language. The right side is best at *detecting prosodic aspects* of language, that is the rate, rhythm, tone, and stress of the words.

Language, Communication, and Culture

How important is the need to communicate? I would venture to say that *the ability to develop effective communication skills is a basic need, much like the need to seek food, shelter, and comfort.* Not only are feelings, ideas, and information all conveyed through communication, but language and communication are very much a part of the culture in which one is brought up. We use communication to pass down family stories; folklore, experiences; record our past; and plan for our future.

Language is one of the most important skills we can develop to be successful in society. But there are things that need to line up in order for humans to have a verbal communication system. The words "speech" and "language" have similar connotations, but they are quite different. Read on to find out.

Speech—That's the Same Thing as Language, Right?

Well, not exactly. *Speech refers to the sounds that come out of your mouth and take the form of words.* To speak, many things must happen, often at the same time, at a rate of up to fourteen sounds per second! Speech requires the coordination of more than seventy muscles and body parts. Speech is one of the most sophisticated, complex, dynamic, and highly skilled human movement.

A person first has an idea and wants to communicate it to others, and then...

The brain:
➤ Must formulate the idea it wants to communicate in the form of words
➤ Needs to send that message to the mouth
➤ Must tell the mouth what sounds to make to say the word(s)
➤ Needs to send the correct signals to the muscles that control the tongue, lips, jaw, and palate—all structures/muscles needed to coordinate and produce speech.

The muscles in the face:
➤ Must have the strength and coordination to do what the brain is asking

The respiratory system:
➤ Must be able to orchestrate air flow into and out of the lungs
➤ Must use the muscles of the abdomen to drive the diaphragm
➤ Must direct air with enough force so the vocal cords vibrate and produce sound. Air must be going out—not in—for speech to occur.

The auditory system:
➤ Needs to hear correctly and monitor what comes out of the mouth to make sure it's being said "correctly"

The interpersonal connection:
➤ Must be made—that is, someone else must be a part of the conversation. If no one is communicating (listening and reacting) with us, what's the point in talking?

What Is Language, Then?

Language is the content of what is spoken, written, read, or communicated through gestures. You've heard someone say, "I don't like your language." And that usually means, "I don't like the words you're using." But it can also be in the form of body language or sign language. There are a few signs and gestures that typically mean the same thing across cultures. For example, rubbing one's belly after a large meal usually means you've had enough to eat, crossing your arms across your chest might indicate that you are closed off (or simply cold—look for goose bumps). Placing your hands on your hips might signify that you are angry or showing authority (sometimes both).

In a basic sense, language is divided into two categories: *receptive and expressive.*
➤ *Receptive language is the process of receiving and comprehending language.* It involves a significant amount of listening and observation.

If receptive language is not developed properly, then the entire language system sort of stalls. In other words, we must be able to understand and correctly hear the words before we can produce (express) them.

➤ *Expressive language is the process of producing (expressing) words, phrases, and sentences, along with gestures, to convey a message.* Sign language is considered a form of expressive language, although no actual speech is occurring.

In order for children to understand and use *spoken (expressive) language*, a few things need to happen:

The brain:
➤ Must have the cognitive capabilities to process and understand what is being said
➤ Needs to have a system of storing communicated information, and be able to retrieve it later
➤ Needs to have a method to communicate ideas to someone else

The muscles:
➤ Must "fire" and coordinate properly; the child must have the physical ability to talk

The auditory system:
➤ Must have ears that "work" (or the child must learn a visual system such as cued speech to compensate for the lack of hearing)
➤ Must be able to hear differences in tone and accents, as well as detect changes in sentence structure (such as raising the pitch of one's voice at the end of a sentence when asking a question)
➤ Must be able to distinguish words from nonspeech sounds and extraneous stimuli

The interpersonal connection:
➤ Must be made by parents and significant caregivers who use and model words
➤ Springs from a psychological and social need to communicate with others
➤ Must be strengthened through listeners who are interested in what the child is saying to reinforce communication.

Are You Listening to Me?

Most parents ask their kids this all the time. But really, the act of listening is a little more complicated than it may seem. Again, a series of events must occur to hear and be heard:

➤ Sound waves carry sound (perhaps spoken words, or other noise) to our ears.

➤ For the sound to travel efficiently through the outer canals of the ears, there must be *nothing* in the way (physical abnormality or obstruction of some kind).

➤ Sound vibrates the eardrum, which connects to three little bones in the middle ear. (If there is fluid in the middle ear (*otitis media)* due to colds, infection, or allergies, the sound will be distorted or muffled at this stage. The middle ear needs to be healthy for sounds to move through clearly.)

➤ Sounds move from the middle ear to inner ear; the inner ear needs to be "working" and healthy, too.

➤ The inner ear takes sounds directly to the auditory nerve and the brain.

➤ The brain makes sense of it all (or tries to). A message is deciphered.

Talking Is a Two-Way Street

Communication is a two-way process. It involves a speaker and a listener. Both "speaker" and "listener" have important jobs to fulfill if they are going to communicate effectively.

I am sure you have been in the position where you have "heard" someone but you weren't really listening. You didn't "get" the message they were trying to convey. The speaker may have felt misunderstood or unimportant. It's frustrating, to say the least.

Think of how your child with apraxia must feel. While he is trying so hard to communicate with you, you struggle to interpret his message. He gets more frustrated, and so do you. If you are frustrated, then chances are that he is *more* frustrated; after all, he doesn't have the experience and coping skills under his belt like you do to work through such frustrations.

I facilitate a support group for parents of kids with CAS called Small Talk: All About Apraxia, and asked members to share their experience with frustration. One mother commented: "I get so frustrated sometimes trying to decipher what my son is trying to tell me. I feel bad even admitting this. He will fuss, and grunt, and point. I know he's trying really hard to tell me what he wants, but I just don't get it sometimes!"

Another mom mentioned a similar scenario when her son was trying to get her attention about a Buzz Lightyear toy [*Toy Story* character] on the top shelf of a bookcase in his bedroom: "I couldn't figure out what he wanted. This went on for a long time [his grunting and pointing], he kept saying 'oy, oy.' I had no idea. He was in tears and I was close to them, too. Finally, it dawned on me that he wanted his Buzz Lightyear toy. 'Oy oy' meant "toy" in his language."

What's a parent to do?

Sometimes, it helps to simply say: "Whatever it is you want to tell me is really important, I can tell. I am having a hard time understanding your words, can you *show* me what you want instead?"

Parents Cope

A child's frustration can lead to negative behaviors such as aggression, anxiety, and attention problems, and he or she may even be stereotyped as "dumb." We'll touch on stereotypes and stigma later in this chapter. If you are interested in learning more about your child's coping and socialization, look at Chapter 14. We will discuss your child's feelings and coping skills in greater detail there.

What Causes the Glitch in Childhood Apraxia of Speech?

Ah, the million-dollar question: what is the glitch that causes CAS? There are conflicting theories; no one really knows for sure. One thing is clear, however: *Parents are not the cause of their children's apraxia!*

Some folks believe that kids with CAS have difficulty creating, transmitting, and storing speech movement plans. Of course, all we "see" is a child who is frustrated because he can only produce limited or unclear speech. The even bigger question is, why? We'll discuss this more fully in Chapter 6. However, one theory indicates that not all systems of the brain mature at the same time. This might explain, in part, why children with CAS have a hard time learning to communicate in early childhood.

Consider this idea: could it be that the right side of the child's brain is right on schedule in *understanding* language, but the left side is behind in terms of *producing* it? Eventually, most systems "catch up." Language development occurs throughout childhood, but it continues throughout life.

Myths, Feelings, and Unwanted Advice about Speech Development

I am sure you have heard your fair share of speech myths and the grandmotherly neighbor's advice along the lines of this:

➤ Einstein was a late-talker.
➤ Some very bright children won't talk because they are bored with "baby talk."
➤ He'll talk when he has it all perfected in his mind.
➤ He just doesn't have anything to say.
➤ You (or big sister) do all of the talking for him.
➤ He has all of his needs met and doesn't "need" to communicate.
➤ He'll talk when something really interests him, or he really wants something.

These statements can be reassuring when you first notice signs that your child's speech development is lagging. And it's true—some children "just" have a delay in speech development. A *delay*, by the way, is defined as a "slowness." Delays *could* occur in *both* receptive and expressive language *at the same time*. Everything related to speech and language could be lagging behind, but generally occurring together. Then suddenly your very quiet two-year-old grows into a totally chatty three-year-old. Those things happen. Other times, they don't. Children have their own unique growth patterns with growth spurts in different areas of development at different times.

It's common for parents to second-guess themselves and wonder, "Does he have a problem, or not?" You may be quizzing your own parents about when you started talking (they likely won't remember—unless there was a problem) and whether there is a history of late-talkers in your family. You might even be a teensy bit defensive. When was the last time Grandma called and asked whether her little Angel Cake was "talking,"only to hear you sigh, "Not yet?"

"Wait! What If He *Is* Just a "Late-Talker?"

According to Becca Jarzynski, a pediatric speech-language pathologist and blogger of Child Talk (www.talkingkids.org), "If a child reaches 24 months and isn't yet using 50 words and/or isn't yet putting two words together into short phrases (e.g., "more juice," "bye mama"), we typically recommend that [parents] talk to their pediatrician about an evaluation by a speech-language pathologist."

That, however, isn't the full answer. Here are some other considerations a pediatric SLP would look at when evaluating toddlers who aren't yet speaking as much as expected:

➤ *What does the child understand?* Can he follow a wide variety of directions? Find objects when Mom and Dad ask him to do so? Point to pictures in a book? Show off some body parts when they are named? Follow silly directions like "put a cup on your head?"

➤ *How he is communicating with gestures and facial expressions?* Is he nodding and shaking his head no? Pointing at things that he wants or that interest him? Waving "hi" and "goodbye?" Clapping with delight?

➤ *How he is using the words he does have?* Is he using them appropriately? Does he have inflection in the right places? Can he articulate well?

➤ *What kinds of sounds is he using?* Does he use his voice to get attention? Does he vocalize often throughout the day? Did he babble often as a baby? Does he use his voice in a way that sounds like he's having a conversation, even if there are no real words involved in that conversation? (At 24 months, for example, a child should be using a variety of sounds such as p, b, m, n, t, d, h, and w—and using them in a variety of words).

➤ *How is he playing?* Does he use pretend play in some very simple ways? For example, does he give a bottle to a baby, or feed a stuffed bear with a spoon? Is he able to play simple rolling or fetching ball games with others, and starting to imitate housework?

➤ *How does he imitate actions?* Will he clap when an adult does? Does he imitate stacking blocks? Will he imitate you if you do something silly and unexpected, like place a block on top of your head?

➤ *How is he hearing?* Any concerns with hearing should be evaluated to rule out a hearing loss. Some kids can hear some sounds but not others.

What if the child were doing all those things just described but still wasn't talking as much as we'd expect? "Then he'd be what we call a 'late talker,'" according to Becca Jarzynski, CCC-SLP. As she explains, "The benefit of getting an evaluation for a 'late talker' is that parents have a professional speech-language therapist looking specifically at all those areas and helping them to figure out what's really going on. If nothing else, this can ease a parent's mind. The SLP can also give parents some simple suggestions that can be woven into their day to increase the odds that their child will start using more words. A really good speech-language pathologist will shed light on what comes next in child development and help parents figure out how they can get their child to that next level."

Ms. Jarzynski continues, "Opinions are mixed about whether or not speech therapy is truly needed for children who are just late talkers. Some studies seem to indicate that as long as late talkers are in supportive, nurturing, and responsive families, they will catch up on their own. Other studies suggest that late talkers can potentially have lingering difficulty with reading and spelling when they enter elementary school."

If you'd like some tips and ideas on working with a late-talking child, please visit Becca's blog, at: www.talkingkids.org/p/strategies.html.

"He Don't Talk Right": Dealing with Stigma

We seem to attach a stigma to folks who are quiet, reserved, or nonverbal. You think this person is dumb, stuck-up, brainy, unfriendly, goody-two-shoes, an observer, shy, reclusive, reticent, introverted, indifferent, ambivalent, aloof, upset, bored/boring—you get the idea. Most of these descriptors have a negative vibe to them. Who really wants to be known as the "Unfriendly, indifferent, brainy recluse?" Um, that's right—no one.

What's a Parent to Do?

If you are dealing with some less-than-supportive folks when it comes to your child's speech concerns, you'll want to respond to them as diplomatically as possible. I know; it's hard at times. Try some of these "nip-it-in-the-bud" statements:

➤ "He's just slow to warm up."
➤ "We all develop at different rates."
➤ "Quiet and cautious, and I couldn't be more grateful."
➤ "He's more of an observer, like his dad/mom/you."

- ➤ "I'm glad you mentioned that. I have been meaning to ask you about it." (This works especially well if the person has a background in child development or speech-language pathology. It can also provide a great opening for digging deep into familial connections.)
- ➤ "Gosh, I don't know. What would you recommend?"
- ➤ "I appreciate your concern. Thank you."

How Communication Skills Typically Develop

As we covered in earlier sections, humans need both receptive language (the ability to comprehend what others are telling us) and expressive language (the ability to use speech or another system to transmit our messages to others) in order to communicate. The development of both receptive and expressive language is quite complex. It's easy for something to go awry in the development of either. Everything must fall "magically" into place. Let's take a quick look at the processes involved for a child to develop speech and language.

The Development of Speech (Expressive Language)

The ability to talk is developed in a gradual way. Consider this formula:

mental growth + neuromuscular maturation + imitation of speech sounds = speech [talking]

Many children are at different stages of this process, which is especially true for children with CAS. Some may move quickly through the speech development stages; others may linger or get stuck in one or more stages. Child development is an individual process. The sections below explore what is involved in each of these elements of the speech equation.

Element #1 in the "Speech Equation": Mental Growth

We humans are pretty darn amazing. It is mostly because of our brain's left cortex that we are able to communicate using a complex system of words. Language itself has its own neuronal apparatus, like a computer, that evolution has inserted directly into the human brain. But it's grammar that really sets language apart from other forms of communication.

When I mention grammar, I am not referring to those boring rules you learned in middle school. Instead, you can think of grammar in this case as syntax, or the ability to arrange words and phrases into sentences that make sense in a particular situation.

Most of our speech and language abilities are housed in the left hemisphere of the brain. This is true for the majority of people, but like everything, there are always exceptions to the rule.

The left hemisphere of the human brain sorts out the sounds of the environment (the vacuum cleaner, dishwasher, and birds chirping), from the human speech noises. (Typically, the left hemisphere knows how to do this from birth.)

Wernicke's area is in charge of understanding the meaning of words and remembering and applying the rules of grammar. It is the part of the brain that is necessary for speech **comprehension.** Wernicke's area is located in the temporal lobe of the brain.

Image retrieved from the National Institute on Deafness and Other Communication Disorders, a division of the National Institute of Health.

Broca's area is in charge of **speech production.** This area, located in the left frontal lobe of the brain, is anatomically a long distance from Wernicke's area, relatively speaking.

Fluid, easy communication depends on these two areas working together without much effort. For that to happen, your child needs to develop strong neural connections (pathways) between the areas. It is through listening and communication experiences that your child develops strong connections between Wernicke's and Broca's areas, just as he might strengthen his biceps by lifting dumbbells.

Element #2 in the "Speech Equation": Neuromuscular Maturation

Learning to speak clearly and correctly is complicated. First of all, you have to have an idea. Then the muscles in your face, mouth, tongue, and soft palate have to work together. You need developed pathways in your brain to "communicate" with those muscles. You also must have the right timing and coordination (which is part of motor planning) in order for your brain to orchestrate this event.

All of these changes involve *neuromuscular maturation.* That is, the brain and nerves must develop in tandem with the muscles required for speech development.

To help you understand the complexity of the neuromuscular development needed for speech, consider these facts:

> ➤ *Speaking requires about 5,000 neuromuscular events per second.* These events must be coordinated in time and space to produce fluent speech.
> ➤ *There are only a few nonspeech movements that are faster than speech.* For example, your eyes move faster than you can talk. Both eye movement and speech are forms of what is called "fine motor function."

Element #3 in the "Speech Equation": Imitation of Speech Sounds

You might think that developing speech is instinctive, but it's not. Without models to listen to and imitate, a baby would not learn to produce words on his own.

Kids learn to do a lot by imitation. They watch and listen and see how you do things (also known as "modeling"). For example, they watch you walk all day—to their bed, to the refrigerator, out the door. And since they are watching you do this, they naturally want to do the same thing. But there are steps (so to speak!) before that can happen, especially when you are a fifteen-pound baby lying on a quilt, happily gnawing on toys. You will need to learn to roll over, sit up, crawl, pull to stand, stand alone, and then coordinate the movements to alternately move the right foot, then the left foot, and so on. It's challenging work to control all of those muscles in the feet and legs.

Of course, walking and talking are not the same, but the *idea* is the same. Talking requires a sequence of events to take place, just as walking does. To illustrate the role that imitation plays in learning to speak, let's look at how babbling typically develops.

Babies around the world—from vastly different cultures, languages, and dialects—will babble similar sounds—and all right around the same age. Babies everywhere produce vowels before consonants and are sensitive to sound and tone differences. (However, the latest research suggests that there may be more differences between cultures and languages than we once thought.)

Babies begin to babble at around three to four months of age. Babies raised in English-speaking households babble in English sounds. Meanwhile, Japanese-reared babies are babbling in Japanese, and bambinos in Italy are beginning to mimic the sounds of the Italian language. All because they are imitating the speech sounds they hear in their daily lives.

For a child to be able to imitate speech sounds, he needs to:

➤ develop the neuromuscular abilities to physically move the muscles in the precise and coordinated way needed to produce speech sounds, and also to get the message from the brain to the muscles involved.

➤ be able to hear well and accurately (without distortion from middle ear fluid or anything interrupting the passage and interpretation of sound from the ear to the auditory cortex in the brain). *If you are concerned about your child's hearing, have an audiologist evaluate him.* Your child should have his hearing screened on a regular basis. This is routinely done during well-child visits and in school.

➤ have the capability and motivation to imitate others (which can be delayed or lacking in some conditions such as autism).

More information on imitation is found in Chapter 7 on speech therapy strategies.

Slow and Steady

Remember, learning to communicate is a *gradual* process. It requires general intelligence and mental development to **identify** ("Yes, I know what a ball is"), **associate** ("Oh, the words ball and roll are related?"), **remember** ("Yesterday we played with the ball. I threw the ball. Yay!"), and finally, **reproduce** ("Ball?").

Say That Again?! Chapter Summary

This chapter was designed to be an introduction to speech, language, and listening, but all in all, it was a bit complex, wasn't it? It gets easier, I promise. This chapter provided a background on receptive and expressive language, the brain anatomy, and physiology for speech and language, and also provided some ideas to gauge your child's speech and listening development. We touched briefly on myths, stigma, and nay-sayers, including some tips for how to cope.

Read On! Recommended Resources

➤ *The Late Talker: What to Do If Your Child Isn't Talking Yet* by Marilyn Agin, MD, Lisa F. Geng, and Malcolm Nicholl (St. Martin's Griffin, 2004) is a clearly written resource with charts on reaching language milestones, as well as some warning signs to look for.

➤ **The ChildTalk blog by Becca Jarzynski, CCC-SLP,** is a parent-friendly and very helpful resource if you are looking for strategies for working with your child and gaining valuable speech-language information: www.talkingkids.org.

➤ *Nobody Ever Told Me (or My Mother) That!: Everything from Bottles and Breathing and Healthy Speech Development* by Diane Bahr, an SLP with over 30 years experience (Sensory World, 2010). This book is designed primarily for parents of typically developing kids to help keep them on track in feeding, speech, and mouth development beginning at birth. It gives great tips so parents can make feeding, early sound play, and the journey to better speech easier.

➤ Laura E. Berk is a distinguished Professor of Psychology at Illinois State University, where she has taught child development for over 30 years. She has published several books. My favorite is *Awakening Children's Minds: How Parents and Teachers Can Make a Difference* (Oxford University Press, 2001). You will find lots of good information on why and how children talk to themselves and classroom learning, as well as a chapter devoted to helping children with deficits and disabilities.

➤ *What's Going on in There: How the Brain and Mind Develop in the First Five Years of Life* by Lisa Eliot, Ph.D. (Bantam, 1999) is one of my favorite books on child development. While the illustrations and format remind me of something you might see in medical or nursing school, the writing is pretty easy to follow. It covers the basic biology of human brain development, prenatal influences on the fetal brain, milestones, memory, and intelligence.

➤ Debbie Feit's book, *A Parent's Guide to Speech and Language Problems* (McGraw-Hill, 2007) is another one of my favorites. It gives you real-world advice from a mom who has been there, as well as charts, tips, and advice from parents on met or missed speech milestones.

➤ *The American Speech-Language-Hearing Association* is *the* professional organization for speech-language pathologists and audiologists in the U.S. Their website offers many valuable resources for parents as well: www.asha.org.

➤ You may also appreciate *Speech Therapy Information and Resources (STIR),* a UK online resource that's all about speech and language. You may find the sections on play, communication, and anatomy particularly helpful: www.speech-therapy-information-and-resources.com.

Chapter Three

When You Suspect Childhood Apraxia of Speech

Where to Go and What to Ask

As first-time parents, we didn't want to appear "delinquent," so when Kate was 15 months old, *exactly*, we headed to the doctor (the same one who delivered her) for her scheduled well-child check-up. I say "we," because *both* doting parents were off work for the occasion. We came armed with our wiggly daughter; along with thoughts, questions, and toddler antics to relate to our doctor.

The Nuts and Bolts of This Chapter

➤ Determining the "right age" to get help for your child

➤ The different modes of receiving a diagnosis of Childhood Apraxia of Speech—from your pediatrician or your speech-language pathologist—as well as a review of some of the specialists in the medical, psychological, and educational settings

➤ What early intervention is and is not, how to get involved, and what to expect

➤ How and where to look for an SLP; the qualities you'll want to seek, and the questions to ask a potential treating clinician

Here's Our Apraxia Story

Kate was meeting all of her developmental milestones right on target. Except one: talking. She had only one word, "Hi." I was excited that she had such a friendly and outgoing first word and proud that it was the one I had predicted she'd say first. When I told others my prediction, they would all say, "You might be right—she really likes people." It seemed I had a natural extrovert (how did that happen with two self-proclaimed introvert parents?). She was smiling and saying "hi" to strangers in the grocery store, on the playground, at the library.

In the exam room, Dr. Baumgartner asked a series of questions…was Kate doing this, doing that? Yes, yes, and yes, we nodded and smiled proudly. "Is she saying 'mama' and 'dada' and a few other words?" Nope. We held our breath, awaiting her response.

Sure, I was slightly concerned. I had friends from childbirth class whose toddlers were jabbering up a storm. As a first-timer, however, I didn't want to jump the gun. Kate *was* only 15 months old after all. She still wore diapers, took a pacifier when distressed, and was rocked to sleep. In many ways she was still a baby, and babies don't talk, do they? Plus, I *knew* kids—through my years as baby sitter and as a child psych nurse.

We told our doctor that all Kate was saying was "hi," and that she started saying that around 13 months. Wasn't that good enough? Our caring doctor probed a little further and eventually referred us to a local speech-language pathologist (SLP). "You can do it now, if you want to be aggressive, or wait until she is 18 months, if you want to take a conservative approach."

I took the conservative approach. I finally made the call at 18 months. Kate still wasn't saying "mama" and I wanted to hear my little girl call my name, instead of grunting when she needed me.

I'll admit, I was totally skeptical of the capabilities of a speech-language pathologist at first. What could she possibly do to get my kid to talk that I couldn't? But we

Introvert vs. Extrovert

Generally speaking, an introvert is someone who is more reserved and receives her energy from within. An extrovert can be described as someone who is outgoing and gets her energy from being around other people. It has little to do with speech disabilities or disorders, but is more of an inborn personality trait. Says one mother of a son with CAS:

"It is soooo interesting that apraxia kids tend to be extroverted by nature! Mark always is quiet when meeting new people; he watches and waits…and he slips in the odd witty comment to show his nature. Then once he is confident others have accepted him, he gets more chatty. He has a fabulous vocabulary, as he is a 'reader' and this also promotes his wit to others."

stayed the course—taking Kate to speech therapy weekly after the SLP determined there was a "delay."

We'll talk more about what therapy consists of in the next chapter, but in this one, you will get a good overview of how to go about getting the help you want and need. There are lots of different routes to reach the same destination: diagnosis and treatment.

"Wait a Minute—That Seemed Way Too Easy!"

I'll admit, our example does make it seem easy: you show up at a well-child appointment with your M.D. and he or she detects a delay and sends you to the right professional. You have great insurance and there is a speech clinic down the street with no wait list. Voila—you're in, problem solved. I am not sure if there is a "typical" sequence of events that occurs. From others I have talked with along this journey, however, I have learned that it usually takes longer to figure out what is going on. Many families seem to have a journey to diagnosis similar to this one:

> *"We worried and wondered what was going on with our daughter for years. Her pediatrician thought maybe autism. She had an evaluation and it wasn't autism. My parents told me not to worry—kids talk when they want to; you can't force it. My neighbor thought it may be auditory processing disorder like her son had. The preschool was suggesting a learning disorder. I didn't know what to believe. Finally, an SLP started to rule out [childhood] apraxia [of speech]. We finally received a diagnosis at 4 years and 2 months."*
> —Small Talk: All About Apraxia Participant

Whatever your story is, it doesn't matter. If you are concerned about your child's speech and language development, it is never too late to pursue a diagnosis. And whether or not you have good healthcare insurance, you're in luck: every state has some kind of early intervention (EI) program that will provide an evaluation if your child's speech concern is great enough. We'll touch more on EI later in the chapter.

The "Right Age" to Seek Help

Appendix D at the back of this book presents some typical developmental charts on childhood speech and language development. Go back to them and highlight or mark the milestones you are concerned about. Now look over your list of concerns and determine just how concerning you think they are.

If you want a number here, you aren't going to get one. Here's why: kids are developmentally unique; no one child will develop at exactly the same speed. I know, that's frustrating to hear. If you are concerned that your child might have apraxia, then I would aim for getting your child an initial assessment at 2 years and 3 months (27 months). Okay, I fibbed. There's your number. Most SLPs won't give you a diagnosis for CAS until your child is closer to 3 years old. My daughter Kate was diagnosed at 2 years, 6 months, which was considered on the early side. It took just over a year to get a diagnosis for Kate after I first took her to an SLP. She had some very classic symptoms of CAS (more on that in the next chapter).

Here's something else to keep in mind: if you are concerned that a *younger* sibling may have CAS (your older one has already been diagnosed), then get an evaluation even earlier. CAS tends to run in families, so if one sibling has it and another is exhibiting similar features, then by all means, don't hesitate! (The same advice goes for anyone in the family whom you *suspect* has—or had—a speech-language issue, even if it wasn't formally diagnosed. More on that in Chapter 5.)

Case in point: Kate's little sister, Kelly, wasn't saying much at her 12-month check-up. By 15 months, she only had three words. She was assessed by Kate's SLP who found "characteristics consistent with CAS." At 18 months of age, Kelly started therapy. By the time she was 27 months, little Kelly was no longer showing any symptoms of a motor-speech disorder. She was dismissed from speech therapy. Of course, we were thrilled. Meanwhile, Kate—who was older and perhaps had a more severe form of CAS—continued with speech therapy, much to her dismay. Try explaining *that* to a Type A oldest sibling!

Why Not Wait Until School Starts?

If you wait until your child starts kindergarten to take the reins regarding your concerns about the possibility of apraxia, that is probably too long. Your child will likely be at a distinct disadvantage for academics and participating in classroom activities. *Do not put off pursuing a diagnosis if you are concerned about CAS!*

Here are some reasons to convince you to get early and aggressive treatment:

➤ School at this age is all about the group setting. Kids are expected to sit still, listen, have a good memory for spoken language and a decent attention span, and be able to articulate their basic needs, such as "May I use the bathroom?"

➤ Kindergartners learn to sound out sounds, associate sounds with letters, and understand that sounds make up words. In "fancy" talk, this is called phonological awareness. Chapter 12 is devoted completely to phonological awareness and CAS.

➤ Another skill that emerges in kindergarten is the ability to tell and retell stories. Sequencing becomes a big theme in the classroom. Your child will need to describe *in words* what comes first, middle, and last in a story.

➤ Finally, for a child to explain something as simple as what he brought in for show and tell requires the ability to put words together and communicate them intelligibly to others.

I remember our goal for Kate was to "have her ready for kindergarten." We wanted her to be on par with her peers by then, in hopes that no one would ever know she had apraxia. At this writing, I am happy to report that she is in full-day kindergarten and doing fantastic verbally.

But I need to throw in this monkey wrench: **getting help before kindergarten does not guarantee a trouble-free school experience.** Kids with CAS often have other academic concerns that could pop up in later school years (difficulties with reading, sequencing, executive functioning, even math and science). Chapters 11 and 12 discuss these concerns step by step. However, the earlier you start getting your child the appropriate help for apraxia, the sooner you will see positive results.

Doctors & Specialists

Let's jump right in and start reviewing those professionals who could point you in the right direction when you are seeking a diagnosis.

Pediatrician/Family Practice Physician (M.D.)

Just as in our situation, your child's treating physician could detect a concern and give you a referral to a SLP (more on this later). If you do get a referral, call the member services number on your insurance card to verify coverage and amount of benefit. Your child's doctor won't and can't treat CAS. It's just not in-scope for an M.D.; that's the role of a speech-language pathologist. If there are other concerns, your doctor may give you a referral to a pediatric neurologist (see below).

If your pediatrician doesn't think there's anything to be concerned about, follow your gut instinct. Please, be an advocate for yourself and your child. You can always ask your pediatrician for a second opinion or a recommendation to see a specialist. Try saying it this way, "I know you treat many children and you'd tell me if there was a problem. But I am still feeling uneasy about my child's speech develop-

> **Parents Share...**
>
> *Pediatricians*
>
> *"We saw a wonderful pediatrician who agreed with most everything I said, was impressed with the research articles I brought along, and told me that I was doing a great job being a parent. Wow. You don't get that every day."*

ment. Do you know of another physician, SLP, or organization who may be able to give me another opinion?"

Pediatric Neurologist (M.D.)

A medical doctor by education, a pediatric neurologist typically spends two additional years gaining general experience treating children and then three *more* years training in child neurology. That's nine years of post-college specialization.

Pediatric neurologists can rule out other causes of speech delay through medical exams such as CAT scans, EMGs (electromyography—determines muscle disease), and EEGs. Take your child to a pediatric neurologist if she has a serious neurological history such as seizures, hydrocephalus (unusual amount of fluid in the ventricles of the brain), or progressive muscle weakness.

On occasion, a neurologist will suggest brain-imaging studies such as an MRI. This test is typically done for children who have "focal" neurologic findings (like weakness on just one side of the body, loss of coordination, and speech/language difficulties among others).

An EEG (electroencephalography) may be ordered if your child has a history of seizures, episodes of "zoning out," autistic-like symptoms, or a regression in language skills. An EEG measures the tiny electrical currents generated by brain activity. It's possible to analyze these findings to determine which is responsible for certain cognitive tasks—like talking and understanding speech.

Parents Share...

Neurologists

One mother of a daughter with CAS shares her experience with a pediatric neurologist:

> "I was so disappointed in my appointment with the [pediatric] neuro [logist]. I had this appointment on the calendar for four months. I wanted to have my daughter evaluated. We went right after Christmas. I was frazzled. All [the doctor] did was confirm that my daughter had apraxia. I was hoping for more, especially after that long wait."

Not all experiences with a pediatric neurologist end like this. Like everything, there are some experiences that are better than others:

> "We had a great experience with a pediatric neurologist. We took our son because we wanted to have another look [at his apraxia]. Owen responded well to the doctor's bedside manner and we left the appointment feeling hopeful. He told us, 'a child that has no other delays outside of verbal apraxia and is able to comprehend what others are communicating has a high probability of developing normal speech communication.'"

All of these scans are painless, but can be anxiety producing. But it's not all about imaging scans. There are some laboratory tests than can rule out metabolic diseases that can occur in children with a speech delay or hypotonia. Tests may include:

> *Chromosome analysis for Fragile X Syndrome*—which is an inherited disorder seen almost exclusively in boys. It generally causes intellectual disabilities and sometimes autistic features, as well as speech and language delays and differences. Women and girls who are "carriers" and don't have the disorder themselves can also have some speech differences.

> *CPK*—which is a muscle enzyme that is increased in instances of muscular dystrophy. If muscles aren't firing correctly, it can be difficult to produce intelligible speech.

> *Lead screening*—will likely be done to determine if increased blood lead levels have resulted in behaviors that look like autism or developmental (speech) delays.

Developmental Pediatrician (M.D.)

A pediatrician who has completed four years of medical school, two years in a pediatric residency program, and then an additional year in developmental-behavioral postgraduate training is a developmental pediatrician. A children's hospital in your area should be able to help you find a developmental pediatrician. They are known best for looking at the "whole" child within the context of the family. They can provide guidance on development, eating, sleeping, and behaving. These professionals are able to diagnose ADHD and learning disabilities and may be able to advocate for your child at the school level. Of course, it goes without saying that you should consult one who has interest and experience in childhood speech issues.

Some SLPs believe that developmental pediatricians and pediatric neurologists give the diagnosis of CAS when the child is making no attempt to talk whatsoever. Not attempting to talk is *not* a criterion for the diagnosis of apraxia. ***Typically, kids with CAS want to communicate and try to do so.*** Please keep in mind that while there are some developmental pediatricians out there who are well versed in childhood speech-language problems, the diagnosis of CAS is in the scope of practicing SLPs. ***Always have a diagnosis confirmed by a speech-language pathologist.***

Pediatric Physiatrist (M.D.)

Not a psychiatrist, but a *physiatrist*…a *what*?! This doctor is usually board certified in pediatrics and physical medicine and rehabilitation (physiatry). These docs work closely with occupational therapists, physical therapists, and speech-language therapists. Because a good number of pediatric physiatrists specialize in motor disabilities such as CAS and feeding issues, you may find some treatment options here. Look for a qualified professional through a rehab facility or a major university hospital.

Psychologists and Psychiatrists

Neuropsychologist (Ph.D., Psy.D.)

A psychologist who has received further training in brain-behavior relationships is a neuropsychologist. These professionals typically have an intense background in psychology and neurology. "Brain-behavior relationships" is simply how the brain and body connect, like learning and memory, and not "bad behavior."

A neuropsychologist is helpful if you want to determine your child's areas of weakness, as well as strengths. He or she can provide a detailed profile of brain functioning related to language, spatial skills, memory, attention, executive functioning skills (organization), and problem-solving, to name a few. This might help in terms of determining your child's best ways of learning in a school setting. For example, assessments may be able to determine if your child learns best by seeing, hearing, doing, or reading.

Interestingly, learning and behavior styles of children can affect kids' academic achievement, behavior, and social adjustment. The assessment and evaluation provided by a neuropsychologist is typically more in-depth than that of an educational psychologist.

Why it's important if your child has CAS: Often kids with CAS have difficulty with academic achievement, attention, and organizational skills. A neuropsychologist can provide information to help optimize these day-to-day functions at home and school. See Chapter 10 for more discussion on how a neuropsychologist can be beneficial.

We took Kate to a neuropsychologist when she was exhibiting more and more symptoms of what looked like ADHD in addition to her already confirmed CAS diagnosis. Dr. Kelly was fantastic with Kate! When the comprehensive testing period was all over (a total of six hours over three weeks), our neuropsychologist sat down with my husband and me for a full hour and reviewed her findings and recommendations. She provided a wonderful written report for us to pass along to the school to help Kate focus and also supported us through the diagnosis.

Educational Psychologist or "School Psychologist" (M.Ed., Ph.D., Psy.D.)

These professionals focus mainly on how students learn in educational settings. They study student attributes, instructional processes directly related to the classroom, how effective that education is, and the psychology of teaching. They might act as a consultant to a special needs teacher who is directly responsible for your child's education. Further, educational psychologists commonly administer IQ tests, as well as achievement tests and can diagnose ADHD, executive function problems, and learning disabilities, as well as autism. They can figure out whether a child's academic struggles are due to a disability, and whether difficulties communicating are due to cognitive problems. You may encounter this professional when your child is being evaluated for EI or special education.

An educational psychologist may also be referred to as a school psychologist, thus found at your child's school. Although some psychologists employed by schools have master's degrees, if you are hiring someone to do a private evaluation of your child, you will probably want to look for someone with a Ph.D. and experience working with students with speech-language disorders. They can choose different tests (that require little or no verbal response) for your child if she can't answer the questions verbally.

Another caveat: if you suspect a problem, consider getting an "outside" or third-party evaluation rather than one within the school system. This way, your school—and you—can be objective about the results. Same thing goes if the school does testing on your child, you would be a good consumer if you got a second opinion. Keep in mind, however, that schools often like to do their own evaluations, as they often have different standards than private practice clinicians.

Child Psychologist (Ph.D., Psy.D.)

A child psychologist can help you and your child cope with the diagnosis, as well as work with her on social issues, frustration, impulsiveness, anxiety, and aggression—all of which may be related to CAS. He or she may or may not also do testing for cognitive and behavioral disorders such as ADHD, learning disabilities, autism, or mood disorders. However, a psychologist cannot diagnosis a child with CAS.

Child and Adolescent Psychiatrist (M.D.)

A psychiatrist is a medical doctor who has received specialized training in child/adolescent development, behavior, and mental health. They are a great resource if your child has a co-occurring behavioral or mental health concern such as ADHD, an anxiety disorder, or obsessive compulsive disorder (OCD), among others. Unlike a psychologist, a child/adolescent psychiatrist can prescribe medications to treat certain conditions. As far as *diagnosing* CAS, a child/adolescent psychiatrist isn't the "go-to" professional. They may, however, understand what it is and be able to help you understand how to cope with it.

Speech-Language Pathology

The "gold standard" to getting your child diagnosed and treated for Childhood Apraxia of Speech is an evaluation by a speech-language pathologist (SLP), according to the 2007 Position Statement from the American Speech Language Hearing Association (ASHA). Please keep in mind that if you live outside of the United States, your therapist may have a different professional title than SLP. This section will help you understand the process of referrals and selecting a SLP, and will give you some encouragement on taking that first leap to your first appointment.

Getting to a Speech-Language Pathologist (SLP)

If you are lucky enough to have a doctor who catches a concern on a well-child visit, consider yourself blessed. If not, you may contact your doctor's office and explain that you are interested in having your doctor make a referral to a SLP because your little pumpkin isn't progressing like you think she should. If your doctor knows and re-members you and your child well, he or she might just go ahead and write that referral without troubling you to come in for an office visit.

Most likely, you will have to make an appointment—maybe even a couple of weeks out—and go in when the time rolls around.

The appointment will probably go something like this: The doctor will look at your precious offspring and say, *"Your mom tells me that you are having trouble talking—is that right?"* Your child will nod and smile and won't say anything when prompted (as do most kids when they are in a new/unfamiliar setting).

Your child's doctor will likely ask you to describe your child's *attempts at communication* (sounds and gestures commonly used). If they seem remarkable, you'll get a referral to a SLP.

But, what should you do if your doc doesn't think a referral to a SLP is in order? Be polite but persistent. Come with some research or a list of symptoms of CAS; present them to your doctor. Remember, you know your child better than anyone else. If you feel there is something more going on, please be proactive. You do not necessarily need a referral from your doctor to take your child to an SLP (unless your insurance requires it, or you want to see an SLP whom your pediatrician especially trusts/respects). You can find lists of SLPs on the ASHA website: www.asha.org. Worst case scenario: you go to the SLP only to hear that nothing is wrong. It's better to be safe than sorry, right?

What Is a Speech-Language Pathologist (SLP), Anyway?

Simply put, the SLP is the key player in your child's progress with speech and a sounding board for you. He or she is also a professional with a master's degree (some may have a Ph.D.) with a background in communication disorders. SLPSs complete a practicum—usually a year in length—following their graduate program. SLPs are re-quired to be licensed in the state in which they practice and must complete continuing education criteria to maintain their licensure. They are also accredited by the American Speech-Language-Hearing Association (ASHA). They perform evaluations, deliver a diagnosis, carry out therapy, and recommend "homework" for you. They are also there to field questions and concerns and give you resources for additional information.

By the way, *SLPs are the only professionals qualified to treat CAS.* And while this is a subjective piece of information, you may also hear that an SLP's diagnosis of CAS is more respected than that of another professional.

SLPs work hard with your child to model and support developmentally appropri-ate communication. It takes patience, persistence, humor, and creativity, along with organization and good interpersonal skills to be an effective child SLP.

Qualities and Qualifications to Look for in Your Child's SLP

If you are fortunate enough to be able to choose your therapist, consider yourself lucky. Not all SLPs are created equal and you are going to want the one who meshes best with you and your family, has flexible (accommodating) hours, and is very knowledgeable about CAS. Here's a list of qualities and characteristics you'll want to look for:

➤ *Educational background should include at least a master's degree.*

➤ *Certification by ASHA, as indicated by "CCC" after their name (Certificate of Clinical Competence).* Why is this a big deal? It shows that the SLP has met a minimum level of training and has agreed to ASHA's code of conduct and ethics and has committed to continuing education. This is similar to being a "board-certified" physician, but for speech-language pathologists.

➤ *Years of experience is a bit of a gray zone.* Some may think that the more experience, the better. But, that's not always the case. Some seasoned therapists can get set in their ways, may lack excitement and passion, and may be a little too "old school" for your taste. On the other hand, a new graduate may not have the necessary experience. Ah, yes the conundrum of how to get experienced if you lack experience....

➤ *Your therapist should* like *working with children.* Does she have experience working with kids in your child's age group? Does she have experience with CAS? Keep in mind that not all therapists are trained in pediatrics.

➤ *Ask directly, "How many children with CAS have you worked with?"* Hopefully, he or she will tell you five to ten, or more

➤ *Ask how therapy will be carried out.* Will you be in the room or observing from a one-way mirror or sitting in the waiting room? This is important. *Therapy will be most effective when parents and therapists work as a team.* In the beginning, it is ideal if you are in the room. This way you can see what the therapist is doing and how your child is responding, and you will be able to ask questions. It is also helpful if your child is not comfortable being left alone with strangers.

➤ When we first started therapy, I was in the room. Hectic—yes—with a two-year-old and a baby, but I felt more confident and eager to replicate some of the techniques she was using in therapy. On the other hand, your child may be less likely to perform with you in the room; you might be a distraction. Your therapist may ask that you *not* sit in the room. If this is the case, ask if you can at least sit outside the door (leave it open slightly) and listen in.

➤ *Ask how updates will be handled.* Will the therapist give you a blow-by-blow account of the session and your child's performance? Will she do routine reevaluations? How often will you know if and when your child has reached a goal set by the therapist? Will you have access to what those goals are? Will you get regular written reports?

➤ *Your therapist should give you "homework" and instruct you on how to do it with your child.* Simply handing you a piece of paper and telling you to work on it for the next week isn't very beneficial. As a parent you'll want to reinforce whatever your child is doing with the therapist.

➤ *Do you feel accepted, valued, and respected by the SLP?*

➤ *Does the therapist work from an office or come to your home?* Pros of the office: it's a new environment; work feels "important." Cons of the office: it may be too far away; may feel too clinical. Pros of at-home therapist: you and your child are comfortable in your own setting; no driving. Cons of the at-home therapist: "Too comfortable" can prevent progress (therapy no longer feels important), and can be too distracting (toys, TV, dog, siblings, phone). What do you prefer?

➤ *Don't be afraid to ask how much the SLP charges for therapy.* Better to know than to get a surprise bill. How is billing done—expected at time of service, once a month, billed through insurance? How are co-pays handled? Some clinics only take check or cash. Know your financial facts before moving forward.

A Speech-language Pathologist's View on Selecting an SLP

"In addition to providing a warm and supportive environment for children, one of the best things that families can do for a child with CAS is to locate a therapist who understands the unique needs of children with motor-speech challenges. Request that your SLP explain the goals and methods, as well as the types of things you can do at home to support your child's communication skill development. It is encouraging as I travel around the country to meet so many SLPs who are interested in learning more about helping children on their caseloads with CAS. *I am hopeful that increasing knowledge and supporting new research will serve to improve communication outcomes for children with motor speech challenges.*"

—Margaret (Dee) Fish, CCC-SLP and author of
Here's How to Treat Childhood Apraxia of Speech

If you have choices when it comes to selecting the best speech-language pathologist for your child, don't waste any time in finding one. Be systematic and efficient, and don't be afraid to change therapists if you feel like your child isn't progressing, isn't happy, or it just isn't a good fit for your family. If you don't have choices (because you don't have insurance that will pay for speech therapy), see the section on early intervention, below. Remember, a "good" therapist is flexible (adjusts to the needs of the child), eager to learn and research better ways to help *your* child, attends continuing education events and conferences, and is able to admit that she or he "doesn't know," but is willing to help find an answer.

"Cheat Sheet" for Interviewing a Potential SLP

1. Tell me about your areas of interest in the field of speech pathology.
2. What types of kids do you usually see...their ages? Their diagnoses?

3. Have you worked with many kids with CAS?
4. What can you tell me about CAS? How is it diagnosed? How is it treated?
5. What can you tell me about your specialized skills, knowledge, and experience related to CAS?
   (The ASHA strongly recommends special knowledge in CAS and motor learning theory, differential diagnosis, and experience with a variety of intervention techniques to be "qualified" to work with a child with apraxia—so look for his or her answer to include a high number of patients with CAS and lots of continuing education classes.)

Apraxia-Kids/CASANA has an online list of qualified SLPs who can diagnose and treat CAS at www.apraxia-kids.org.

Parents Share...

Reevaluating Your Child's Progress and SLP

Amy, the mother of a daughter with CAS, says this:
"*Basically, it's a constant reevaluation process. Consider asking yourself these questions, 'Is the therapist a good fit for my child? Does she or he have the experience necessary to treat my child? Is my child responding and making progress? Are there other factors—financial, educational, insurance-related, family status—that require us to change SLPs?'*

[My daughter] Brooke is getting ready to switch for the fourth time total. We've jumped ship for a variety of reasons: the SLP didn't have the 'right' experience, not a good fit for my child's personality, transitioning to an educational setting, and pending family move."

Where SLPs Work

Oh, but *where* to find a speech-language pathologist (SLP)? You can look in the phone book or hop on the Internet, but the *best* way is to ask for a recommendation.

Talk to your friends with kids or your child's pediatrician. You'll find that SLPs work in a variety of settings. Here are places where you may find an SLP:

➤ *University Clinic:* Some universities provide students with an extensive training ground and give you reduced fees in return. But the "therapist" is a student. This can be a good thing—he or she is energetic and motivated and eager to please. Most students are closely monitored by a seasoned SLP (but not always), and will almost always "rotate off" your child's case, whether or not therapy is "done."

➤ *Hospital Outpatient Clinic:* Hospitals accept your insurance and submit claims on your behalf, which is like heaven to a stressed parent. If your child has additional medical needs or requires physical therapy (PT) or occupational therapy (OT), this is ideal. Hospitals have high hiring standards, so you are likely getting a "really good" therapist as well. However, hospitals can feel cold and clinical and have that "hospital smell." If this bothers you (or your child), this isn't the place for you.

➤ *Private Therapy:* If flexibility and personal service have a good ring to your ears, you may want to go this route. SLPs in private practice offer one-on-one therapy (sometimes group therapy), accommodating hours so you can get there after work if need be, and offer continuity through the whole year—not just the school year. You can also work directly with your therapist to determine how long and how often you should bring your child to therapy. But all of this comes at a price. Private clinics can charge $100 and up an hour. Multiply this by 2 or 3 (or 5!) sessions a week and you've got a hefty bill. Most health insurance will pay for therapy through a private clinic, but your insurance will likely cap off at some point. *How* speech-language pathologists work (provide therapy) is covered in Chapter 7.

➤ *Early Intervention (EI):* You may have heard of **IDEA** (Individuals with Disabilities Education Act). It is a federal law in the U.S. that allows kids with disabilities (including speech and language impairments such as CAS) to have free special education services from birth to age 21 years (referred to as **F**ree **A**ppropriate **P**ublic Education, FAPE). Early Intervention (EI) is designed for kids up to age three.

Early Intervention 101

There's a lot to know about early intervention. In fact, I could probably dedicate an entire chapter to the topic. I'll give you a brief overview of the processes involved, some first-hand experiences, and resources, if this is a route you'd like to pursue.

Your first step is to determine whether your child qualifies for early intervention. Under the law, early intervention is only available to infants and young children who are found to have delays in development or who are diagnosed with a disability that is likely to cause delays in development. (The amount of delay that qualifies a child for services varies from program to program and state to state.)

To find out whether your child qualifies, contact your local early intervention office. You can find a state-by-state guide for locating an EI office in your area at: www.earlyinterventionsupport.com. (Look for it under "Contacts in Your State.) You'll be referred to an early intervention coordinator (sometimes referred to as an intake coordinator), who will coordinate the evaluation and become your contact person. All of this coordinating takes time, so try to be patient.

Resources on Early Intervention

For more information on what is involved in early intervention, consider visiting these websites, even if they are outside of your state.

➤ Missouri's program is called *First Steps*. Check them out at: www.dese.mo.gov/divspeced/FirstSteps
➤ California has *First Five*: www.ccfc.ca.gov
➤ In Pennsylvania, it's *Achieva Early Intervention*: www.achievaearlyintervention.org
➤ The National Center for infants, toddlers, and families is called *Zero to Three*: www.zerotothree.org

The coordinator will likely come to your home at a prescheduled time. You'll get the chance to chat and she'll meet your child, take some notes, and leave you with a mountain of paperwork to complete.

Next, the coordinator will probably get a speech-language pathologist lined up to come to your home to evaluate your child. In some cases, your child might be evaluated by another professional, such as an early intervention specialist or infant educator, or you may be asked to bring your child to an office or center for an evaluation. Don't be surprised if your coordinator recommends additional evaluations from the EI staff—physical therapist (PT), occupational therapist (OT), or psychologist. Again, this takes time and patience. You may be put on a waiting list for your child to even get an evaluation.

Once the evaluation is complete, you will be notified as to whether your child qualifies for early intervention services. If so, the next step will generally be to meet with all of the professionals who will be on your child's early intervention "team." There you will develop something called an Individualized Family Service Plan (IFSP). The IFSP is a legal document that sets out:

➤ Your child's present level of performance (results of tests detailing her strengths and needs)
➤ The goals that you and your child's team want her to work toward (for a child with CAS, these may include being able to say a targeted sound/word/phrase, make approximations for commonly used words, or learn sign language until she can use speech to communicate her needs)
➤ The services that will be provided to help your child meet her needs (such as speech therapy or OT)
➤ Whether your child needs any assistive technology (low tech or high tech equipment such as a communication book, special software, or an electronic communication device)
➤ The setting where the services will be provided (in your home, at your child's daycare or nursery school, at a center)
➤ The amount of time anticipated for the process, including when reevaluations might occur

Be aware that the evaluating SLP may not be the *treating* SLP. After your child's evaluation is completed, it may take some time for her to be assigned to an SLP or other therapists/educators.

Other plus-sides to early intervention:

➤ It's free or reduced-cost. This will depend on several factors: your state, your income (some states provide services on a sliding fee scale), and how your EI office operates (some services may be offered free of charge; others may not).

➤ The service providers almost always come to your home or to your child's daycare or preschool, if that is more convenient for you.

➤ They are there to help you, the parent, understand the disorder and learn to become your child's advocate, as well as teaching you positive coping skills.

➤ They will become very familiar with you, your child, and your family.

➤ They help you navigate the transition between the early intervention program and the next steps of sending your child to preschool (around age three).

Parents Share...

Experiences with Early Intervention

"We love our early intervention [SLP]! She comes to our home first thing on Wednesday mornings. I don't have to rush around getting myself and my son ready to go out—in fact, sometimes we do speech therapy in our pajamas! Marcus is happy to be in his own home where he is comfortable with the environment, and I like the fact that it's free."

—Mom to Marcus, 2.6 years with suspected CAS

"I am nervous about when Henry turns three [and we no longer qualify for services]. I hope the therapist walks me through the next steps. We've had a hard time coordinating schedules. At first she came at 8:00. That was too early. Now she's coming at 11:30, which isn't working well, either. Henry is getting hungry and cranky at that time. But, really, he has made some progress."

—Mom to Henry, 2.6 years with 1-year speech delay.

"I got the sense that the therapist [speech pathologist] wasn't really doing any therapy with my son. She was teaching me how to do it while my son just sort of sat there. I wanted her to work directly with my son. I felt guilty when she came back next week and asked me if I did any of the things she suggested and I told her I simply hadn't had the time."

—Mother of a son with CAS who has outgrown EI

What Are the Downsides to Early Intervention?

Programs vary by state and sometimes also by county, so look into what's available in your area. As with anything, there are downsides. Here are the few I uncovered:

➤ You have to "catch the wave" early in order to qualify for EI before your child is too old for it. Some parents (especially first-time parents) aren't sure what to look for, or deny that their child is exhibiting any problems with speech. You could miss the boat as we did (see text box). We got the EI boat rolling too late for our daughter to benefit from the therapy. If so, you can look into special education services instead (see Chapter 11).

➤ Chances are, if school is out of session (for summer break), your child will be out of therapy. We already know that frequent and intense therapy is crucial to success in CAS—so you'll want to find out if you can secure therapy for summers and holiday breaks, either through special allowances through the early intervention program or privately. You'll also want to take costs into consideration—expect to pay out-of-pocket or higher rates for summer therapy.

➤ Another potential downside is heavy caseloads for SLPs. There is a huge demand for speech therapy in early intervention programs, which equates to decreased time and attention you may desire.

➤ Unlike with private therapy, you probably won't be able to pick your therapist. One will likely be assigned to your child.

Whatever you decide is best for your family is best. There are many merits to an early intervention program. Don't overlook them.

Our Experience with Early Intervention

When my family first started down this CAS path, I looked into our local EI program. We had the coordinator come to our home and I was inundated with papers and forms and acronyms—at the same time I was dealing with a clingy ten-month-old and an indifferent toddler. My head was spinning when she left. Plus, I was discouraged to hear that there was a waiting list for a SLP. Then, I learned that Kate would age out of their services in six months—she was two and a half at the time. (Typically, when kids turn 3 years old the school district takes over.) We went the private route instead.

Say That Again?! Chapter Summary

As parents, we are the ultimate experts on our kids. Who else spends 24/7/365 with, or thinking about, them? While there are lots of darn good specialists out there, you'll want to stick with a certified speech-language pathologist to evaluate, treat, and diagnose CAS. It's your job as a parent to be on the look out for a really dynamic speech pathologist—someone you like who meshes well with your child's personality.

Your therapist will likely be your hero once your child reaches some developmental verbal milestones with her help. She will become your friend, your support, and your child's cheerleader. Pick him or her wisely. And don't be afraid to switch if you are no longer feeling the vibe.

This chapter also covered the basics of early intervention programs. Please find out about the services in your county or area if this is a route you'd like to pursue.

Read On! Recommended Resources

➤ When *shopping for a speech pathologist* to treat your child for CAS, you may want to look to the Apraxia-Kids website. They have a list of qualified SLPs by region: www.apraxia-kids.org

➤ *Parents' Guide to Speech and Language Problems* (McGraw-Hill, 2007), by Debbie Feit, a journalist and mother of two children with CAS (now resolved), does a great job of compiling information on related speech disorders in an easy-to-use guide, complete with tips for finding a speech pathologist.

➤ *Does My Child Have a Speech Problem?* by Katherine Martin, SLP (Chicago Review Press, 1997) takes an in-depth look at this weighted question, with tips on where and how to get the help your child needs.

➤ *Childhood Speech, Language & Listening Problems: What Every Parent Should Know* by Patricia McAleer Hamaguchi (Wiley, 2001) offers a good overview of basic questions about where to go and what to ask, understanding IEP jargon, and common speech-language problems.

➤ *My Brother Is Very Special* by Amy Glorosio-May (Trafford Publishing, 2004) is a picture book designed to help kids understand the need for speech therapy. Ms. May, a nurse and "apraxia mom," wrote the book to help her daughter understand why her little brother was going to speech therapy.

➤ If you are looking for a book about the speech therapy process in general to share with your child, consider the fully illustrated *Speech Class Rules* by Ronda M. Wojcicki, SLP (The Speech Place Publishing, 2007).

➤ *The Early Intervention Guidebook for Families and Professionals: Partnering for Success* by Bonnie Keitty (Teachers College Press, 2009) provides a good overview of what early intervention is all about.

➤ ***Working with Families of Young Children with Special Needs*** by R.A. McWilliam (Guilford Press, 2010) is a user-friendly guide designed for professionals, but can give parents an inside view of the early intervention model. Expert contributors, tools, and checklists included for kids ages birth to 6 years.

Chapter Four

- - - - - - - - - - - - - - -

At the Speech Clinic

- - - - - - - - - - - - - - -

Your First Appointment with a Speech-Language Pathologist

So the day had rolled around. We were scheduled to be at the SLP's office in just fifteen minutes. I really had no idea what to expect, but I imagined it would be no big deal. As a nurse, I was used to assessing kids and being in a clinical setting. I knew that the more nervous I felt and acted, the more Kate would think this was a big deal. I wanted her to be relaxed and happy, like usual, so I tried very hard to be natural and at ease, but, in reality, I was feeling a little unsure myself.

The Nuts and Bolts of This Chapter

➤ The continuation of our story of working with a speech-language pathologist (SLP, sometimes referred to as "therapist") for the first time

➤ Everything you can expect to discuss with the speech-language pathologist at the initial appointment—demographics, family history, medical concerns, prenatal and birth history, social history

➤ How your SLP will "get to work" with your child, assessing things like receptive and expressive language, pragmatics, gestures, behavior, play skills, and oral-motor and feeding skills

➤ Tips on how to read your child's first speech report—because these things can be pretty dense!

Our Assessment Story Continues

I tapped on the sliding glass partition between the waiting room and the receptionist's office, signed in, and showed her our insurance card. Meanwhile, Kate made her way to the child-sized table and chairs—and reached for a crayon. I was amazed and impressed that at only 19 months old she was eager to create something artistic. Immediately, I engaged with her—partly because I wanted to—and partly because I wanted the therapist, or the receptionist—*anyone*—to hear that I really *was* a good mom and that yes, I *did* work with my kid to help coax the sounds and words out of her.

It appeared as though my tactic worked, at least to some degree. I sensed the SLP "spying" on our interactions from the hallway. Darn...she caught me being an engaging mom! She invited Kate and me back to her office with a nod and smile, and I found that she was quite friendly and pretty good with kids, even though I knew she had none of her own.

Her cramped office was stuffed with books, toys, and a computer. Kate was impressed with the dry erase board and I was impressed with the vast assortment of toys. I crammed my very pregnant self into a desk chair, and searched for a stool to prop up my swollen feet.

The therapist asked a bit about Kate's developmental history—my pregnancy, her birth, medical concerns, and illnesses. I mentioned that I fell on the ice when I was about six months pregnant and required oxygen during labor, as Kate's heart rate decelerated when I pushed. Neither seemed to raise an eyebrow, although I considered both occurrences "remarkable."

The SLP leaned her body back as she searched for something on her over-stuffed bookshelf. Flip-charts. My heart raced a bit, because this definitely felt like Kate was being "tested."

Kate was asked to point to simple animals and objects like pig, cup, and house. She did so perfectly. I smiled, thinking, "she doesn't really have a problem, does she?"

A shiny red toy barn appeared from under the desk. Kate found the cow first, picked it up, and inspected it. She presented it to the SLP as a sort of peace offering.

"Moo," the therapist said. "The cow goes 'moo.'"

Silence from Kate.

I began to feel nervous. "Come on, kiddo, you can do it," I cheered in my mind.

"Can you say, 'moo'?" she asked. Silence again. And then Kate lost interest in the cow and gravitated back to the dry erase board.

Together, Kate and the speech pathologist tried blowing bubbles and saying, "bubble" and "pop." The big grin on her face told me that Kate enjoyed blowing bubbles, yet she didn't have a single thing to say about them! *Why not? Come on, Kate, I want you to talk.*

The SLP asked Kate to find a toy and "take it to Mommy." She did. I clapped and smiled and praised her up the wa-zoo.

The SLP asked, "Who's that?" and pointed to me. I so badly wanted to hear Kate call me "Mommy," but nothing. I choked back tears. I didn't expect this strong sense of emotion to overcome me. I felt Baby Kelly kick from inside of me and tried to chalk it up to pregnancy hormones. But, no—these feelings were real and painful. It was as though I was "hearing" for the first time that my sweet little girl *couldn't* talk.

For the next twenty or thirty minutes, we continued with toys and prompts while the SLP crouched on hands and knees trying to elicit a sound or a word from my daughter. Kate couldn't care less, although she *was* interested in mouthing the toys and showing me what she had discovered with her customary "eh?"

I feigned interest with bright eyes while saying, "Oh! Wow. A truck." But in reality, I was tired. I was scared. I was not comfortable with my pregnant body crammed into a tiny room. And most of all, I was fearful of what the speech-language pathologist was going to tell me. I was beginning to see that Kate's language—or lack thereof—was concerning.

The SLP caught my eye and pulled her lips into a tight line as she nodded, "Well," she began, "Kate definitely has a delay. It's hard to say if there is anything more at this point. She's probably three or four months behind her peers. We could do therapy once a week or so, if you want to."

I sucked in a deep breath and let my eyes wander around the room. I bit my lower lip and then looked down at Kate. I smiled halfway and nodded ever so slightly.

When my husband heard there was a "delay," he thought an hour of speech therapy a week couldn't hurt. And that's when he 'fessed up that *he* had been a "late-talker."

His first word was "clop-clop" for helicopter and that wasn't until he was *three*! I had known about his trouble saying "s" words and his experience with speech therapy through third grade, but *late-talking*—this was something he hadn't shared during those "tell me about your childhood" date discussions.

After I mulled over my husband's late-talking "confession," I followed up with our pediatrician, who said, "Leslie, really, what can it hurt? I know you want the best for Kate."

It took some time, but I warmed up to the idea that Kate *did* need speech therapy. But I was skeptical that playing with toys could *really* get my kid to talk. After all, she played with toys all the time at home, at playgroups, and in the daycare at the gym—and this was *structured* play, often with me at the center of it all. The only utterances we were hearing was "eh?" and "hi." *(Later I learned that play-based therapy is very good for kids; it taps into their innate need to discover and manipulate objects).*

Needless to say, we went back. On visit #2 or #3, The SLP told me that motion activates the vestibular system—which is responsible for the body's balance and coordination—and suggested that movement might get Kate to say more.

So we tried the large swing in the clinic's "gym." After about fifteen minutes of swinging and repeating the words over and over, something resembling "mama" popped out of Kate's mouth.

You'd think I'd grin from ear to ear as my eyes welled up, but actually it was a bit anticlimactic, "Did she really just call me 'mama' or was that what I *thought* I heard?" But the SLP was convinced Kate was saying 'mama' all because of the swing.

Swinging Kate as often as possible—with prompts to make sounds and say words—was strongly recommended on our departure from the clinic that day. But this was November in Minnesota, too cold for the playground.

"Hang a plastic swing from a rafter in your basement," the SLP chirped on several occasions. We considered her suggestion, but with a finished basement, decided against it.

We eventually heard Kate say, "mama," "dada," and "ball" over the course of the next six weeks. *Six long weeks.* Of course, I was pleased, but I couldn't help but be worried, "Is this normal for it to take *so long and feel so hard*—on both Kate and us [parents]?"

The SLP made no formal diagnosis besides a "delay." With Christmas around the corner and a baby sister due in three weeks, Kate was released from therapy with a promise of a follow-up phone call in January. The call never came and neither did any more words.

But, baby sister, Kelly, did and so did a job offer for Dad—out-of-state. The house went on the market, the boxes got packed, and speech therapy went on hold.

Bear in mind that our first experience with a speech-language pathologist was not the "one and only" we worked with throughout our journey. We started in Minnesota—where we learned Kate had a "delay." Then we moved to Illinois—where the formal diagnosis occurred and therapy followed. Over the course of being at the *same* clinic in Chicagoland, we had three different speech-language pathologists. Therapists come and go for a variety of reasons (job change, maternity leave, back to school, etc.).

Parents Share...

My Resistance to Speech-Language Therapy

To be honest, I really didn't want to take my daughter to speech therapy, at least not at first. "Why," I wondered "would it do Kate any good to sit in a small cubicle of an office jam-packed with toys for $100 an hour (granted, insurance paid for all of it) when we could easily do the same thing in the comfort of our own home *for free* and no appointment to disrupt our tidy routine?" Later, I learned that in order for Kate to be a typically speaking child by the time she entered kindergarten (a goal we had established early on based on her severity, attention span, willingness to engage), I really needed to get her to speech therapy as often as possible. **Kids with CAS respond and make the most progress when they receive frequent, intense therapy and plenty of home practice.**

Forms, Forms, and More Forms!

At this point, there may be an SLP you have done a bit of homework on. You know a bit about his or her experience, philosophy, and background. Or, maybe you were like me: you knew nothing and just showed up at your appointment.

Every clinic and every therapist is going to have a different approach. But there is a general recipe all SLPs follow.

After you have made your appointment (perhaps some weeks, or even months out, depending on the availability of SLPs in your area), you will likely receive a stack of paperwork from the evaluating clinic.

These forms will ask you to detail everything about your little one from the moment of conception (well, not quite—but almost)!

➤ *General information* will include demographics, insurance, and your occupations.

➤ *Overall language problem* is *your* description of why you are bringing your child to an SLP; what you believe the concern/diagnosis is (Childhood Apraxia of Speech), what caused it, what helps, and what makes it worse.

➤ *Family history* will be covered—speech, language, and academic difficulties. Pay close attention to relatives you may have never met, but have heard about through other family members. For example, Uncle Pete used to stutter or Great-grandma Effie struggled with finding the right word. Perhaps there is a history of learning disabilities or late-talking children. Make sure you note any and all relatives who may have contributed to your child's genetic make-up.

➤ Another section will cover *medical concerns* such as surgeries, major accidents, hospitalizations, medications your child is currently taking (include vitamins, supplements, as well as anything over-the-counter) and be sure to mention if your child has any negative reaction(s) to medications.

➤ There will likely be a section on *prenatal and birth history*—covering things like mom's general health during pregnancy (illness, accidents, medications) and how long the pregnancy lasted. Make sure you mention everything you can think of: the fall on the ice in your fifth month counts, as does your diet and exercise routine. You will need to note how long you were in labor and if there were any complications. Be sure to mention the use of oxygen, forceps, whether a C-section was necessary (these concerns could indicate a child in distress). Your SLP may also be interested in knowing your child's birth weight. In addition, you'll want to make special note of any complications your child had immediately after birth. Please don't panic as you read this—just because these things were part of your child's birth does not indicate they caused your child to have apraxia—it's just worth noting.

➤ Your *child's developmental history* will be detailed in yet another section. Dust off—or find—that baby book. When did he crawl, sit, stand, and walk? What about feeding himself, dressing himself, and using the toilet? When did he first use a single word? What are the words or approximations he attempts? Does he commonly use gestures to communicate his needs or wants? What are they? (Guess on these dates if you are unsure; just make note that you don't recall specifically. Can you think back to the season or what was going on with the rest of your family as you review these milestones?)

➤ *Social history* will cover things like shy vs. outgoing, your child's general level of cooperation, whom he spends most of his time with, his preferred style of interaction, and whether preschool or daycare are part of his life.

➤ *"Anything else you would like to share"* will come last. No doubt you are tired and just want to be done with these forms. Try not to overlook this section. Your SLP will know what to do with this information. Here are some examples:

  • "Carter loves his pacifier. He won't go or do anything without it."
  • "Olivia loves her baby blankie. I hope you won't mind if she brings it to therapy."
  • "Anthony is very afraid of dogs. Talking about or playing with them will not be effective."
  • "Ava has separation concerns right now. It's probably just a phase, but if I could stay in the room, it will make things much smoother for all."
  • "Gavin's great-grandmother died recently. They were pretty close."

What If Your Child Was Adopted?

If your child was adopted, it will no doubt be challenging to complete these forms. Every adoption, like every child, is unique. If you know the answers to some of these questions, then great. If not, do what you can. If you have just partial knowledge of the birth mother and her family, indicate what you do know.

After you have filled out this tedious paperwork, you'll have a major case of writer's cramp and need a breather. Go ahead and indulge in something that makes you feel better. You need to take care of yourself, too.

Make sure you mail or drop this "book" off at the clinic prior to your appointment so the therapist can review it.

At the Appointment

You're there. You might be excited, nervous, indifferent, or in complete denial. Depending on the type of SLP you have—and how she or he prefers to work—you'll likely see a combination approach to formal and informal testing at your first appointment. If your SLP is completely informal, you may wonder, "How can playing with Play-Doh and blowing bubbles really help?"

Your SLP should have enough toys to hold your child's attention for a good hour or so. You'll *want* to feel like you just walked into a toy superstore. But on another note, it should be organized and well maintained, and not too overwhelming. A good SLP will know this and perhaps only bring out a few items at a time.

Besides developing trust and rapport and assessing your child's behavior, your therapist is busy evaluating. Remember how your child's job is to play? Well, your SLP's "play" *is* her work. Here are some components of a typical speech-language evaluation:

➤ **Behavioral Observations:** How your child engages in play, whether or not the play style is developmentally appropriate/similar to other kids this age, alertness/attentiveness/excitability. Be sure to point out to your therapist if the behavior is an accurate representation of your child's abilities.

➤ **Pragmatics:** Your therapist is evaluating how your child uses language to communicate with others in his environment. Examples of pragmatics include: responding to other's vocalizations, point to/show/give objects, making eye contact, responding to greetings, and controlling behavior.

➤ **Gesture:** How does your child use gesture to express thought and intent without spoken language? Examples of gestures include taking on/off articles of clothing when asked, "dancing" to music, pushing a stroller/shopping cart.

➤ **Play:** Time for fun! Really this piece of the evaluation determines your child's development of representational thought. This is really a fancy way of saying, "your child's ability to think in analogies; to understand symbols and infer meaning." Can he show how to play with a toy in different ways? Hand a toy to an adult for assistance? Group objects together? Use two toys together? Put toys away when asked? This is also an opportunity to see your child's temperament and personality; important for planning future speech sessions.

➤ **Language Comprehension (Receptive Language):** Determines how well your child attends to, processes, understands, retains, and integrates spoken language with and without linguistic cues. This may be tested by asking your child to pick just one object from a group, follow two-step commands, identify body parts/clothing items on himself, and perhaps follow novel commands.

➤ **Language Expression (Expressive Language):** Examines how easily your child can put words together to express himself verbally to others. If your child is able to sign certain concepts such as "more" or "thank you"—it's still considered "expressive language," though not verbal. Your therapist is looking to see if your child can shake his head yes/no, name an object, say several meaningful words, consistently identify 5-7 familiar objects when asked, or use single words correctly and frequently. (See Chapter 2 for more information about receptive and expressive language.)

➤ **Speech and Articulation:** What speech sounds are in your child's repertoire, and how accurately and meaningfully does he produce them? Does "down" sound like "done?" If so, he is unable to differentiate his speech. Does your child have one word that represents several different concepts? (Kate's word was "nanni." It meant "Grandma," "pacifier," and "blanket.") Does your child appear to be looking for the right word, but come up empty-handed (groping)? Does he grunt, squeal, and scream to get his needs met?

➤ **Motor-Speech Examination (MSE):** An essential tool for speech pathologists faced with diagnosing CAS is the MSE. The child is asked to imitate utterances of increasing length and complexity. Your SLP is looking to see if your child can make the same sounds in different contexts. When the SLP makes modifications to the MSE by slowing down the rate or by giving the child cues (by touch or gesture), she can begin to determine severity, and even get clues for determining the prognosis.

Parents Ask...

Isn't there just a simple test that can determine if my child has CAS?

The evaluation consists of several components: clinical observation by an SLP, your observations as a parent, and *some* test batteries. However, for these tests to "work," children need to be able to talk; that is, they need to be able to repeat words/phrases/sentences and use spontaneous conversational speech. If your child can't, then the evaluation depends on just observation. Here are some tests that may be used:

➤ *The Apraxia Profile.* Two versions exist: the Preschool and School-age Profile. Both include an oral motor exam, words, phrases, and sentences, and connected speech. A checklist of common apraxia characteristics is used. The Preschool Profile is shorter and less complex. The School-Age Profile includes rhymes, counting, and sentences with a rhyme.

➤ *The Kaufman Speech Praxis Test for Children (KSPT).* A standardized test that can be used for initial evaluation and re-evaluation. This test includes subsets for oral movements, syllables, vowel sounds, and conversational speech.

➤ *Verbal Motor Production Assessment (VMPAC).* Helps to identify the "best" method for treatment: auditory, visual, or tactile (hands-on). It measures speech and nonspeech skills at different levels of child participation. Best for children ages 3 to 12 years.

➤ *The Verbal Dyspraxia Profile (Jelm).* Observational checklists help structure what the SLP "sees" through your child's patterns of speech and feeding.

➤ **Oral Motor Skills:** Do your child's tongue, lips, jaw, and facial muscles work together to formulate words? Are facial and oral features symmetrical? Can he smile, frown, and press his lips together? Your SLP might use a flavored tongue depressor and gloves (mention if your child has a latex allergy) to examine his mouth. This can be tricky—some kids hate the idea of having someone's gloved hand in their mouth and some kids are painfully reminded of the dentist or doctor. Your SLP should ask you and your child if this is acceptable. Some therapists will allow your child to play with the instruments used for this examination.

➤ **Feeding:** Your child may be asked to eat something like a cracker or cookie and take a drink of water (or juice). This will assess whether your child has any difficulty drinking, swallowing, chewing, or aspirating (drawing in air and liquid at the same time—choking). Your SLP will also ask if you have observed any eating difficulties at home. Pay close attention to the texture of foods that your child eats well and those he doesn't (does he hate applesauce, but eat yogurt in earnest?). Mention them to the SLP, as well as any food allergies or insensitivities your child may have.

Impression and Initial Comments

At the end of your child's evaluation, the SLP will likely give you his or her impression and initial comments. You may even receive a diagnosis. But keep in mind that most SLPs will need some time to look over the results of the standardized testing (if used) and review their notes from the session.

Others may hesitate to give a diagnosis until they have worked with your child for a length of time. Perhaps they will suggest therapy once a week to rule out CAS. They may give a *suspected* or *working* diagnosis of CAS. This will ensure that the diagnosis is accurate. **It is worth noting that CAS cannot be diagnosed if your child is completely nonverbal.** Once your child attempts to communicate verbally, the SLP will be looking for any inconsistencies and patterns in your child's speech that may indicate he has apraxia.

Many SLPs may be reluctant to give a formal diagnosis of CAS until your child's third birthday. Some parents and therapists feel that waiting until three is too long. Others may tell you that a diagnosis prior to three years sets you up for an emotional rollercoaster. What if you worry and curse and cry, lose sleep, spend hours online, and then learn it wasn't CAS after all? This happened to one of my blog readers:

> *"We were told that Ryan had apraxia [CAS] when he was just about 27 months. I was a wreck. I didn't know what to make of it. He started a special preschool and they couldn't get him to talk for a long time, either. Finally, they told me they thought Ryan had autism and some other neurological issues. It wasn't apraxia, after all. I felt cheated. I took him to this school, read so many books, spent hours on the Internet. I want that time back."*

Finally, another word of caution: school-based SLPs may not diagnoses CAS. There are various reasons they may not give the official diagnosis, including being less familiar with CAS, being told not to give a medical diagnosis ("Speech Impaired" or "Sound System Disordered" are educational diagnoses), and believing that young children, in particular, may make quick progress in therapy and outgrow the label. Instead, a school-based SLP may use the term "suspected motor concern."

If this is the case for you and your child, you may consider having an evaluation conducted by an SLP in private practice to confirm the suspicion of CAS.

Parents Share...

Experiences with Learning the CAS Diagnosis

As you can see from the mothers' comments below, when and how children receive the official diagnosis of Childhood Apraxia of Speech (CAS) varies. SLPs, children, and parents are all unique individuals. It is often this combination of uniqueness that determines how and when you get a diagnosis.

"Our SLP didn't come right out and say that Marcus had apraxia. It wasn't like it was a secret, it just was never really discussed. I continued to take him to therapy knowing that things were improving [with his speech], but I never really knew what to call it until she mentioned it casually to me one day."

"I was mad when my therapist told me that she had been treating Finley for apraxia all along. Never once was this brought up to me. Finley has other issues as well [cri du chat syndrome] and everything is delayed. But when our therapist [SLP] said she codes for apraxia, I was dumbfounded."

"We didn't know at first. Our EI [early intervention] therapist was calling it a 'delay' for a long time. I was okay with that. As soon as she called it Childhood Apraxia of Speech, I went bonkers. Somehow 'delay' felt safe and fixable."

"Our daughter wasn't diagnosed until kind of late. She was seven. She has some other issues, too and we just thought her communication skills—or lack thereof—were related. It was all sort of a hoax about how and when she was diagnosed."

A Label?! I Don't Want My Child to Have a Label

Another concern I am sure you have is the label: Childhood Apraxia of Speech. Perhaps the idea that your child has a "problem" is worrisome, or you just can't stand the idea of your child being labeled. Or perhaps you have a completely different concern. Hang tight—we'll be sure to touch on some of those concerns you have. For now, having a label means you know what you're dealing with, there are ways to help your child, it may qualify your child for early intervention or other special help through the school, and it helps in terms of insurance reimbursement (more on that in Appendix B).

You may actually be pleasantly surprised by what happens after you get a label, as Amy of St. Louis was:

> *"As the months tick by since Brooke was officially diagnosed with CAS (she was 2 years, 3 months at diagnosis), one thing that I have routinely noticed throughout all of our doctor visits, therapy appointments, and developmental evaluations is that they were all hesitant to label a child. Which is really outstanding for so many reasons!*
>
> *"One of our biggest fears when we first noticed Brooke had developmental delays was that she was going to be labeled—correctly or incorrectly— and that it would "stick" and forever change the way people see her. And it has been nothing short of amazing to see that the exact opposite has happened. Labels are not slapped on without significant thought, and even when they are applied, it does not impact how people treat her."*

With the exception of a formal diagnosis to secure services or insurance funding, a label doesn't really matter. What matters is that each child is getting the right amount and type of support to help them reach their greatest potential.

Don't worry about the label; instead ask yourself, *"Is there anything else my child needs to be successful?"*

After the Evaluation

Whether or not your SLP gives you a diagnosis immediately after the evaluation, you should most definitely be advised *on what type of therapy* would best serve your child and how often he'll need it. I hope you are provided some resources such as the *Hope Speaks* DVD (see Resources), parent support group contacts, website guidance, or this book!

A written evaluation from your SLP should appear in your mailbox in the next several weeks. Please remember, speech clinics are busy. You may have to place a follow-up call to ensure you will be receiving a written report. Consider asking for it to also be mailed to you electronically. That way you always have a back-up if your paper copy gets misplaced.

Parents Share...

Keep Track of Your Evaluation Reports

"Remember where you keep your paper copies, you'll need to access them from time to time—when your child goes to preschool or when working with insurance."
(Refer to Chapter 11 for tips and hints on organizing all of that paperwork).

How to Read That Report

The report of a speech-language evaluation is exciting in some ways, hard-to-hear in others, and excruciatingly boring and cumbersome all at the same time.

The written report you'll open will likely be long—5 to 7 pages—and very detailed. You will come across words and phrases you probably aren't familiar with and nearly each one of them will cause you some alarm, question, or anxiety.

Reading about your child's problems in black and white composed by a "stranger," yet also a professional, is often a wake-up call. Brace yourself. You may choose to hold onto the report—unopened—until your spouse or significant other can be there with you. You may think it's easier to read the report if you already suspect CAS and are looking for validation and justification by a professional. Just be warned, even in that situation, it's not easy. No parent wants to be faced with the fact that their child is struggling.

Here are some other tips that may help you make heads or tails of the report:

➤ *Remind yourself: I am the parent.* "I am concerned about my child's developing speech. I want to help my child and so does this speech pathologist."

➤ *Take turns reading the report out loud to your spouse, partner, or trusted friend.* This sort of depersonalizes the words. At the end of each section, pause to ask questions, clarify, make notes, etc.

➤ *When making notes about the report, refrain from writing directly on the report.* You never know when you'll need to provide a copy of the report to the school or another medical provider. Keep your originals "clean." Use a Post-It note instead.

➤ *If you don't understand a word, phrase, or some terminology specific to speech pathology, make a note of it and look it up later.* You will likely see lots of words you aren't familiar with. (Refer to the glossary located at the back of this book if you'd like.)

➤ *If you notice something inaccurate in the report, bring it to your SLP's attention immediately.* Give her a call or send an email and explain your concern in a diplomatic manner. You may not agree with everything your SLP observed during your child's evaluation; if you feel a particular observation is not a true representation of your child, kindly ask if your SLP can add a statement to the report indicating something along those lines. For example, "Mother indicates it is not typical for Kate to drool during speech." (Kate really *did* drool during her evaluation and I was sure to tell the SLP that it wasn't typical.)

➤ *Take time to digest the information.* You've learned a great deal about your child's communication difficulties. You need time to absorb it all.

➤ *Do what you need to do to cope with it.* Reading the report is going to dredge up some feelings you may or may not be ready to accept. You may be in denial, you may be angry, you may seek to receive a second opinion, or you may just want to cry. Go ahead and let it out. Do something proactive, though. What have you done in the past to cope with unpleasant news? Do it now.

➤ *When you're ready, begin sharing the results with those who love, support, and encourage you and your child.* You will need to pull from various sources as you and your child cope with CAS.

What's a Treatment Plan?

A treatment plan ("Tx Plan") is typically about a paragraph or two of detailed recommendations for therapy generally printed at the end of your initial report. It may include a target date for a re-screen or reevaluation. Your SLP will list *specific initial goals*, along with possible recommendations for additional therapy (OT, PT), and suggestions for family and educational professionals.

When I practiced as a Child and Adolescent Psychiatric R.N., we often used this acronym for setting treatment goals: **S**pecific, **M**easureable, **A**ttainable, **R**ealistic, and **T**oward dismissal [from speech therapy]. Keeping this acronym in mind can give you a quick and easy way to remember ways to create goals and keep tabs on your child's treatment place. The acronym also works for speech-language therapy, with one addition. SLPs always need to keep the reason for the goal in mind, whether or not they include it in the written goal. The following sample illustrates how SLPs may write their goals with SMART in mind:

➤ **S**(pecific): To improve articulation, Josh will produce target CVCV [consonant-vowel-consonant-vowel], CV, and VC syllables with correct articulation in structured therapy.

➤ **M**(easurable): 80% accuracy on target words even if he needs visual cues, and during therapy time, not necessarily in his spontaneous speech.

➤ **A**(ttainable): An SLP will likely describe the circumstances under which Josh was expected to produce the targets (during structured therapy in which notes are being taken)

➤ **R**(ealistic): "To be realistic, I would never take a child who couldn't do CVCV, CV, and VC syllables and expect him to be producing three-syllable words in spontaneous speech in a year's time," says Rhonda Banford, CCC-SLP. "In my goals, I also want to tell the circumstances under which I expect him to produce the targets—e.g., during structured therapy, which is when I am taking data. Of course, if the child made quick progress, I would adjust my goals to reflect higher level skills. If the child is truly apraxic, however, we have to be cognizant of the fact that it may take him quite a while to truly establish basic motor movements with consistency. As he progresses and internalizes new motor movements, I would anticipate his therapy to start moving along with greater speed."

➤ **T**(oward dismissal): Remember that CAS is a dynamic disorder, meaning it changes over time, so it is challenging to pinpoint a specific date for dismissal. SLPs often have time constraints imposed upon them, particularly when they work in hospitals and schools. Many children with CAS will be seen for therapy in the schools. School IEPs typically cover a period of one year, so goals must be attainable in that period of time (in effect, when children are dismissed for summer break).

[**Reason:** To improve articulation.]

You likely won't see your child's goals written out next to the SMART acronym. Instead, you will see all the elements combined into a paragraph along these lines:

➤ In order to improve articulation, Josh will produce early developing consonant phonemes /p, b, m, t, d, n, w, h/ in target CVCV, CV, VC, and CVC words during structured conversation, with 80% accuracy over 3 data days.

OR:

➤ In order to improve expressive language, Emily will produce target CVC words with correct articulation in four carrier phrases (I want ____, I have ____, I see ____, I need) during structured therapy, with 80% accuracy over 3 data days.

The treatment plan is something you will hear mentioned often. Know it well. Ask for revisions if you find that things aren't progressing as they should, your child has reached some goals, or a new concern has cropped up.

Say That Again?! Chapter Summary

This chapter presented you with an initial-speech-pathologist-visit-in-a-nutshell scenario. Do your homework ahead of time by filling out the appropriate forms and getting them to the speech clinic ahead of time. As you read the final report from the SLP, it's important to remember that he or she is there to help your child. Reading that first report is never easy. No parent wants to admit that his or her child has a concern that is best dealt with by someone else. Reach out to supportive and helpful individuals as you make sense of the treatment plan and the recommendations of the speech-language pathologist.

Bottom line: if you *suspect* there is a *potential* diagnosis of CAS, get your kiddo to a SLP ASAP!

Read On! Recommended Resources

➤ The Greater Baltimore Medical Center has a nice online guide to *Pediatric Speech-Language Pathology* that you may find helpful: www.gbmc.org/home_voicecenter.cfm?id=1568.

➤ You may also appreciate Speech Therapy Information and Resources (STIR), a UK online resource that's all about speech and language. You may find the sections on play, communication, and anatomy particularly helpful: www.speech-therapy-information-and-resources.com

➤ *Assessment of Speech-language Disorders in Children* by Rebecca McCauley (Psychology Press, 2000) is a great resource, although it's not exactly written for parents. You may find it tedious because it's so comprehensive—and designed mostly for a professional or graduate student audience.

➤ At 800 pages, this is a huge volume of information, but you will find plenty of examples, assessment styles, and treatment plans in *Language Disorders from Infancy Through Adolescence: Assessment and Intervention* by Rhea Paul, Ph.D. CCC-SLP (Mosby, 2006). Most definitely a textbook or desk reference for speech pathologists, this text can be found (or requested) through your public library, as can the book listed above.

➤ *Parent's Guide to Speech and Language Problems* (McGraw-Hill, 2007), by Debbie Feit, a journalist and mother of two children with CAS (now resolved), does a great job of compiling related speech disorders in an easy-to-use guide, complete with tips for finding a speech pathologist, as well as assessment and intervention.

➤ *Hope Speaks: An Introduction to Childhood Apraxia of Speech* (2005, DVD) is a half-hour documentary that is both educational and inspirational. It is designed as an introduction to parents of children who have recently been diagnosed with apraxia. You can order your copy through the Apraxia-Kids Store at www.Apraxia-Kids.org

➤ *Here's How to Treat Childhood Apraxia of Speech,* by Margaret (Dee) Fish (Plural Publishing, 2010), is mostly written as a textbook, but is readable for motivated parents as well. It covers a substantial amount of information about assessment, but is mostly concerned with treatment.

➤ The Apraxia-Kids/CASANA website has an article written by Thomas Powell, Ph.D., CCC-SLP, that you may be interested in checking out: "A Brief Overview of Language and Approaches to Assessment: One Professional's Perspective." Look for it at: www.apraxia-kids.org (type Thomas Powell in the search box).

Section Two

. . . .
Now What?!
. . . .

Chapter Five

· · · · · · · · · · · · · ·

Getting the Apraxia
Diagnosis

· · · · · ·

Initial Reactions

"Well," she began, "I think she has Childhood Apraxia of Speech (CAS)." I sat there looking at Kate and then at the speech-language pathologist who had just completed the intense hour and fifteen-minute assessment.

"OK," I thought, "At least we know what to call it." But just what exactly *is* Childhood Apraxia of Speech? The only words I caught in the therapist's answer were "neurologically based" and "motor-speech disorder." Yes, of course—that makes perfect sense. I was stumped and I had questions—lots of them.

I was tempted to just scoop up my children and our belongings and hustle on to the next stop: the craft store. Being the creative mom that I am, I figured I needed some themed scrapbook pages for the next milestone: "Kate Riley—The Apraxic Years."

You may think I wasn't taking this seriously. Rest assured, that wasn't the case. At the time, I wasn't sure what to make of this information. I had never heard that term before. I was tired and drained after the evaluation. I had been entertaining a wiggly baby in a new environment. And there were plenty of things floating around on my mental to-do list.

I had no knowledge and no past experience with speech disorders, so I asked the therapist if she had any handouts or pamphlets on the diagnosis she had just handed my daughter. She didn't. But she did offer a website, the Childhood Apraxia of Speech Association of North America (CASANA), which can be found at www.Apraxia-KIDS.org.

"I'd just get online when you get home and look it up," she suggested. And that was it. I was also encouraged to stop at the front desk to make an appointment for Kate's first speech session.

Therapy was recommended twice weekly for one hour until Kate reached "age-appropriate speech milestones." Again, I had no idea what that meant either. The speech-language pathologist said she would type out a full report and mail it to me, complete with therapy goals.

Indeed we did go to the craft store afterwards. They had no stickers or embellishments for CAS—I looked—but they had plenty of holiday-themed ones. I grabbed a handful, determined to keep my newly diagnosed daughter as normal as possible. So what if she had a speech disorder? I still needed her help making invitations for a family holiday get-together.

Any "good" mom would have gone right home, plopped her kids in front of a video, and logged on to the Internet to do some hardcore research. I didn't. Instead I told my husband how the evaluation went as he flipped through the mail and kissed his family.

"So, it's called Childhood Apraxia of Speech. That's why Kate isn't talking yet," I informed him. He had questions similar to mine…. What does that mean? What caused it? What can we do about it? What's the prognosis?

I wasn't a complete slacker-mom. That night, after the girls were off in dreamland, I pulled out my laptop and did some research. Not a lot. Just enough to get a few of my most pressing questions answered. I still needed time to digest all of this information. Plus, there were invitations to create.

It may sound as though I was taking this news about Kate's CAS all in stride. In reality, I was confused, yet relieved that we finally had something to call "it." I was worried, yet trying to remain hopeful for her sake and mine. I cried and yelled at my parents on the phone, "My kid can't talk—this is a *big* problem!" The story that I relate above really did happen pretty much as I tell it here. It took time and energy to muster up the courage to learn more about apraxia. Once I did, I realized just how serious it was.

The Nuts and Bolts of This Chapter

➤ You're on an emotional rollercoaster—we'll talk about that

➤ A trip back in time to 1891 when we *believe* the first case of CAS was identified

➤ Information on prognosis, or the likelihood that your child's CAS will resolve

Learning the Diagnosis

You may have been searching for years for some term to identify why your child isn't talking like every other child. Perhaps you weren't that concerned in the first place, but took your child to a speech-language pathologist because your friends, your mother, or a concerned neighbor or teacher urged you to. In either case, you now have a term to describe the phenomenon: *Childhood Apraxia of Speech (CAS).* What's next?

Common Reactions

If it took you awhile to arrive at a diagnosis, you may be feeling like your competence as a parent has been challenged.

"Gosh, I knew there was something wrong.
Why wouldn't (or couldn't) anyone tell me what it was?!"

You may feel some resentment toward any professionals you consulted who shooed you away, assuring you everything was "fine."

"I knew I was right! Those doctors were so incompetent.
Their lack of competency and time wasted really irks me!"

You might feel like I did: relieved.

"Now I know what to call this thing that was preventing
my little sweetie from saying much more than 'eh?'"

But you could also feel discouraged, as I did.

"What now? What does this mean for my kid?
Will she ever be able to talk? Where do I go from here?"

Case in point: One of my playgroup mom friends said, "Oh, apraxia…that's a tough one. I was so glad when Jackson didn't have it after all. Call me if you want to talk about it." I didn't. Not to her, anyway. If Jackson didn't really have CAS, I didn't want to get stuck talking with someone who would make it sound like the end of the world. Plus, I wanted to believe that it would be an easy fix.

Another mom friend of mine—who also has a daughter with apraxia—indicated she felt naïve when she first got the diagnosis: "I just didn't know what to think. Maybe one or two months of therapy and then she'd be talking normally."

Really, the "fix" is somewhere in the middle. Receiving a diagnosis of CAS *is* pretty serious, but it's not the end of the world, and it's certainly not a quick fix. We'll cover therapy approaches in Chapter 7.

Other feelings and emotions you might be experiencing after learning the diagnosis of CAS:

➤ Disbelief /uncertainty
➤ Confusion
➤ Denial
➤ Information overload
➤ Numbness
➤ Isolation
➤ Loss

> ➤ Shock
> ➤ Anger
> ➤ Guilt
> ➤ Sadness
> ➤ Yet, you may also feel acceptance, and even a proactive sense of duty.

Here's a blurb from my journal at the time, expressing my mishmash of feelings:

"I am feeling a bit dumbfounded about Kate's diagnosis. I used to be in speech & debate [club]. I wrote and performed an oratory at a competition level; how could I possibly have a kid who couldn't talk?! Maybe I have been 'chosen' to help a little person—my Kate—navigate the road of apraxia… with my public speaking skills and child psych background, perhaps this is a perfect fit for parent and child. But I can't help feeling like this is all too un-fair—for me and for Kate."

Some folks have a more positive reaction from the outset. They may even say they feel "blessed" or as though they were "chosen" to have a child with such a diagnosis. For example, here's how one mother I spoke to came to terms with her child's diagnosis:

"I'm a nurse in a neuro-rehab unit. We see a lot of patients who are suffering from brain injuries, stroke, and such. I know CAS isn't really the same, but there are a lot of similarities. I have a good knowledge base of neu-rological issues, so learning about apraxia isn't so out of my comfort zone."

For now, sit tight with your feelings about your child's diagnosis. Listen to them, accept them, and talk them over with someone such as a friend, your spouse, or your child's SLP.

Parents Share...

Early Feelings after the Diagnosis

"It is a funny thing, apraxia. It just CONSUMES you as a parent when you are at the worst of it. I can remember wondering what Allison's voice even sounded like. And wondering what she would say when she started talking. Would she talk? I remem-ber when a friend's son, who was a year younger than Ally, started talking preco-ciously and—I hate to admit it—it filled me with despair that took my breath away."
—Susan, mother of Ally

More on Denial

Chapter 2 covered some common remarks that others may make to you to ex-plain your child's speech delays. For example: You do all the talking for her, so she doesn't need to talk. Or: she'll talk when something really interests her. Sometimes when parents get the diagnosis of CAS, they don't believe it, and may actually wonder if the comments that others made to them are true.

Along those lines, you or your spouse may wonder, "Is she just shy?" In reality, there is a big difference between having a speech disorder like CAS and "just being shy." A shy child might have genetic tendencies to be more introverted (that's perfectly okay), or might not have developed the social skills, confidence, or maturity to speak up in uncertain or new situations. Some kids (and adults) need time to "warm up" before they feel comfortable conversing with others—even those they know well. Shy kids *can* talk, they just prefer not to—at least at that moment.

I am convinced that my daughter is an extrovert at heart whose mouth simply can't keep up with her extroverted thoughts and modes of relating to others.

Having CAS—while not exactly a "good thing"—can be corrected with early, frequent, and intense intervention.

Although feelings of denial are common after the diagnosis of CAS in a child, remember: Before you are given the diagnosis of CAS, everything else that it *could* be should have been ruled out through the process of *differential diagnosis*.

What is a Differential Diagnosis?

In fancy talk, you may hear folks refer to the "differential diagnosis." What this really means is the process that professionals use to tease out other disorders or factors that may be contributing to what *looks like* CAS. "It is difficult for SLPs to diagnose CAS when a child has little or no speech because many of the characteristics of CAS

Parents Ask...

Is verbal apraxia (CAS) and oral apraxia the same thing?

No. While these two disorders seem to have the same connotation, they are actually quite different. **Oral Apraxia** is the impaired ability to voluntarily perform nonspeech tasks with the mouth and tongue, such as kissing, puckering, puffing out cheeks, licking lips, sticking out the tongue. To clarify further, a child might be able to lick an ice cream cone without any problem, but when asked to stick out her tongue, she might be unable to. If asked by her SLP to "pucker your lips like you are going to give someone a kiss," she might not be able to, but she might be able to kiss her mother good night without any delay. These children may be late-talkers, but can often speak normally, *if* they don't also have CAS in addition.

CAS (sometimes referred to as verbal apraxia) is the impaired ability to voluntarily perform speech tasks with the mouth and tongue. The child may have no problem imitating or producing nonspeech mouth movements (sticking out tongue, puckering, etc.) on command, but *sometimes* a child has *both* CAS and oral apraxia.

However, verbal and oral apraxia are not the same thing! Apraxia of any kind is a motor programming problem, not a muscle function problem. For more information on the other types of apraxia, see Appendix A.

involve speech," explains Di Bahr, CCC-SLP, and author of *Nobody Ever Told Me or My Mother That!* "For example," she says, "kids with CAS often leave sounds out in words, or make the same [consistent] speech errors in spontaneous speech but make different [inconsistent] errors when *asked* to imitate. In order to observe these characteristics of CAS, the child must have some speech."

Also, SLPs will consider whether your child may actually have word finding problems, an autism spectrum disorder (ASD), social anxiety (shyness taken to an extreme), hearing loss, auditory processing disorder, or something else.

To use the CAS label with utmost confidence, the practitioner(s) must find evidence that the child has the symptoms characteristic of children with CAS that are listed on pages 7-8 in Chapter 1.

Coping with Bad News

We all deal with bad news in a uniquely predictable manner. As I came to terms with my daughters' CAS I recalled my clinical experience in hospice care with the grief process. One of the best known theories as to how people cope with loss comes from Elizabeth Kubler-Ross, the author of *On Death & Dying,* published in 1969. Her theory is a continuum that looks something like this:

→ **Denial** → **Bargaining** → **Anger** → **Fear** → **Acceptance** →

She indicates that individuals who are confronting the loss of a loved one can vacillate between the stages, finally ending at acceptance at some point.

Although Kubler-Ross developed her theory to explain how people manage the loss of a loved one, her theory has been extrapolated to explain how people cope with other types of bad news, as well. When it comes to parents dealing with grief related to a child's disability, it's a similar, yet different route one takes, mostly because that child is alive and with us every day. As a parent, you won't neatly arrive at the final level of "acceptance" after going through the prescribed stages above. Instead, CAS feels like a roller coaster—perhaps feeling "up" about the diagnosis, then feeling "down" about it, and finally coming to terms with it as the ride nears its completion. The discussion about the completion of this process (resolving apraxia) is found in Chapter 15.

Another take that may help you understand the adjustment process comes from Holly Olmsted-Hickey, parent leader and moderator of Windy City/Chicagoland Apraxia Network (whose teenage son has struggled with CAS):

"There are three ways I've described the process of learning about a child's development:
1. Peeling an onion: discovering something new with each peeled layer. Like an onion, sometimes those new discoveries make you cry.
2. Playing a game of whack-a-mole: with great fervor and determination, whacking at the mole only to discover something new popping up in the process.

3. Wandering in a dark, underground maze with a candle and a key to a door: sometimes your candle goes out and your key doesn't fit the door, but you always find someone on your path to light your candle and point you in a new direction."

What's a Parent to Do?

We all cope in unique ways. I am sure you have a few "favorite" coping techniques you can pull from. This list may get you started:

➤ Get support by seeking out an online support group such as the Apraxia-Kids listserv (www.apraxia-kids.org) or the Windy City Apraxia Network listserv (serving areas of suburban Chicago, NW Indiana, SE Wisconsin, and Eastern Iowa). You can subscribe by emailing windycityapraxia-subscribe@yahoogroups.com. You can find other online groups throughout the U.S. and Canada by going to www.yahoogroups.com and typing "apraxia" in the "Find a Yahoo Group" search box.

➤ Apraxia-Kids/CASANA has a state-by-state (as well as Canadian, Australian, and South African) guide for finding local in-person support groups. Go to apraxia-kids.org, click on "learn about apraxia," then "library," and "resources & support."

➤ CHERAB Foundation, a "world-wide nonprofit organization working to improve the communication skills and education of all children with speech and language delays and disorders." Their emphasis is on CAS and oral apraxia. Visit them at www.cherabfoundation.org.

➤ Try to connect with others in your community with a similar diagnosis. A good starting point is to ask your child's SLP or school for contacts.

➤ Seek out other information you need to feel empowered to help your child. You may find other books, magazines/newsletters, or online resources helpful.

➤ Express and acknowledge your emotions, whether in a journal, by talking to friends, your spouse, family members, with your child's SLP, a counselor, or clergy.

➤ Balance all of this with a healthy diet and exercise. Sometimes, a quick jog can clear your mind and help you feel empowered.

My Feelings Are All Over the Place!

If you feel like you might need a little extra time or TLC to absorb all of this information, you are not alone. Consider seeking out a therapist—the counseling kind. It's not wrong or bad if you feel the need for professional help. Remember, it's a *process* of accepting and coming to terms with a diagnosis. It's not supposed to happen overnight, and everyone deals with it in their own unique way.

Coping Advice

I interviewed "apraxia mom" and music therapist Katie Eshelman on my blog, Leslie 4 Kids (www.leslie4kids.wordpress.com), and asked her: "What would you tell parents just learning their child's diagnosis of apraxia." Here's her response:

"Personally, I just needed time. Time to process, time to cry, time to share, and finally time to make a plan. I also needed to remember that [my daughter] was the same mischievous, sweet, funny little girl regardless of the CAS. Therefore, when the diagnosis comes up, I tell them I have a daughter with CAS, not an 'apraxic daughter.'"

Of course, since Ms. Eshelman is also a music therapist, I had to ask her if her career choice was a natural extension of helping her daughter communicate.

"Although my education and experience in the field [of music therapy] gave me some of the technical knowledge and theory to support my musical techniques, there is such an emotional component to working with your own child. I often tell people I am the kind of music therapist I am because I am a mom and I am the type of mom I am because I am a music therapist." (You'll find more references to music and music therapy in Chapters 7 and 8.)

If you look for coincidences like these in your own life, you just might see how you are the best parent for your child with apraxia of speech, too.

Families adjust and perceive a diagnosis of CAS in different ways. It depends on the family's cultural background, resources (financial, insurance coverage), religious beliefs, social supports, and temperaments (of individuals within the family). Your response may be different than your spouse's and even different than your mother's response. Just because someone isn't responding in the manner you think they should doesn't mean they aren't affected.

Your Child's Prognosis

Probably one of the first questions you had after you learned your child's diagnosis was something along the lines of "Will she ever be cured?" Or "will she have speech problems her whole life?" In other words, you wanted to know your child's prognosis—or the likelihood of her getting "better."

Unfortunately, that is not something that anyone knows at diagnosis. At most, your SLP may describe your child's CAS as mild, moderate, severe, or profound. Of course, you probably want to know, "What does it mean to have *moderate* CAS?"

"The terms 'mild, moderate, severe, and profound' are related to a scale of goodness," according to Di Bahr, CCC-SLP. As she explains, "A scale of goodness has to do with the percentage of characteristics exhibited by the child. If a child has few characteristics of a disorder, the child has a mild disorder. If the child has many characteristics of a disorder, the child may have a severe to profound disorder. Disorders like CAS (where there is a list of behavioral characteristics) are often evaluated with a scale of goodness."

At present, there are no commonly accepted definitions of the various degrees of impairment in CAS. As Rhonda Banford, CCC-SLP, explains, the use of mild vs. moderate vs. severe vs. profound is a subjective decision made by the SLP:

"If a child has an extraordinary number of speech errors and is almost entirely unintelligible, I would probably characterize him or her as having profound difficulty. If she is largely unintelligible but is able to say a few things correctly, I would characterize her speech as severely impaired. If she is intelligible about half of the time, I would call her speech moderately impaired, and if she only has a few difficulties, I would use the mild designation. The terms are rather arbitrary.

"A child who has a profound speech problem has just as good a chance of becoming intelligible as a child who has a lesser speech problem. It will just take her longer to get there, especially if she has apraxia, and it will take therapy with a professional who has a good understanding of her speech concerns and the most effective ways to address them. This is assuming that she has good cognition, adequate receptive language, appropriate attention and task focus, etc. If she does not have these precursors to good speech, it will be difficult for her to attain the same level of proficiency."

The authors of *Developmental Apraxia of Speech: Theory and Clinical Practice* concur that severity ratings of CAS are quite subjective. They note that some SLPs base it on only one observation, while others may predict severity with improvement over time. So, if a child is progressing quickly, her apraxia may be judged as "not as severe" as another child's who doesn't progress as quickly. However, one characteristic that differentiates CAS from other speech disorders is *relatively* slow progress in speech treatment. Here are some other factors that authors Penny Hall, Linda Jordan, and Donald Robin take into account when assessing the severity of CAS:

➤ Does the child's speech get worse with longer words? (more severe)
➤ Does the child have the ability to control the environment through speech? (if so, less severe)
➤ What is the child's developmental lag (usually given in months)? (Less lag = less severe)
➤ How well can a listener understand what the child is saying (intelligibility)? (Better intelligibility = less severe)
➤ Finally, there is the impact of co-occurring problems (additional concerns/diagnoses = more severe)

Although nobody can predict today what your child's speech will be like when she is older, a variety of factors can affect how well and how quickly she is able to overcome her speech difficulties. I have summarized an article by Lori Hickman, CCC-SLP,

"What Does the Future Hold," for you to follow as you track the variables considered in the prognosis of apraxia:

Factors That Affect Prognosis

Cause of the Child's Apraxia (often called, "etiology," the fancy way of saying "cause" or "origin")	Is the cause of your child's speech problem primarily motor or linguistic? The cause of apraxia is unknown, as is the prognosis. The difficulty for the SLP lies in the differential diagnosis of CAS vs. other types of speech disorders. (A "motor problem" can be due to a muscle function problem or a motor programming issue, sometimes both. Phonological disorders are "linguistic problems." **CAS is a motor-speech disorder.**) See Chapter 6.
Family History	When other family members have a similar speech history, it is likely the child's long-term outcome/prognosis may be similar to that family member's outcome (providing, of course, that their causes are truly the same). See Chapter 6.
Severity of Apraxia	In general, the more severe a child's apraxia is, the longer treatment is needed.
Verbal Apraxia (CAS) with or without Oral Apraxia	Children who exhibit **oral apraxia** (difficulty puffing cheeks, licking lips, sticking out tongue on command) *in addition* to CAS often require treatment longer than children who have only CAS. **Remember, oral apraxia and CAS are not the same thing!**
Overall Health	Children whose overall health is good are more available to speech therapy than kids who have periods of time when they are less "learning available" due to illness (middle ear infections, upper respiratory infections, etc.).
Cognitive Skills/ General Intelligence	Children who score in the average to above average range in intelligence testing have a better prognosis than children with cognitive and intellectual delays.
Attention & Ability to Focus	Children with concerns such as ADHD often require intervention for longer periods than children without these concerns, as attention, focus, and concentration are *required* for motor learning. The SLP can focus on the child's sound productions rather than working to maintain her attention. Children with attentional concerns tend to have more difficulty monitoring their own speech.

Child's Reaction to Their Intelligibility Deficit	Children who seem unaware of—or less bothered by—the difficulty other people have understanding them often require longer treatment. See Chapter 14 for information on coping skills.
Ability to Self-Monitor	Children who are able to monitor their own speech tend to progress more quickly. Children who are unable to "self-monitor" continue to need their SLP or others to comment on their speech. Self-monitoring occurs when the child begins to "hear" his/her own speech and "edits" it as necessary. If a child doesn't "hear" an error, it will be nearly impossible for him/her to correct it.
Age at Which Intervention (Treatment/ Therapy) Begins	The younger the child is when treatment begins, the better the long-term prognosis.
Appropriateness of Therapy	The therapeutic approach used in treatment ought to be tailored to each child individually. ***A "one-size-fits-all" approach does not work for children with apraxia.*** The child's SLP needs to be able to adjust sessions according to the child's needs.
Frequency of Therapy	The more frequently the child receives appropriate therapy, the better the long-term prognosis.
Comorbidity (other diagnoses that *may* occur along with CAS, co-occurring).	Children who have other disorders in addition to apraxia (dysarthria, autism, ADHD, Down syndrome, etc.) generally have a poorer prognosis than children whose primary disorder/delay is CAS. See Appendix A.
Motivation	A child who is happy and enjoys working with an SLP has a better outcome than a child who is resistant or indifferent toward therapy.
Parent Involvement, Education, and Support	Informed parents can encourage a child's communication skills. They are also much better equipped to advocate, network, and seek out additional resources.

Information taken from "Prognosis for Apraxia: What Does The Future Hold?" by Lori Hickman, M.A., CCC-SLP, copyright Childhood Apraxia of Speech Association of North America (CASANA). Adapted with permission from CASANA: www.apraxia-kids.org.

Generally, when children are neurologically different in one area (in the case of CAS), other neurological conditions/concerns (such as learning, motor, or behavior issues in other areas of development) are usually part of the overall "package."

Parents Ask...

Is there any research about the prognosis of CAS?

There are no definitive studies on the outcome of children with apraxia. Since there is a lack of agreement/identification of this group of children, it is hard to design studies that would measure this. Kids with CAS vary quite a bit in terms of their apraxic characteristics. Therefore, it is nearly impossible to establish a control group to determine efficacy and results of long-term speech therapy.

In a nutshell, the prognosis for the average child with CAS is that she will likely learn to use speech as the primary method of communication and will eventually be able to communicate in complete, grammatically correct sentences. Most people will not even realize that she ever had a speech disorder when she was younger. But this will take time, regular speech therapy, and plenty of practice at home. Each child with CAS progresses at a different rate, but you can probably count on at least one year of speech therapy. Kids with more severe apraxia or additional disabilities may continue to receive speech therapy through adolescence. Please defer to your SLP for a more specific range for *your* child.

If you are interested in learning more about resolving/recovering CAS, stay tuned. It will be covered in Chapter 15.

Cultural and Social History of Childhood Apraxia of Speech

Have you ever wondered what would have happened to your child if she had been born with CAS-like symptoms a hundred years ago? Would she have been labeled as "dumb and mute?" Would she have been institutionalized? Would she have "outgrown" it? Well, I did a little historical research. History Buffs—rejoice!

The first case of CAS published in the medical literature was not called CAS at that early date, but was referred to as "aphemia. This case appeared in literature in 1891 by English physician W.B Hadden. Dr. Hadden made a house call to see eleven-year-old Charles M. to assess his lack of intelligible speech (intelligible meaning "understandable," not a reflection of one's intelligence). Young Charles hadn't attempted speech sounds until he was three years old. His older sister was the only one in the family who could understand him, thus becoming his interpreter. After some work with Dr. Hadden, Charles was able to produce short, automatic words and phrases better than he produced longer, more spontaneous speech. Today we know this as a symptom of Childhood Apraxia of Speech.

An 1897 edition of *The Lancet* included an article by neurologist H.C. Bastian. His conclusions about the disorder were more organic in nature than Dr. Hadden's. He wrote, "Speech has now become a truly automatic act for human beings...and if children do not speak at birth...its main cause is due to the fact that their nervous systems are too immature." His century-old statement (along with additional theory and research in the last 100 years) is now driving researchers to infer that CAS is a delay or inadequate development of those neurological pathways required for speech and not a result of a cortical (brain) lesion.

A progressive woman by the name of Muriel Morley first described the condition of Childhood Apraxia of Speech in the late 1950s. She didn't call it CAS at the time, but instead referred to it as "defective articulation," and also "developmental apraxia/ aphasia." Children began to be labeled with these diagnoses sometime in the 1960s, most likely in response to the most severe cases. However, today we know CAS as a continuum from mild to moderate to severe to profound cases.

I was curious enough to do a little biographical research on Dr. Muriel Morley. I invite you to join me as we travel through speech pathology history.

More about Muriel Morley's Theories

Dr. Morley concluded that kids with the disorder she called developmental apraxia/aphasia failed to develop the central processes of speech to begin with. In other words, the child has never had normal speech and therefore has not "lost" it somewhere along the lines as brain injured (aphasic) adults have.

Here you'll find a list of Muriel Morley's findings/symptoms from her study conducted in 1947 (published in 1957), Children with Developmental Apraxia/ Aphasia:

➤ [Have] poor expressive language (delayed neurological maturation for motor processes in verbal expression)
➤ Can understand other's speech with no problem (good/normal receptive language)
➤ [Are] friendly and cooperative; making every effort to communicate with others, but unable to do so through speech
➤ [Have] little or no interest in imitation of sounds of speech, even making animal sounds like "moo" and "baa" is difficult
➤ [Have] little or no vocal play or babbling as a baby
➤ [Are] quiet children—they rarely use sound and voice
➤ May show signs of frustration when they can't make requests known
➤ Rely mostly on gesture to achieve needs/wants
➤ [May have] one or two isolated words may be used during first 2-3 years of life (ages 12 to 24 months)
➤ Have a slowly developing vocabulary
➤ Have a sudden growth in vocabulary around 4+ years of age

Muriel was born in 1899 in Halifax, England. She studied physics and biology and taught at a girls' school for ten years. In 1932, she answered a newspaper ad from a plastic surgeon looking for an "educated woman" to assess the speech of children before and after an innovative surgery to correct cleft palate. For the next five years, Muriel read all she could about cleft palates and speech. She began studying speech-language pathology by working with colleagues in Liverpool and London. In 1938, she received a certificate from the British Society of Speech Therapists.

Muriel founded The College of Speech Therapy in 1945. She insisted that speech and language be studied and taught at universities and that is should include studies of pathology based on normal developmental behavior. She also insisted that students complete a clinical rotation with supervision. It wasn't until 1955 that speech-language pathology was recognized as a college major.

Even before Muriel published her work in the 1957 edition of *The Development and Disorders of Speech in Childhood,* the subject of apraxia (adult apraxia and acquired apraxia, *not just* CAS) had been controversial for over 130 years. The characteristics, the explanations underlying the disorder, and the very label itself have been debated for a very long time.

As I read Morley's list of symptoms, I thought, "This is it! This is exactly what my daughter has…and this is the woman who identified it. Amazing." If your child has CAS, you will also probably feel as this if this list of symptoms describes your child well. Your child may not have *all* of these traits, but she will probably have most of them.

Today, SLPs and researchers continue to tweak the diagnostic criteria for CAS. Perhaps a few traits that are missing from Ms. Morley's early criteria are: "saying words out of the blue," difficulty following sequenced directions (e.g., "Put your shoes on and then grab your backpack before going outside"), errors with vowel usage, and decreased intelligibility as phrases get longer.

Some Advice for the Road

Here are some points to keep in mind as you set about your apraxia journey:

➤ *CAS is dynamic and can change over time.* Most kids with CAS have difficulty making sounds. As these children get older, their motor planning improves. Yet they will still have difficulty making the *correct* sounds, even though—in theory—they are able to. It may *appear* as though a child previously diagnosed with CAS now has a phonological delay, but in reality she just has a more sophisticated version of CAS. (A phonological delay/disorder is a language-based disorder. It has to do with difficulties underlying the sound system of a given language, not the neuromotor connection, as in CAS.) *Keep in mind that not all features will be present at the same time; some may not be present at all. CAS is complex and individual.*

➤ *If there is a "problem area" or a breakdown in your child's speech output, it's important to begin to understand where in the system that breakdown is occurring.* A child could have *a breakdown in the retrieval system*, for example. Think of it this way—your Golden Retriever can locate the stick you threw into the lake and bring it back to you for another round of fetch without any problem. But your child with apraxia…well, she's no retriever. You throw a word out to the lake and she can't plan the path to find/form it. She *knows* the word, but she just can't find it when she wants to use it. Please refer to Chapter 7 on speech therapy for more information on this.

➤ *Another little snag your child with apraxia may encounter is that she has difficulty producing certain speech sounds and sound patterns.* Let's face it, some sounds are just harder to produce. What can we do? Practice, practice, practice! I don't want to sound patronizing, but that practice piece of it is the hardest part of CAS. It's got to be done and it's anything but glamorous (more on that in Chapter 9: What You Can Do at Home).

➤ *Speech learning can be interrupted as the brain learns new things and tries to figure them out and make sense of new knowledge—be it cognitive or motor.* I am sure you have heard this theory on child development before—"your baby isn't babbling because she is working really hard at learning to roll over or sit up or crawl. Once she masters that motor skill, she'll get back to babbling." One thing at a time, right? Well, there is some truth to that, but don't latch onto this as the one and only reason your child isn't talking yet.

➤ *Once your child with apraxia does start talking more, she may start to mumble, stutter, self-practice, or grope for words.* (Self-practice simply means that she is working on speech sounds on her own, without any suggestion or direction to do so. It may sound as though your child is babbling, but this is a very important step to being a more effective communicator.) Don't lose heart—She may just be learning a new aspect of speech production, developing a word retrieval system, or learning to combine words into sentences. It might look like a regression in her speech-language skills, but in reality, it's probably just your child's brain working faster than it can produce the sounds. This may become more apparent as your child gets older.

Help! I Need a Dictionary!

No doubt you will continue to come across some new words on your quest to learn about CAS. Please refer to the glossary (Appendix F) for more detailed definitions and additional words and phrases you may come across along your apraxia journey. No worries—there won't be a test!

Say That Again?! Chapter Summary

You may have never heard of apraxia. Don't despair—get busy learning about it. Reading this book is a great first step. Applaud yourself for seeking out resources and information. Your feelings and emotions will change once you learn the diagnosis. There is no right or wrong way to feel. Seek therapy from a professional who has experience with disabilities if you feel like it's too much to adjust to.

This chapter also presented a history of early accounts of CAS (or suspected CAS). The idea of apraxia has been under much controversy for nearly 200 years. Please refer to Appendix D for additional information on this topic.

Finally, rest assured that *children with CAS can and do get better.* As a parent, the best thing you can do is to provide your children with frequent and intense therapy at an early age.

Read On! Recommended Resources

If it's truly CAS your child is struggling with, it's unlikely she'll "outgrow" it. Instead, your child will need the professional services of a speech-language pathologist. Check out this *educational/informational video* by Teri Peterson, M.S., CCC/SLP: www.youtube.com/user/ChatterboxBooks#p/u/0/7C6NAXvljpw.

➤ *Reflexes. Learning, and Behavior: A Window into the Child's Mind, a Non-Invasive Approach to Solving Learning and Behavior Problems,* by Sally Goddard (Fern Ridge Press, 2002).

➤ Lori Hickman, M.A., CCC-SLP, is a practicing speech-language pathologist and author of the *Apraxia Profile,* an assessment and therapeutic tool. The original article from which the chart on pages 80-81 was adapted can be found on the Apraxia-KIDS website, www.apraxia-kids.org (type "Lori Hickman" into the search field).

➤ For more guidance and support in your apraxia journey, try *You Will Dream New Dreams: Inspiring Personal Stories by Parents of Children with Disabilities* by Stanley D. Klein and Kim Schive (Kensington, 2001). It includes inspiring personal stories collected from parents around the U.S. It's like "a support group in a book."

➤ *Shut Up about Your Perfect Kid: A Survival Guide for Ordinary Parents of Special Children* by sisters Gina Gallagher and Patricia Konjoian (Three Rivers Press, 2010) is another great resource—funny, too—in which you will see these parents' frustration, sadness, and stigma as they share frank accounts of raising children with special needs.

➤ *A Different Kind of Perfect: Writings by Parents on Raising a Child with Special Needs* by Cindy Dowling (Trumpeter, 2006) provides 50 personal essays written by parents of children with special needs. Here, you'll find heartbreaking honesty as these parents grapple with grief and despair to gratitude and laughter.

➤ Speech-language pathologist Dr. Ruth Stoeckel addresses the question about degrees of severity in a YouTube video from a 2011 Charleston, WV workshop in a series entitled *Questions on CAS: Levels of Severity and Therapy:* www.youtube.com/user/ApraxiaKids#p/u/2/nXOfruNY3Dk.

Chapter Six

· · · · · · · · · · ·

So What *Caused* All of This?

· · · · · · · · ·

Theories and Medical Diagnoses Related to CAS

You'd like to blame someone, *anyone,* for the misfortunate combination of luck and biology that lead to your child having Childhood Apraxia of Speech. But chances are, there is nothing or no one who can take the blame. There is a lot of conflicting information out there about what causes CAS. To date, the professionals can't agree on a cause—but there are lots of theories. I am certainly no expert in CAS theory, so if you really have an interest in this topic, I urge you to seek out additional resources.

The Nuts and Bolts of This Chapter

➤ A review of the ASHA 2007 *Ad Hoc Technical Document on Childhood Apraxia of Speech,* which summarized what is known about CAS and advanced three theories about its causes

➤ Familial factors, infectious diseases, and medically based diagnoses that may be involved with a CAS diagnosis

➤ Some theories about causes proposed by parents, including traumatic birth experiences and environmental toxins

➤ A discussion on the possibility of an "apraxia gene"

Of course, you are wondering why *your* little one has CAS. As mentioned before, CAS is a relatively "new" diagnosis (not used for children until the 1960s) and much research is still going on. In fact, some practitioners and researchers say that we are still at "square one" in identifying this disorder. ***There are no clear-cut answers as to what caused your child to have CAS.***

But there are theories—several of them. Some theorists believe that CAS is based on underlying language issues. Others believe that the brain isn't formulating and sending the correct "message" to the muscles involved in speech. Still others think that children with CAS have problems listening to and interpreting speech. Genetic experts point out that CAS runs in families—that members may have a history of apraxia, another speech concern (late-talking or stuttering for example), or other learning differences. Recent research findings point toward this genetic perspective.

Starting at Square One: The ASHA Technical Report

We already know that it is hard to define CAS. If it's hard to define, then it's hard to identify its cause, right? CAS has been defined mostly by its characteristics, which has led to theories of its cause.

In 1994, Edythe Strand and Shelley Velleman (both speech-language pathologist/researchers) suggested that CAS is a disorder of the "hierarchical organization of elements of the language/speech system into larger organized patterns." My interpretation of this is: Children with CAS may be able to say some isolated speech sounds, but the more difficult words and phrases become, the harder it is for children to articulate what they want to say.

Velleman and Strand also asserted that kids with CAS may be impaired in their ability to organize and analyze information from their sensory, motor, and linguistic systems for spoken language. In other words, kids with CAS may mentally receive and store information, yet they don't have the skills to organize and sequence that information into movements needed to make words and phrases. Much of what Velleman and Strand suggested in 1994 is still considered true today. But, a lot has happened in the world of speech-language pathology since then—perhaps most importantly, the publication of the 2007 ASHA *Technical Report on Childhood Apraxia of Speech*.

In terms of the "discussion of apraxia," 2007 marked a pivotal point for the speech-language pathologist community. ASHA convened a committee of highly respected SLPs to study the available information on CAS. ASHA's Technical Report was an important matter to the members of the committee, and the SLP community at large. It is now a respected "go-to" document for caregivers, speech-language pathologists, and a variety of other healthcare professionals when they need detailed information on childhood apraxia. I am certainly no expert in discussing CAS theory, so I encourage you to take a peek at the 74-page ASHA Technical Document on your own at www.

asha.org/policy. If you have questions, concerns, or need more direction, please ask your child's SLP.

Let's go back to the 2007 ASHA *Technical Report on Childhood Apraxia of Speech* and start at square one. The definition of CAS proposed by the ASHA Ad Hoc Committee was this:

> *"Childhood apraxia of speech (CAS) is a neurological childhood speech sound disorder in which the precision and consistency of movements underlying speech are impaired in the absence of neurological deficits....CAS may occur as a result of neurological impairment, in association with complex neurobehavioral disorders of known and unknown origin, or as an idiopathic neurogenic speech sound disorder....The core impairment in planning and/or programming spatiotemporal parameters of movement sequences results in errors in speech sound production and prosody"* (pages 3-4).

Possible Causes of CAS Addressed in the ASHA Technical Report

With the exception of cases of *acquired apraxia of speech*—in which a child has a specific damage to the motor programming area of the brain (e.g., stroke, brain injury)—CAS typically does not show up on common brain scans. Therefore the possible causes of CAS are mostly theoretical. The ASHA Ad Hoc Committee that studied CAS suggested three theoretical perspectives: 1) Suprasegmental, 2) Sensorimotor, and 3) Auditory Processing. As discussed below, all three perspectives take into account that the timing and coordination of speech is "out-of-whack."

Suprasegmental Perspective on Childhood Apraxia

Suprasegmental refers to the way in which a word is formed, the syllables involved, and the rate, rhythm, and stress [of the syllables] of the word. Most theorists agree that *both* syllables *and* prosody are affected in "more profound, distinctive ways in CAS" than they are in other speech problems (ASHA Technical Document).

As a parent, you may notice this as:

> *"My child seems to really struggle to find the right sounds when he speaks; when he finally 'gets it out,' his message sounds choppy." ("Choppiness" is part of prosody, as is rate, rhythm, stress, and intonation.)*
> Or:
> *"He can say simple things just fine, but when he learns new, bigger words, it's really hard for him to say them." (Bigger words have more syllables = harder to communicate.)*

Perhaps the "cause" in this perspective is an unidentified glitch underlying the motor-linguistic system that results in difficulties putting syllables together and producing them smoothly.

Sensorimotor Perspective on Childhood Apraxia

You may be wondering if apraxia is *just* sensory or *just* motor, or could it be a combination of both—*sensorimotor*? Well, the ASHA Ad Hoc committee had similar questions. They suggested that the core problem of CAS is in the relationship between perception (sensory processing) *and* some part of motor processing.

In 2002, Dr. Ben Maassen suggested that kids with CAS may have "poor sensorimotor learning" which can lead to weak "auditory mappings," which makes talking more difficult. ASHA's 2007 Technical Document says, "… a sensorimotor deficit could also underlie proposed difficulties in automating motor programs, such that each word production needs to be planned anew" (pages 16-17).

As a parent, you may recognize this as you think, *"He really struggles to find the right sounds in words when he is talking."* (You may also think of this as, *"He can't find the 'mental map' or 'program' to say the word."*)

Parents Ask...

Did I do something to cause my child to have apraxia?

The short answer is "probably not." It's a completely natural and normal reaction to blame yourself, however. Parents I spoke with who shared their speculation and feelings about where their child's apraxia came from offered these theories about possible causes:

➤ The top of the list included "traumatic birth." Moms mentioned umbilical cords being wrapped around their babies' necks (thus, decreasing oxygen to the brain), emergency C-sections, low muscle tone noted at birth, and decreased heart rates during labor and delivery as potential concerns. One mother shared that her baby was born with poor suck reflexes, paralyzed vocal cords, and a need for tube feedings.

➤ Others mentioned premature birth followed by a stay in the NICU. Some had babies with jaundice and wondered if that had anything to do with CAS. Other families mentioned that their child with CAS had chronic ear infections as an infant.

➤ Many mothers were concerned that a glass of wine or a fall while pregnant did something to the developing neurological system of the embryo.

➤ Finally, some theories from "apraxia moms" had to do with the environment and the food we consume. A mother in one of my "Small Talk: All About Apraxia" groups commented: "There's got to be some environmental connection here…pesticides or processed foods and preservatives that we are consuming as a nation."

➤ While some of these factors may contribute to CAS, we don't know what causes CAS, according to theorists. Eventually we will have a better idea of what does cause CAS. In the meantime, try not to blame yourself. **Focus on helping and loving your child instead.**

Auditory Processing Perspective on Childhood Apraxia

While many children with CAS have "normal" results on hearing tests, they may have *some* subtle hearing/listening (auditory) deficits. If that's the case, then it could be that kids with apraxia aren't able to correctly detect and encode speech sounds from conversational speech, as Maggie Snowling and Elizabeth Bridgeman found in 1988. ASHA's 2007 Technical Document says, "... a few studies have addressed the hypothesis that children suspected to have CAS have deficits in auditory perception, auditory discrimination, and/or auditory memory" (page 19).

As a parent, you might note a problem along these lines if you observe, *"Even when I model the word correctly, it's as though he doesn't hear me right."*

Genetic Disorders

A genetic disorder is one that is caused by a *difference* in the child's genes or chromosomes. Some genetic disorders are inherited (passed on from parent to child), while others occur spontaneously or randomly during conception or pregnancy. There are several noninherited and inherited conditions that are sometimes associated with CAS or CAS-type symptoms. If you are concerned that your child may have one of these genetic disorders, you should visit a geneticist to see if genetic testing is warranted.

Galactosemia

One group of CAS researchers—Donald Nelson and colleagues— have found some connection between kids with CAS and a condition called galactosemia. It's an autosomal recessive inborn error of metabolism. Autosomal recessive means that it's an inherited genetic condition that is passed on through a particular type of chromosome (an autosome; not a sex chromosome) and that both parents have to have the gene for the disorder in order to pass it along to their offspring. Approximately 1 in every 60,000 kids in the U.S. have this condition. Basically it's when the body has a deficiency in the milk enzyme that converts galactose to glucose.

These researchers did a study of 24 kids and found that 54 percent (13/24) had some *characteristics* of CAS, specifically syntax and word retrieval problems requiring extensive therapy. Two other kids in this study had speech problems, but not CAS.

It didn't seem to matter if these kids were compliant with their diet, were boys or girls, old or young. It also didn't matter if their galactosemia symptoms were considered mild or severe as infants. It's interesting to note that babies who had classic cases of galactosemia and were treated early still had a risk for potential problems in the future, including speech sound disorders (SSD). In 2009, SLP researchers Edythe Strand, Larry Shriberg, and Nancy Potter presented findings at the national ASHA convention in New Orleans. They estimated the prevalence of CAS in children with galactosemia to be 24 percent (a conditional prevalence estimate); that is 8 of 33 participants with galactosmia with a prior diagnosis of speech sound disorder (SSD) actually met Dr. Strand's criteria for CAS.

If you suspect this could be your child's problem, it's best to get the professional guidance of a physician and dietician. In the meantime, be sure to mention to your SLP any dietary issues such as milk intolerances.

Fragile X Syndrome

Fragile X syndrome is another inherited genetic disorder that can be accompanied by CAS. It is the second-most common cause of intellectual disabilities.

For some unknown reason, these individuals—usually males—have a "fragile" long arm of the X chromosome. (The X chromosome is one of two chromosomes that determine an individual's sex. Girls are born with two X chromosomes; boys, with one X and one Y chromosome.) When there is damage to this area of the X chromosome, moderate to severe intellectual impairment results. These individuals often have large ears and testes, an elongated jaw, prominent forehead, double-jointed joints, autistic-like behavior, heart defects, and speech delays. Girls and women "carry" the genetic material that cause fragile X syndrome (they can pass it along to their sons), but do not often have symptoms themselves. Sometimes, though, they have difficulties with speech and language, anxiety, or learning disabilities.

By no means all kids who have CAS also have fragile X syndrome. And not all kids with fragile X have CAS—there is just a correlation.

For more information on fragile X, please visit the National Fragile X Foundation at www.fragilex.org. The organization offers support for families and sponsors research toward improved treatments and possible cures.

Parents Share...

"[My son] has fragile X syndrome, but has never been officially diagnosed with apraxia. But the things I have read about it indicate we're also dealing with apraxia. Even his SLPs have said that he has it. He seems to understand what is said to him but he is unable to express verbally what he wants to say. And the few words he does say aren't very clear, or it may be just the beginning of a word."
—Beth, mother of a child with fragile X syndrome

Down Syndrome

Almost every child with Down syndrome has some speech and language delays and difficulties, but there is a subset of children who have bona fide CAS symptoms on top of the usual speech-language delays in Down syndrome. Often the diagnosis is missed because SLPs will say, "Oh, it's just the Down syndrome [low muscle tone]." But children who have Down syndrome *plus* apraxia need different treatment than those who have Down syndrome alone.

One mother of a child with Down syndrome shared this: "Lily's therapist has always said she has 'motor planning issues' but blamed it on decreased tone. That makes it tricky—is the motor planning a result of the hypotonia or a disconnect with the brain?"

Lily's mother isn't the only person who has wondered about motor planning issues in children with Down syndrome. In 2003, Dr. Libby Kumin, CCC-SLP, completed a survey study in an effort to determine whether CAS was a widespread problem for children with Down syndrome. Over 1500 families completed her survey.

Dr. Kumin found that 16 percent of the children with Down syndrome in her study had either been diagnosed with CAS or had been told that their child had difficulties with oral motor skills. Even when parents *had not* been given a diagnosis of apraxia, survey respondents often said their children were experiencing many symptoms consistent with CAS (most notably: more difficulty being understood than their peers with Down syndrome, sound reversals, and sound errors). The survey also showed that children with Down syndrome and apraxia tend to begin speaking at a later age—around 5 years—than kids with "just" Down syndrome.

Yet children with Down syndrome historically have not been identified as having Childhood Apraxia of Speech. That's because early studies describing and identifying CAS were of children who had "normal intelligence," as well as hearing within normal limits, and absence of muscle weakness (or paralysis).

If you have a child with Down syndrome and suspect CAS, please look for an SLP who has knowledge and experience in both disorders. One test an SLP can administer to a child with Down syndrome who has *some* verbal ability is the Kaufman Speech Praxis Test (KSPT). If the child *cannot* imitate words, CAS is often assessed with pictures such as those in the Kaufman Speech Praxis Treatment Kit (Basic Level) and a CAS characteristic checklist. At home, consider reading predictable books with your child, "singing" daily routines, and using scripts and phrases repeated throughout the day ("Hi. How are you? What are you doing? See you later"). Picture clues to enhance communication can also help. These techniques can give your child with CAS and Down syndrome some experiences of success.

Prader-Willi Syndrome

Prader-Willi Syndrome (PWS) was first discovered by Andrea Prader and Henrich Willi in 1956. It's a rare genetic (inherited) abnormality in which 7 genes on chromosome 15 (q11-13) are missing or unexpressed ("switched off"). While these children have a whole host of concerns, some of the most significant are: often a breech presentation resulting in a C-section birth, lethargy and low tone at birth, and, nearly always, decreased muscular tone, decreased suck reflex (feeding issues in infancy) leading to failure to thrive as an infant, delayed infant/childhood milestones, crossed-eyes/wandering eyes (strabismus), and intellectual delays. Children with PWS also have *speech delays, perhaps presenting as dysarthria and CAS.* As these children get older, they seem to "overcome" their infant feeding problems and become obese because they develop insatiable appetites.

Potocki-Lupski Syndrome (PTLC)

PTLC is a "contiguous" gene syndrome—meaning that there is an abnormality of two or more genes located next to each other on the same chromosome, thus carrying an extra copy of a tiny portion of a chromosome (in this case, it's a part of chromosome number 17). The condition is not inherited; it's due to an error in the formation of egg or sperm and cannot be prevented. PTLC is a newly discovered syndrome—the first case study appeared in 1996 and a detailed clinical description was published in 2007 by Drs. Lorraine Potocki and James Lupski of Baylor College of Medicine. Only about 50 individuals in medical literature have been identified. However, it's predicted to be present in 1 out of 20,000.

One of the many symptoms present in this condition is *CAS*. Other symptoms include: low muscle tone, poor feeding, failure to thrive as an infant, delayed development of verbal and motor milestones, mild intellectual disabilities, autistic-like behavior, ADHD, heart defects, sleep apnea, and possible crowding of teeth.

Infectious Disease Hypotheses Related to CAS

● ● ● ● ●

Yet some theorists and researchers point to an infectious disease theory. *An infectious disease is a clinically evident disease that results from pathogenical microbial agents.* Those agents can be a virus, bacteria, fungi, protozoa, parasites, and prions. They are highly communicable (contagious) and often are spread through bodily fluids, the respiratory system (coughing, talking, kissing, sneezing), directly through skin to skin contact, or through fomites—inanimate objects that have become contaminated. Other times they are transmitted via a mechanical or biological vector. There are *some* infectious diseases associated with the brain. It's hard to know if *any* relate to CAS at all. Here's a list of some possibilities:

1. *HIV:* a possibility only if the area of the brain affected with HIV is also involved in the motor speech circuits.
2. *Encephalitis:* the high fevers associated with encephalitis could affect brain functioning enough to cause damage to the circuits that help in the motor programming of speech.
3. *Meningitis* also neurological in nature, causing swelling of the meneges and other brain structures that could affect speech circuits.

It would be really hard to determine whether any of these cause CAS; at this point in time they are just theories that may contribute to CAS. It is still important to include any of these diseases, should they be a part of your child's medical history.

Familial-Genetic Theories

Many children with CAS do not have one of the named genetic disorders discussed above. And yet there may still be a genetic component to their speech and language difficulties. That is, speech-language problems seem to run in their family. The idea that families may pass along the predisposition to have CAS is also known as the familial-genetic theory.

In fact, science backs up this idea. In various studies conducted between 1957 and 1990, researchers have found that there is a frequency and severity of speech problems within families of kids with CAS, at least according to Penny Hall's 1993 text, *Developmental Apraxia of Speech. And* in 2003, a study of family pedigrees of children with suspected CAS was published in the *Journal of Communication Disorders.* This study determined that speech-sound and language disorders tend to "run" in families with CAS (this is referred to as the "affection rate"). However, this study couldn't distinguish between environmental and genetic influences, nor could it ignore the fact that our historical memory can fail. ("Was it Aunt Mimi who had a stuttering problem, or Aunt Molly? Did Uncle Pete always have problems finding the right words—or was it just after he had that stroke?") The "Apraxia Gene" section below summarizes some more scientific studies on the family link.

The Missing Link

Have you thought about the family members—extended and immediate—who may have had a speech disorder? I hadn't thought much about this until my husband

---

Could a Genetic Problem Run in Your Family?

Without being too intrusive, take a look at your relatives—immediate and extended. You might want to refer to family photographs or just notice the next time you are all together at a family event. Is there a physical trait that everyone seems to have? Maybe they all have similarly spaced eyes or maybe all of the folks who have red hair also have a speech issue? Is there a family history of heart defects?

Look at any "odd" behavior(s) they may share. Do all of the women blink their eyes when they are trying to think of a word to complete their thoughts? Does everyone over a certain age have a noticeable shake in their hands or face? Is anyone in the family particularly restless to the point of being hyperactive?

Of course, you are not applying a formal scientific method to this homemade experiment. But, you may find that your observations add up to something meaningful for you. If so, you might mention your observations to your child's doctor or SLP.

piped up and told me that he had a lisp as a kid, "Everyone used to think it was cute, but I was sort of embarrassed by it, especially as I got older." I learned he received speech therapy through the third grade. And then I began asking more: did your parents have a speech disorder? How about your grandparents?

Of course, it's hard to bring this up in an everyday situation. Ever had a Thanksgiving conversation in which you shoot the breeze, talk about the weather, politics *and* religion and *then* ask, "So which one of you lovely relatives gave my kid Childhood Apraxia of Speech?"

Suddenly everyone looks down and gets quiet—so quiet you hear the swallowing of the sweet potatoes. There. You asked. Someone sets their fork down and says, "Why do you ask?" Folks might get a teensy bit defensive. But the fact is, there is often some genetic connection to CAS.

My Daughters' Genetic Legacy

I was more than curious. I was downright nosey. I asked my in-laws about the apraxia connection in our family. Here's what I learned:

Aside from **my husband's** lisp, he reportedly didn't talk until he was three years old. He has no idea if he started speaking in full complete sentences at this time, or if he just started with a few words. Unfortunately, his mother has passed away and his dad just doesn't remember. My husband will tell you that he believes he had apraxia as a child, but this was never formally diagnosed. He would have been three—the typical age for a CAS diagnosis—in 1973, and we know that was a bit early in the development of diagnosing CAS. At best, he had a speech delay. Today, he's still introverted, but he can speak quite intelligently when he needs to.

And so I probed a bit deeper. I wanted to know about **his mother's speech history.** He told me that he felt his mom often had a difficult time finding the right word (dysnomia) and confirmed that his maternal aunts also sometimes groped for words. Interestingly, two of these sisters are very extroverted, while the other is quite reserved. I would assume that if they truly have trouble finding words, they have adapted quite well. (CAS and word-finding problems are often confused. One SLP I talked with treated a bright child who had been unsuccessfully treated for word-finding. She actually had moderate to severe CAS. Keep in mind that there are separate tests for these disorders.)

As for my **father-in-law**—well, he's a man of few words. Smart, yes—he worked for the Army Corp of Engineers for his entire adult life—he can build a great dam, crunch some mathematical formulas—but communicating verbally is not one of his strong suits. To this day, he's the quiet one listening and soaking up family trivia at the Thanksgiving table. He's an only child, so no siblings to compare with him. He did mention, however, that he had a cousin who stuttered.

My outgoing **brother-in-law** seems to have no problems whatsoever with his speech. He loves to talk and make jokes and has the most contagious chuckle you've ever heard. He doesn't have biological kids, so it's hard to tell if he would have passed along an "apraxic gene."

At our last Thanksgiving gathering—really—I learned that my *husband's cousin's children* had been treated for speech problems (though not CAS). Yes, pieces of the puzzle were starting to come together! They are the same generation as my girls... wonder what the connection is? Could it be those maternal genes coming into play?

OK, I'll be brief with my side of the family. *My dad* is a friendly, outgoing sort of guy who can play a game of golf with a stranger. But he would identify himself as an introvert. *His two brothers* have no problems communicating, although they all have a bit of a southern drawl thanks to their wholesome upbringing in Southern Missouri. *His mother* had difficulty finding the words to communicate. As did *his father*—everything was a "whatch-ya-call-it" or a "thing-a-ma-jig." My father would say this was because they weren't very educated and just didn't know the proper names of certain objects. Perhaps he's right, or maybe there's more to it.

On *my mom's side* there was a late-talking cousin, who we believed received speech therapy in the 1960s.

No apparent problems with *my younger sister.* She spoke on time and was a bit precocious. She did see a SLP at the urging of her orthodontist; apparently she needed training to know where to rest her tongue when it wasn't busy talking!

Me—well, I was a shy kid, but I could talk when I wanted to without any problems. I said my first words when I was supposed to but generally was a quiet child—engaging in my own creative world of art and literature. When I was in high school, I was active in speech and debate. But I can't carry a tune in a bucket.

Learn about Your Own Family

I give you this background so that you may begin the process of learning more about your family. It may give you an excuse for bringing the topic up: "I was reading this book about CAS and the author mentioned several relatives with speech issues within her own family and now her two daughters have CAS. What can you tell me about our family?"

When you do ask, keep in mind that there are lots of speech and language disorders to consider. Here's a list, though not exhaustive:

➤ Late to talk
➤ Stuttering
➤ Stammering
➤ Selective mutism (choosing not to speak in certain social situations)
➤ Trouble finding the right words (groping and silent posturing)
➤ Lisp
➤ Trouble with certain sounds (e.g., "r" words)
➤ Unintelligible and imprecise speech (others cannot understand his or her speech)
➤ Volume of voice
➤ Quality of voice (whispery, high-pitched, grating, hoarse, nasal)
➤ Strange rhythm to voice

➤ Mumbling
➤ Chewing/swallowing/eating difficulties
➤ Learning disability
➤ Writing/reading disability
➤ Dyslexia

Remember, accidents from traumatic brain injuries (TBI), paralysis, or stroke (CVA) causing some kind of speech impediment are not "passed down" and should not be considered in this equation.

Parents Share...

Talking about Possible Causes of CAS

One mother in a *Small Talk: All About Apraxia* group volunteered: *"I agree that it must be genetic. It shows up in my father's side of the family. My parental grandfather did not speak until he was five and my dad is very hard to understand in either of the two languages he speaks fluently (English and Spanish). All of my sisters had speech therapy but are fine now. I never did myself, but I do have trouble pronouncing certain words for some reason. I somehow work around those hard words. My oldest daughter has no problems with speech; my middle daughter has severe verbal apraxia [CAS]. We noticed it at age one, but were in denial. She was diagnosed when she was four. My youngest daughter is only 20 months old. She has some symptoms similar to her older sister, but not as severe. I guess it is genetic, but doesn't affect all children in a family."*

A mother of a son with apraxia added: *"I agree that a look into your family might help understand where CAS came from. There is a family connection to my son's apraxia. Now as an adult, I realize that I probably had CAS and so did my uncle, who received therapy in the 1930s. Once I had a child with apraxia, I began to understand why I had problems pronouncing words the same as my peers, in childhood and even adulthood."*

Another parent stated: *"My sons represent the fourth generation of speech disorders on my husband's side of the family, with each generation getting more severe."*

A grandmother who contacted me said: *"I was just at a family reunion. The subject of the grandkids came up and I just learned my nephew was diagnosed with apraxia some 20 years ago. Makes sense now that my grandson has it [apraxia], too. I worry I've passed something on."*

Finally, at a "Windy City Apraxia" meeting I attended, every attendee had at least one family member who had a speech impediment or a strong suspicion that someone in the family had undiagnosed CAS!

What Can You Do at Home? Keep track of your "family speech pedigree"—that is, individuals in your child's family who may have had a speech-language or learning concern. Remember, this is not a diagnostic tool. It's just interesting to you and your child's speech pathologist to see whether there is a family connection. It does not indicate that there is a clear genetic cause for CAS, but it may show a *tendency* for speech problems for your family.

An Apraxia Gene?

You may be wondering: aren't there any *real* genetic studies done on CAS? Yes, there are. We will end with a heady discussion on such matters. Please bear in mind that just as I am not a neurologist, I am not a geneticist. But I can help you understand what these two disciplines have to say about the possibility of an "apraxia gene."

First, in the early 1990s, a group of folks wanted to know if there really was an apraxia gene. Lo and behold, they found a mutation of a gene on chromosome 7 which they believe is strongly linked to CAS in one family—the "KE family" of London, England.

Researchers call this gene the "FOXP2 gene." There is still a good amount of research currently going on to better understand the role of FOXP2 in childhood apraxia. Generally, the family members mentioned in this often-cited study had other differences as well (learning and academic disorders, sensory issues, linguistic and craniofacial (head-face) involvement that is not seen typically with kids who have idiopathic (no known cause) CAS. So, this means that although FOXP2 may be involved in *some* cases of CAS, it's likely not involved in *all* cases.

Needless to say, findings from the "KE family" stirred many researchers into action. The London-Oxford group studied the "KE family" for over fifteen years and found that FOXP2 genes were expressed widely in the cells throughout the brain. That is, the cognitive, speech, and language centers were affected. In fact, they found that the gene mutation affects *both* sides of the brain, which would explain why individuals with CAS tend to have *some* trouble with CAS-like characteristics beyond childhood (finding the "right" [speech sounds for] words when stressed, for example or having difficulty saying larger words).

Other recent case studies are beginning to recognize that there is a specific gene region on chromosome 7—and perhaps some other chromosomes—that appears to be connected with severe speech delay and CAS. For example, a 2005 research group in the United States headed up by Dr. Larry Shriberg found that CAS and dysarthria appeared in a mother and daughter with a chromosome "flip-flopping" (translocating) in a region affecting FOXP2. In Canada, researchers have identified a FOXP2 deficit in a child who reportedly has CAS, as well as a craniofacial difference. However, it's really hard to say whether or not there are other genetic influences at play.

The London researchers were given a grant to study the neural circuits and underlying speech-language development and performance. They are working with powerful techniques in bioinformatics and molecular neuroscience to get to the bottom of all of this "gene talk."

So, yes—it *does* look as if there is a CAS gene out there. We just need to be patient and let the genetic folks do what they do best: discover more.

Point to Ponder: Some researchers believe that there are different factors (familial, genetic, neurological) that contribute to CAS, which would mean that there are subtypes of CAS. This could explain why every child with apraxia shows unique characteristics.

"I Feel So Responsible...and Guilty"

Looking too hard at yourself or your family or analyzing everything about your pregnancy (or your partner's) can lead to guilty feelings. **But there is nothing you could have done to have prevented this condition!** If you *knew, without a doubt,* what caused your child to have CAS, would you suddenly feel relieved? Most likely, the answer is "no."

But you still have questions and concerns. I bet they sound similar to these:

➤ How can I (the parent) help?

➤ What will my child's future academic life be like?

➤ Will it go away...and how?

All of these will be discussed in later chapters.

Although it's interesting to think about the possible causes, it's important not to dwell on them for too long. Believe me, I've been there. To this day, I *still* wonder why Kate had apraxia. I wonder if it was something I did when I was pregnant, or if I failed to use enough "mother-ese" when talking with her. Eventually, I got to the point where I said, "It doesn't really matter. It is what is. I love her regardless. I will do whatever it takes to help her become a better communicator."

Your next step is helping your child be as successful and happy as possible!

By now, you know we need more research. Not to fear, all of the right folks are hard at work trying to make sense of this complex disorder. You are doing your part by questioning and reading about it. Below is a list of more tips and ideas to support research related to the causes of CAS:

➤ **Get an appointment with a geneticist if you must.** Seeing a geneticist is not entirely necessary in order get a diagnosis of CAS. Genetic testing may be recommended if your child has other features or delays (poor motor skills or auditory processing or cognitive problems) that may indicate some other genetic abnormality. Talk to your pediatrician first and then your insurance company to get the green light to enter the "genetic district."

➤ Remember, if you had **amniocentesis or CVS** (chorionic villis sampling), that counts as genetic testing. Review those results before pursuing major genetic studies.

➤ *Read and research what others have done (or are doing)* to help the discipline of childhood speech and language disorders. Consider making a donation to such organizations.

➤ *Help advocate for your child.* Having a genetic diagnosis can open some doors to services such as therapies and educational support through an early intervention program or the public school.

➤ *Don't beat yourself* up thinking that you caused your child to have CAS by passing on "bad" genetic material.

Say That Again?! Chapter Summary

It's a tough call and a loaded question when some well-meaning person asks you what causes Childhood Apraxia of Speech. Short of ripping out this chapter and making copies to distribute to everyone you meet, you can sweetly say, "It could be a number of reasons. Too many to count." That's what the Geek Squad told me when I needed a new hard drive for my computer. That's it in a crude kind of nutshell—your little one's hard drive just needs a Geek Squad (enter the speech-language pathologists, pediatricians, and other professionals).

Otherwise, you could say, "It's idiopathic" (we don't know what caused it)—which is true for the majority of children with CAS at present.

Keep track of family connections as you learn about them. The more often you come across members of your child's family who have a speech-language delay or learning difference, the more susceptible your child is to having CAS.

Geneticists and brain researchers are just beginning to find some links between specific genes and CAS. At this point, nothing regarding CAS and genetics is definitive—it's all speculative. The bottom line: we need more research.

Read on! Recommended Resources

➤ Additional information on fragile X syndrome is available from the *National Fragile X Foundation:* www.fragilex.org or 800-688-8765.

➤ Books by Libby Kumin, Ph.D., CCC-SLP are great resources for learning more about speech and language difficulties in children with Down syndrome. Look for *Early Communication Skills for Children with Down Syndrome: A Guide for Parents and Professionals,* 2nd edition (Woodbine House, 2003) and *Helping Children with Down Syndrome Communicate Better: Speech and Language Skills for Ages 6–14.* (Woodbine House, 2008).

➤ If you want to learn more about genetics, then look to *The Cartoon Guide to Genetics,* by Larry Gonick and Mark Wheelis (Collins Reference, 1991). You just may find yourself laughing as you read it! Another option is **Genetics for Dummies** by Tara Rodden Robinson (For Dummies, 2nd ed. 2010).

➤ You can download an article from the *Journal of Communication Disorders* entitled "Family Pedigree of Children with Suspected Childhood Apraxia of Speech" by B.A. Lewis, L.A. Freebarin, A. Hansen, and G. Taylor: www.waisman.wisc. edu/phonology/pubs/PUB10.pdf.

➤ **Out Came the Sun: One Family's Triumph Over a Rare Genetic Syndrome** by Judith Scott (Academy Chicago Publishers, 2008) is an uplifting, well-written memoir you may find comfort and hope in.

➤ In **What I Thought I Knew** (Viking, 2009), Alice Eve Cohen writes a candid memoir that reads like a novel about her daughter with a genetic disorder. There are plenty of suggestions on coping intertwined.

Chapter Seven

· ·

All About Speech Therapy

· ·

An Introduction to Theories & Methods Best Suited for Kids with Apraxia

Imagine you are in grade school and someone asks you what you are going to be when you grow up. You tell her you want to be a doctor. "But, what *kind* of doctor?" she presses. Well, just as with doctors, there are all kinds of speech-language pathologists, therapy styles, and methods out there.

There are lots of types of speech therapy. Your SLP probably has his or her favorite style—which is likely to be a hybrid of standard models. In fact, it has been suggested that kids with apraxia benefit best from a multimodal approach; that is—a combination approach.

The Nuts and Bolts of This Chapter

➤ What speech therapy consists of, goals of therapy, and how to track progress

➤ Various types and methods of speech therapy, such as natural (play) therapy, directive approach, individual vs. group therapy, as well as modeling and direct vs. indirect instruction

➤ The top eleven things you and your child's SLP should be doing for success in a motor-programming apraxia approach

➤ The importance of imitation

➤ The parent's role in therapy

A SLP ought to be creative and flexible when working with kids. After all, we know kids are unpredictable, have short attention spans, and can be easily frustrated. How an SLP plans treatment sessions is based on your child's age, temperament, and interests, as well as on your therapist's personality and education. Just as a great pediatrician or kindergarten teacher is your new best friend, a skilled pediatric SLP is an invaluable resource. Count yourself lucky if you have found one.

You will likely come across many new terms reflecting strategies commonly used in the world of speech-language pathology. So, let's begin by defining some terms.

The Naturalistic Approach

Remember life sciences in biology? Don't worry, I won't make you relive a painfully boring seventh-grade lesson. Humor me for a moment. Where do frogs naturally spend their time? Are you picturing a pond hidden in the woods? What do frogs do? They hop around and eat bugs with their long sticky tongues. What do frogs sound like? Well, they croak and grunt. This is the natural environment of a frog. If a preschool-aged frog had apraxia, he would likely have therapy in the pond on a lily pad with his favorite stuffed fly as a stimulus for croaking.

SLPs often use a naturalistic approach that involves play, particularly with young children. After all, play is the natural medium for kids to learn. A therapy session may last an hour, and in that hour, there are multiple ways your child will be learning. Your SLP will likely use a variety of stimuli—toys, art, books, games, and puzzles, written work, and old-fashioned "drills," possibly in combination with some gross motor/movement time. All of the activities will focus on your child's predetermined therapy goals. Be sure you know your child's therapy goals beforehand.

Think about it: what are you naturally interested in? Let's say it's architecture. You love visiting display homes and you dream of designing your own house some day. You know the difference between a Doric column and a Corinthian column; dentil molding and crown molding. You can *talk* about architecture because you *like* it, because you have an *interest* in it. Your child is no different, although her interests may be.

Parents Ask...

What's the deal with movement activities?

You may feel that your kid is in therapy to "talk *not* run around!" But according to Diane Bahr, CCC-SLP, and author of *Nobody Ever Told Me (or my Mother) That!*, "Movement activities can encourage vocalizations. Think of how vocal children can become on a playground, even children who are generally quiet. Short movement breaks during therapy can also help a child tolerate relatively long segments of structured speech treatment. Speech work is, after all, a fine motor activity. It can become tedious without breaks for children with speech difficulties."

In figuring out how to work with your child, the SLP usually considers:
➤ The age of your child (language is still—and always—developing)
➤ The severity of the CAS
➤ Your child's overall knowledge base
➤ Your child's attitude and temperament
➤ What motivates your child

You can help with some of these areas. Let your SLP know of any tips and tricks you've used at home, particularly things that motivate your child, even if they're not directly related to speech. For example, you may have found your child is more excited to wash her hands before mealtime when you provide the neat, color-changing soap. She does better staying in bed at night when you offer a prize from the prize box in the morning. You get the idea.

However, if your child needs a lot of motivation to speak, and she is best motivated by food, don't take her to speech on a full tummy; the speech-language pathologist's bargaining power may be lost! (Be sure to tell your child and SLP that snacking during therapy is okay; mention any food allergies.)

Your child will also do better at speech-related tasks when she has something to work for. Sorry, but acquiring the ability to communicate thoughts, ideas, and feelings is not the kind of motivation that will get the job done—at least not for your kid.

Another point to keep in mind is that play—and therapy—should always be child-directed but therapist-selected. Once your therapist knows what your little one likes

What Can You Do at Home?

Before you get to the SLP's office for that first session, make a list of all the things your kiddo enjoys doing:
➤ What are her favorite types of books?
➤ What toys can she play with—independently—for a substantial amount of time?
➤ What activities can she do for long periods of time (create art, play hide-and-seek, climb, assemble a puzzle)?
➤ Does she have a favorite character (from TV, movies, books)?
➤ What does she notice in the "real world?" Babies, trees, dogs?
➤ What frightens or intimidates her? (Make note of this so the SLP doesn't suggest barking like a dog if, for example, she's been bitten by one in the past.)
➤ How does your child learn best? Is she a quiet observer, active go-getter, someone who needs to "warm-up" to a new task first?

An SLP often has about 30 to 60 kids in his or her caseload—most of whom have different interests, learning styles, and speech goals. Your SLP develops a specific lesson plan for each child. Your suggestions for what might work best for *your child* are invaluable.

to do—and is good at—she will likely present several options for therapy that day. It may be that every option is selected by your child (the game, the kitchen play, and the Play-Doh), or the entire session may be devoted to one activity: Play-Doh.

The important thing is, there were options and your child chose the one(s) that excited her the most. Choice-making is an important form of communication. It often pays off when you are attempting to encourage spontaneous speech in "everyday" and new settings. When you think about it, that's what you want for your child—for her to communicate in all settings, not just the SLP's office or the preschool or school program. Your SLP can help you figure out ways to encourage your child's communication at home (see Chapter 9).

"This just looks like play," you may say. Well, remember "play is children's work." It looks unstructured and playful because it is. But, your SLP has a plan. She knows your child's goals and is taking a "backdoor" approach to the anticipated outcome. She is flexible and creative and allowing your child to have some control over the process. This is one key to successful treatment.

Naturalistic Teaching Approaches You Can Try at Home

Technical Name	What It Means for a Parent	Important Points
Milieu Teaching (Alpert & Kaiser, 1992) *This technique uses natural conversations between parent and child to introduce functional words. (e.g., father and child are going to the store. Father waves child's hand and says, "bye-bye, Mommy." There may be a slight pause, then child makes a noise. Father reinforces, "Oh, can you say bye-bye, too?")*	Parent teaches functional language within natural conversations	➤ Uses modeling ➤ Uses time delay (pausing and letting your child think of response) ➤ Uses "teachable" moments in natural environment
Responsive Interaction (Kaiser, et al., 1996) *A program in which the parent first models appropriate language within the context of a conversation and expands the child's utterances. (e.g.,* **Parent:** *"Daddy will be home soon."* **Child:** *"dada?"* **Parent:** *"Yes! Daddy! Daddy will be home soon.")*	Parent models developmentally appropriate language in conversation, and then expands on child's speech.	➤ Follows child's lead ➤ Expands language ➤ Uses turn-taking

Technical Name	What It Means for a Parent	Important Points
Enhanced Milieu Teaching (EMT) (Hemmeter & Kaiser, 1994) *A well-studied program, developed for children in the early stages of language development (although best if child has ~10 words). Prompts require child to make/imitate target language. (e.g., child and mother are playing on the floor.* **Child** *finds a ball in the toy basket and presents it to Mom.* **Mom:** *"Oh, you found a ball! Do you want to play ball? OK!" Child sits and waits for the ball to be rolled to her.* **Mom:** *"Here comes the ball. Can you get the ball? You got it. Yay! My turn."* **Child** *rolls ball to Mom.* **Child** *makes a sound.* **Mom:** *"That's right. Ball! Say 'ball!'")*	Parent uses milieu teaching *and* the responses of the child; works on turn-taking, follows the child's lead in terms of interest.	➤ Uses responsive interaction ➤ Uses natural environment ➤ Child learns language through social interactions
Blended EMT & Behavioral Intervention (Hancock, Kaiser & Delaney, 2002) *Uses the above described method (EMT) in addition to parent providing positive reinforcement to support child's "good behavior." Works well with a child who needs additional support with social skills. (e.g., Father knows child would like a drink. He offers the child milk or juice. Father says, "which would you like? Milk? Juice?")*	Parent uses EMT and gives positive reinforcement (verbal or token) for child's appropriate behavior	➤ Uses responsive interaction ➤ Uses milieu teaching ➤ Supports "good" behavior

What's a Milieu, Anyway?

Milieu is an old French word that means "middle place." It's the social environment in which something occurs. For example, the milieu of the child and adolescent psychiatric unit where I worked as an R.N. was often the lounge where patients tended to congregate for socialization.

The idea behind these naturalistic teaching methods is that kids are learning language in a meaningful way. Language is usually learned in a social context (play *is* social, and so are daily interactions such as meals, bathtime, bedtime, etc.). Remember, speech is not *just* a "task to be learned" or something to be marked off of a to-do list.

Parents, this puts you in the driver's seat as "language educator." You can encourage reciprocity and turn-taking. You can follow your child's lead and expand her utterances, and, finally, you can provide positive feedback during your child's interactions. Although speech and language are functional, they should also be "*fun*"ctional! You'll find plenty of ideas in Chapter 9.

The Directive Approach

This approach may be a little more drill-sergeant-like. It's more structured than the naturalistic approach. The SLP will likely direct the types of activities that take place and when. A large portion of the session may be devoted to drills. For example, the therapist might say a word and then have your child attempt saying it. They may do this several times in a row. It's hard work—for both therapist and child—and it can be a little boring. Drills work best when a child has the maturity to do them. They are used to help a child practice a particular speech skill. Directive therapy is also good for introducing words of increased difficulty, such as words with more than one syllable.

"A child as young as two years of age can participate in drill-like activities when play is incorporated. Speech drill-work provides a child with the practice needed to develop speech-motor plans," says Di Bahr, CCC-SLP.

Bottom line: Try to find a therapist who uses *both* naturalistic and directive styles.

Individual vs. Group Therapy

Speech therapy can be conducted in a couple of different manners. The most frequently used approaches are one-on-one therapy and small or large group therapy. Each of these approaches has its pros and cons, and ideally children would receive therapy in the setting best suited to their needs. But depending on who is paying for your child's therapy (the early intervention program or school vs. you, the parent, vs. your health insurance plan), you may not have a choice as to what setting therapy is provided in.

One-on-One (Individual) Therapy

In this type of therapy, the child and SLP work together closely on the child's specific speech goals. Individual therapy is especially good for beginning therapy with a child and for children with more severe CAS. Children learn comfort and trust. They build a relationship with their SLP. Your child's SLP learns about your child in these sessions, too. He or she can pay close attention to the small utterances your child is making and can closely observe body language.

One-on-one therapy is also good for establishing new skills and learning the rules of grammar, such as usage of pronouns and connectors such as "and" and "or." Think back to when you were learning something new. You may have felt self-conscious at first. Perhaps you didn't want to try playing the piano in a room full of relatives, but you were okay with your piano instructor and your sister in the room. Speech therapy is no different. Kids need privacy to practice something that is new and difficult for them.

One-on-one therapy is best for kids with CAS. The reason is that children and their SLP must focus directly on each other. The child must watch the SLP's mouth and vice versa. It is difficult for an SLP to divide her time and attention between several children while still giving a child with CAS the undivided attention she needs.

Group Therapy

Just as the name implies, this type of therapy involves a group of kids, usually working on common goals. The group could be as large as a preschool classroom of 15-20 kids, or it could be a group of just two children. Group therapy is great for kids working on social interactions related to speech (pragmatics). SLPs can group kids together based on their skill level or based on common goals. Group work can also be used to assess carry-over from private therapy sessions. Problem speech habits that need some extra work in individual therapy may be more apparent in group therapy.

In school settings, group therapy may be the only approach available because SLPs are often stretched to their limits with large case loads. But group therapy can occur in a private setting as well. The kids with whom SLPs are working are usually at the same developmental level and have similar speech goals. Sometimes, however, kids with widely varied goals are put into a group simply because it's the best fit for their schedules. If this happens to your child, and you feel it's a waste of time, speak up. There is no sense in paying for therapy—in time or money—if it's not working for your family.

On the plus side, group therapy can result in peer bonding! If the other members of the group have similar problems and are at a similar skill level, it can also provide a safe place to practice conversational skills. But it can also be nerve wracking for a child who feels shy about revealing her speech difficulties in front of others.

How Does It Work? A Peek Inside One of Our Group Sessions

Kelly, my youngest daughter, attended private speech therapy sessions with another little girl of approximately the same age and abilities. While working individually in private therapy, Kelly seemed very comfortable with the SLP and therapy expectations. But when she was with the other little girl and the other SLP—there were actually two SLPs in the one session—she became quiet and less responsive. She was less likely to initiate conversation. While this may seem less than ideal, this experience gave Kelly opportunities to observe turn-taking, play, and the communicative style of a peer. Kelly didn't receive group therapy *every* time she attended private speech therapy, and it didn't last the full session, but it was a good way to get her to open up.

In preschool, my older daughter, Kate, participated in classroom-wide speech games, as well as "pull-out" therapy with another student or two. She had fun with the games and the work she did with her classmates, leading to increased social interactions and peer-bonding.

We also used another style of combination therapy with Kate. When Kate was working on pragmatics (such as using a "sweet" voice while orchestrating play with others), we brought little sister Kelly into the hour-long session for about 10 to 15 minutes. It was interesting to see how they played and communicated (and fought!) with each other. This gave the therapist an inside view of what we experienced at home. It also gave the SLP an opportunity to facilitate appropriate interactions between our girls.

Parent/Family Participation

You and your family must be actively involved in treatment. It is a partnership between you, your child, and your SLP. Generally, you and your child's SLP will discuss options for how therapy will proceed. If you're not given options, speak up and ask. You know your child better than anyone and can suggest alternatives and ideas your SLP may not have considered. After all, you (and/or your insurance company) are likely paying big bucks to get these little people talking. (If your child is receiving therapy through an early intervention or public school program, see Chapters 3 or 11. You have the right to participate in the development and monitoring of your child's Individualized Family Service Plan or Individualized Education Program.)

Be an active participant in discussing the pros and cons of the various aspects of treatment with your SLP and spouse/significant other so that your child will benefit from everyone's efforts. Also keep in mind that CAS is a dynamic condition—it's always changing—and so should the style of therapy. Maybe you have heard the saying, "If you keep doing what you've always done, you're going to keep getting what you've always got"? Don't be afraid to ask questions, make suggestions, and shake it up a bit.

In *Nobody Ever Told Me (or my Mother) That!,* author Diane Bahr, CCC-SLP, talks about the partnership between parents and professionals: "Many parents seem intimidated by professionals. However, professionals are people too. So try to relax when you are working with them. It is best for you and your child if you can work in partnership with any professional your child may need."

Remember, you'll need to be a team player. That means everyone, including your child, is a member of the team. All members have value. *CAS is a complex condition that requires consistent and persistent work to resolve.*

Therapy Strategies

Before we get into the nitty-gritty details of therapy strategies for CAS in particular, it's good to know that there are two main types of approaches to speech therapy in general:

➤ *The Bottom-up Approach.* The SLP introduces easy to hard (simple to more complex) sounds/words such as vowels (V), as in "oh"; consonant-vowel (CV), as in "me"; vowel-consonant (VC), as in "up"; and consonant-vowel-consonant (CVC), as in "mom."

➤ *The Hierarchical Approach.* The SLP starts where the child is presently performing; that is, she starts with what the child can say already.

Here you will find various therapy strategies with a brief definition:

Therapy Strategy	Definition
DIRECT MODELING	Used in the early stages of therapy, the SLP demonstrates (models) the correct pronunciation of a mispronounced word within a natural conversation. The child looks directly at the therapist's face. There may be immediate or delayed imitation. You may like this example, *"Watch me and say it with me. Now, say it as I mouth it. Now, say it as I give you cues. Now, say it alone."*
INDIRECT MODELING	The SLP provides frequent and correct pronunciation of a target letter. Say the target letter is /b/: "I see a *boat. A blue boat. A big blue boat.* It's *beautiful."* A "back-door approach" from SLP's point-of-view.
PROMPTS/CUES (Prompt is presented in upper-case for the purpose of this chart only. Please do not confuse it with "P.R.O.M.P.T.," a style of therapy developed by Deborah Hayden, CCC-SLP)	Can be verbal or nonverbal. SLP might use this strategy to get the child's attention to focus; e.g., *"Look at my lips as I say kitty."* A visual prompt may involve showing a picture or a card, or some other visual reminder. The goal here is to shape and stimulate articulators (lips, jaw, tongue), improving functional communication.

Therapy Strategy	Definition
SUCCESSIVE APPROXIMATION (May also be referred to as "backward chaining")	Breaking a word or phrase down and asking the child to get closer and closer to saying it correctly over time—works well with multisyllabic words. For example, Kelly had a hard time saying her name. Our SLP started with "say, ly [lee]" and then, "say Keh"—before long, she was saying "Kelly!"
EXPANDING	Rephrasing what was said in a more complex thought. "Cookie?" becomes, "Oh, you want a cookie? Yummy. I love these oatmeal cookies. Here is a cookie for you."
FADING	Fading means eliminating a prompt. Once you have mastered a certain skill, you no longer need that "crutch" to keep you going (think training wheels vs. 2-wheeler). Now your child may only need part of the prompt to respond.
ORAL AWARENESS & EXERCISE	For a child who does not like touch to the face or does not seem aware of her mouth structures, non-speech activities (oral awareness therapy) *might* be useful. If the SLP uses hands-on cues and prompts, the child will need to allow touch. It is a controversial topic, so if your child's SLP works in this manner, ask what she hopes to accomplish by using it. Her answer should be directly along the lines of improving speech or feeding. Oral awareness and oral exercise should be just a small part of each session and should be applied systematically by the SLP. This type of therapy can be just the break a child needs after the intensity of working on making speech sounds. Keep in mind, some kids with CAS also have dysarthria, resulting from a weakness of the oral-facial musculature. These exercises may help to strengthen them.
SYLLABLE FLEXIBILITY DRILLS (using **C**onsonant - **V**owel or **V**owel - **C**onsonant words)	Uses what the child can already say. Sequences such as ba-ba-ba-ba are repeated 4 to 10 times. Then the vowel is changed: "Now say bi-bi-bi-bi." Next, alternate the two sounds: "ba-bi-ba-bi." Finally, throw in something different: "bi-ba-bo-bu." The difficulty is gradually increased over time.

Therapy Strategy	Definition
Awareness through **AUDITORY BOMBARDMENT**	Presents words and phrases with targeted sounds. Similar to indirect modeling, above. Say the targeted sound is /k/. You might read a list of words with the /k/ sound to your child over and over. "I want you to listen as I read these words to you: key, comb, coat, kitty, candy...." You spend a minute or so reading, two or three times a day. We made up silly stories about words:"The kitty wore his coat while he ate candy and carried the key." Make it personal to the child if you can. Help keep it fresh.
MINIMAL PAIR THERAPY	This type of therapy helps kids differentiate between two words that are different in just one way, such as "bay vs. boy" and "cop vs. cot." Minimal pairs can also be used in listening activities as well as speech production activities.
MELODIC INTONATION THERAPY (MIT)	This treatment method was developed with *adults* with impaired motor planning following a stroke— these adults usually have good comprehension, but poor speech. Melody and rhythm are important for the prosodic features of speech such as word stress, inflection, and emotion (a *right* hemisphere activity). MIT has not been very effective for getting speech motor plans/gestures to carry over to functional speech. This is probably because motor planning/ programming is mostly a *left* hemisphere function. MIT has been used with children in combination with other approaches to facilitate the melody of speech.

When Kate was in speech therapy, our SLP used the *Touch-Cue Method* developed by Bahir, Graham-Jones, and Bostwick. This would fit under the category "prompts/ cues" in the chart above. In the most basic sense, it is used for kids who have problems establishing and integrating voluntary oral movements for speech, especially in con- nected speech. It works like this: the SLP provides touch-cues to the child's face or neck. For example, when Kate was learning to say her own name, her SLP would tap on the front of Kate's neck (above the Adam's apple) for the /k/ sound. When Kate had trouble with the /s/ sound, Ms. Jen slid her finger down Kate's arm from shoulder to wrist, while saying /s/. Ms. Jen taught Kate to make these gestures herself, without watching her SLP for guidance. Eventually, Kate could make these sounds without giving herself the cues. In therapy-speak, this is known as "fading."

I had the opportunity to chat with Karen George, CCC-SLP, of Chicago Speech Therapy, who has developed a unique treatment approach in which SLPs perform speech-language therapy in-home. She speaks highly of using integral stimulation in the treatment of CAS. "[Integral stimulation] is also referred to as the 'watch me, listen, do as I do' approach using multimodal cues (gestural modes of body movement, pointing, sign, and conversational gestures) to teach the child new information. What appears to be a natural progression toward more complex speech patterns and movements for a normally developing child is a more effortful, demanding, and slow process for a child affected by CAS. So learning this longer speech routine takes much more practice, just as learning a dance for a recital would take more time for other children."

Ms. George continued on to explain that these important steps should be included for CAS therapy to be effective using integral stimulation:

1. "The child watches and listens and then produces the sound or movement simultaneously with the therapist.
2. The therapist demonstrates, and then the child repeats the sound or movement simultaneously while the therapist mouths it.
3. The therapist demonstrates and provides cues and the child repeats.
4. The therapist demonstrates and the child repeats with no cues provided.
5. The clinician elicits the sound or movement without demonstrating; e.g., asking a question with the child responding spontaneously.
6. The child produces the sound or movement in less-directed situations with therapist's encouragement in role-play or games."

Parents Ask...

What therapeutic intervention is best for kids with CAS?

I wish I had a better answer to this question, because it is frequently asked by parents and discussed among SLPs and researchers. However, the studies that have been completed on the various therapeutic techniques for the treatment of CAS are limited. Therefore, SLPs don't really have a "one" therapy that is more effective than others. Most SLPs will emphasize a motor-programming approach (see below). Remember, CAS is unique and individual for each child. A combination approach developed by your child's SLP is probably "best."

Motor-Programming Approaches

Of course you are aware now that CAS is a neuro-motor disorder of speech. So wouldn't it make sense to start out with a motor programming approach to therapy? *The goal here is to voluntarily, accurately, and consistently control speech articulators.* (Remember, articulators are the jaw, lips, and tongue.) Reaching this goal will enable your kiddo to say words and sounds when she *wants* to, or when *asked* to do so.

Before jumping into an explanation of the motor learning approaches to CAS, it is important to understand what motor learning is all about. First, a child needs *motivation*. Next, a child needs *focused attention*. She needs to be able to focus on the actual movement of saying the words (e.g., "did you see how that felt when you said ____?") while *also* paying attention to the SLP. Finally, for a motor learning approach to be effective, a child needs to practice. The best example I can give to illustrate this concept is learning to ride a bike. The motivation is "I want to ride a bike just like my big sister." The focused attention is, "I feel wobbly when I look down; maybe if I look straight ahead I will feel more balanced." And the child needs plenty of practice before she is independently riding!

Dynamic Temporal and Tactile Cueing (DTTC)

This research-based treatment approach is a very effective method for children with severe CAS. It's a hybrid approach to motor learning developed by Dr. Edythe Strand and colleagues at the Mayo Clinic. It is based on the 1973 work of John Rosenbek on *adults* with acquired apraxia of speech, *not* CAS. It is used with children who have difficulty with verbal imitation—a common characteristic of CAS. Let's break it down:

1. The child and SLP say the word together very slowly with touch cues and/or gestures.
2. Next, the SLP asks the child to increase her rate so that she is speaking at a more normal rate and there is no groping for words.
3. The SLP begins to fade the cue (saying the word with the child) by first speaking in a quieter voice, then whispering the word with the child, and then just mouthing the word with the child.
4. Then the SLP works directly on imitation and asks the child to wait 1 to 2 seconds before the child imitates her.
5. Finally, the SLP asks the child to spontaneously produce the word by saying, "What's this called?" (perhaps pointing to an object, picture, or word).

The key to DTTC is that the SLP works to fine tune the speaking process so that the child can ultimately respond or speak spontaneously (a process referred to as "task analysis"). DTTC is a good example of a multisensory treatment method, as it involves three of the basic senses: seeing, hearing, and feeling.

P.R.O.M.P.T.

The chart on page 113 referred to this treatment approach for kids with CAS. So what is it? P.R.O.M.P.T is a sensory motor-based technique developed by Deborah Hayden, CCC-SLP, in which children develop awareness for verbal communication through multisensory cueing. That is, the SLP acts as an "external programmer" for speech by physically touching—and sometimes moving—the child's facial structures (lips, jaw, tongue, and cheeks) in order to "show" the child the correct way to say something. See page 123 for more information on P.R.O.M.P.T.

Sounds Like a Plan!

You have heard this notion of a "motor plan/programming" often in your apraxia journey. So, just what *is* a motor plan? In terms of speech, it's the development of timing and coordination strategies necessary to produce a series of speech sounds. For example, without the right timing of sounds, words come out as gibberish. Childhood apraxia of speech occurs because there is a *disruption* in a child's ability to learn and control the motor planning aspects of speech, which happens at a neuro-motor level.

There are stages to motor learning. For example, in these are the stages described in 1991 by Richard Schmidt:

➤ **Verbal-cognitive Stage:** The child knows the goals of therapy; makes initial attempts to say target words, but with less attention and effort
➤ **Motor Stage:** *Child begins to develop motor programs* for movement; words become smoother and better timed; more consistent
➤ **Autonomous Stage:** Movement gestures are perfectly performed with less effort/attention.

A motor-programming approach has a few "rules" you should keep in mind for it to work successfully.

The top 11 things you and your SLP should be doing for a successful motor-programming "apraxia" approach to therapy:

1. *Intensive services.* What one defines as "intensive" will vary. Should it be daily? Weekly? Since these kids tend to progress slowly, you will see results faster with intense therapy. Most SLP's suggest twice weekly appointments. These kids will do best with as much therapy as time and money will allow. But beware of burnout. And speech therapy time and money commitments can quickly add up. Remember, you'll need to practice with your child five to seven days a week outside of therapy time. You are helping her develop and change motor habits; doing so requires a lot of practice (and patience)!

2. *Many repetitions and drills.* The goal is for your little one to produce words and phrases without really thinking about *how* to make them. She needs to sequence speech movements correctly, and she needs to develop those neuro-pathways. Let your child "rest" her mouth structures after a certain number of repetitions, especially if she is showing any sign of fatigue. You won't necessarily see fatigue, but you may *hear* it (your child has problems saying words she could previously say well).

Consider this scenario: You are working with a personal trainer. The next day your muscles are sore, so you take the day off from exercise. The next time you meet with your trainer, you remember some of the exercises because you have done them before—and your body remembers them, too. It's the same idea for your child in therapy. But the "resting portion" may be only a minute or two while the therapist jots down some notes before she asks your child to complete another speech task. If you are working on speech at home, you can have your child take a quick gross motor break: "Okay, now show me 5 jumping jacks!"

A couple in the Chicago suburbs gleaned this from their child's pediatric neurologist: *"Using speech therapy for a child with CAS is comparable to using a personal trainer for an exercise program—[SLPs] can show you what to do and provide a roadmap, but the real work comes on your own as you incorporate the lessons from speech therapy at home with your child."*

3. *Be systematic.* Begin with the most simple task and work up to the most complex task. Find out what your child can do first—in terms of words and sounds—and start building on it. (More on this topic in the "imitation" section of this chapter).

4. *Jaw, tongue, and lip strengthening.* Children with CAS or oral apraxia don't need strengthening unless they also have dysarthria. Oral exercise must be chosen wisely and applied only if a child has dysarthria in addition to CAS. *If your child "just" has apraxia, then no strengthening exercises are needed.* Instead, what your child needs is automaticity of movement, and possibly increased (or decreased) movement and greater endurance.

5. *"Motor memory."* Back to our earlier analogy of learning to ride a bike. You remember that it was hard and frustrating at times; once you got the hang of it, you never forgot. That's called motor learning. It involves motor programming and muscle memory. Your goal in taking your child to therapy is to help her learn articulator programming and memory so she can communicate.

6. *Auditory discrimination.* Many children with CAS have subtle problems with telling the difference between words, or auditory discrimination. Talk to your child's SLP to see if this is the case for your child; she will help you determine whether your child needs extra practice in this area. Minimal pair work is often used (see chart on page 115).

7. *Kids with CAS are very aware of what sounds and words they can and cannot say.* Has your child ever flat-out refused to say a word when asked? That's because these kids are smart—if they know they won't be successful, why even bother attempting a sound or word? Instead, work in small increments; let your child succeed at an easier task before making it more challenging.

8. *Self-monitoring.* This is an important skill that your SLP will teach your child. It will enable her to identify when she is correctly producing verbal sounds and

modify those that aren't correct. Your child will learn to monitor her spontaneous speech with the skills of self-monitoring.

9. *Rate, tone, intonation, and stress of speech* (prosody). These are all related to motor planning. Children with CAS have difficulty with prosody. Poor prosody affects the overall intelligibility (understandability) of speech. What helps: practicing rhyming words, tapping out words to a beat, climbing the stairs and saying a word for every step, finger tapping while saying words, and whole body movement while saying/practicing words.

10. *Teach compensatory strategies.* These are similar to the idea of self-monitoring. Your SLP will teach your child to slow her rate of speech, increase the length of vowel sounds in words, or substitute a developmentally easier sound for one that is harder, such as using a /d/ for "th" rather than omitting the sound (phoneme) completely. (For example, a child may say "**d**at" instead of "at," if the word "**th**at" is too hard for her, eventually adding the correct "th" sound).

11. *Give your child some success!* Even little pieces of success feel good! Give positive reinforcement—all kids need it to stay motivated and cooperative.

Parents Ask...

What's the difference between positive and negative reinforcement?

Positive reinforcement is when the entirety of your statement is positive. For example, "Yes! That's right. Daddy will be home soon. You got the word 'daddy' right. Hooray for you!" (Never-minding the fact that the rest of your child's statement was unintelligible.) You may also think of positive reinforcement as adding something of value to the environment that increases the chances that the child will repeat a particular action/behavior. So, you give her a reward or praise when she says a word. Hopefully, it increases the likelihood that she'll say it again.

In contrast, suppose you responded to your child like this: "Nope, that's not how you say 'daddy.' Not even close!" That would be negative reinforcement. Negative reinforcement is when you take away something from the child or her surroundings in hopes it will increase the chance that she will respond "correctly" the next time. (It's the punishment approach—which may work in other situations, such as taking away your child's toys if she leaves them scattered around the living room.) There's not really a token you can take away from a child who is learning to talk; but saying something hurtful or degrading to your child would take away her self-esteem or willingness to speak and most likely make her not want to try the next time around. *Always be positive when reinforcing your child's speech attempts.*

A Look Inside a Speech Therapy Session

No doubt you are wondering what therapy will look like. How soon will you begin to see progress? Keep these pointers in mind before we delve into a therapy session:

➤ *Kids with CAS need frequent, intense 1:1 therapy—at least in the beginning.* Be prepared to be at the speech clinic at least once a week. Most kids with CAS will require some form of speech therapy for at least two to three years.

➤ *Some SLPs recommend at least two sessions a week.* It depends on the severity of diagnosis, your child's age, attention span, and personality, as well as your time and financial resources.

➤ *Some kids with CAS don't respond as quickly and easily to "traditional" therapy approaches; or at all.* That is, they don't respond to the SLP who says, "Look at me. Do what I say. Do what I do." For this reason, a good SLP should use a combination of creativity, flexibility, drill, and engagement in each session.

➤ *Your child is learning to recognize different sounds (phonemes) by ear.* It is also your SLP's job to assist in that process by providing additional cues—visual, tactile, and proprioceptive (the body's sense of movement in space)—to help your child establish motor plans for speech.

Parents Ask...

How often should we really practice speech skills/go to speech therapy?

Should you be doing "distributed" practice (spread out across time) or doing it all at once ("mass" or "blocked" practice)? Mass and distributed practice are used in treatment to help the child establish motor plans/programs for words. In mass practice, a word may be practiced as many as 100 times (e.g., 4 sets of 25). In distributed or random practice, the word is practiced *among* other target words.

In the 1990s, researchers Richard Magill and Jack Fletcher determined that for the development of skills such as speech, distributed practice periods are *best* for motor learning in CAS. According to a 2010 presentation by Dr. Edythe Strand, CCC-SLP, "Mass practice yields quick development of the skill, but poor generalization for incorporating it into other motor skills. Distributed practice takes longer, but [the child] will get better motor learning in the long run."

So, if your SLP recommends two hours of speech therapy a week, the best scenario would be to break those two hours into four thirty-minute sessions. But with busy lifestyles, that may be near impossible. As far as actual "practice" goes—as often as possible—while still allowing your child to be "just a kid." See Chapter 9 for ideas.

Welcome to the Two-Way Mirror, Mom and Dad

Let's assume you are sitting in a therapy room with a two-way mirror. You can see your child at work with the SLP, but she can't see you. Ideally, you are alone, your phone is turned off, and you have pen and paper nearby.

Your little one walks into the therapy room with the SLP and they begin with a brief **warm-up period.** Your SLP may have already selected a few toys, games, and books (stimuli) to work with based on what your child likes to do, and perhaps some target words or phrases that are challenging.

Other therapists like to have kids pick out their own stimuli by leading them to a toy closet (heaven for any child!). This ensures that the child has chosen something she is really "into," with the hope that it will elicit some spontaneous response.

Assuming everything is in the room, your child may begin with some **exploration of the stimuli**—picking it up, going from toy to toy, and perhaps making some spontaneous utterances.

Our therapist often used **"apraxia cards"** during sessions. These cards were like large flashcards that showed pictures of common objects or actions. You may know them as Kaufman cards, created by speech-language pathologist and CAS expert, Nancy Kaufman. (From the *Kaufman Speech Praxis Treatment Kit*, these are just one example of "apraxia cards/materials" your SLP may have access to.)

Our SLP, Ms. Jen, would select a few of these cards from her stash to drill Kate. The aim of these cards is to help children produce correct articulation. But for children who find correct articulation too challenging, it is often enough to allow them to produce approximations—not the whole word and not even perfectly—of the action or object depicted on the card.

Ms. Jen often made two different piles of cards: 1) words that were easy for Kate or "mastered," and 2) words that were a bit more challenging.

My youngest daughter, Kelly, got to where she actually *liked* these cards and would ask, "More cards, please." Needless to say, once she got to this point, we ended therapy!

Parents Ask...

What are Kaufman Cards?

Diane Bahr, CCC-SLP, describes the *Kaufman Speech Praxis Treatment Kits* in her book, *Nobody Ever Told Me (or my Mother!) That,* this way: "[these kits] are designed to help children with speech motor-planning problems say word approximations that get closer and closer to the real word. They build speech from the bottom up. The kits help speech-language pathologists to systematically cue speech and fade that cueing over time as the child develops speech." The Kaufman cards are also large and visually appealing to children. For more information on the Kaufman Speech Praxis Treatment Kits for Children, the Kaufman Children's Center (located in Michigan), and Nancy Kaufman's work please visit www.kidspeech.com.

The Role of Imitation in Therapy

Since a major goal of therapy is to increase your child's voluntary control (automaticity) over the movements for speech, imitation is a huge component to therapy.

You want your child to be intelligible, of course, but don't be surprised if the imitation activities presented in the beginning of treatment have nothing to do with words. Of course the goal is to talk, but sometimes you have to start with something your child will have success with. Here's an example:

Can your child jump? Clap? Touch her toes? Your SLP may have your child watch and learn at first. "I'll jump…now you jump."

Your child and the SLP *may* spend a small portion of the session working on imitating nonspeech movements. Look at it as a way of laying the groundwork so that more complex motor tasks—like talking—can be added in subsequent sessions. This builds trust and rapport, and can be fun. It takes the pressure off talking. If you are quiet and patient, you may even hear a spontaneous word or two. The hierarchical approach would then build on these words.

However, an entire session of gross motor imitation is *not* an efficient use of precious speech therapy time. If you notice that this is all your child is doing in therapy, say something to your SLP. It could be that she chose this method of "warm-up" because your child is particularly young (developmentally, gross motor imitation comes before fine motor oral movements), or if your child is cognitively delayed.

Imitation tasks evolve from easiest to hardest. For a child who is unable to imitate speech sounds and words, this may begin at a gross motor level and progress like this to speech imitation:

➤ **Gross motor activities:** clapping hands or stomping feet

Parents Ask…

Does the P.R.O.M.P.T. technique use imitation?

Well, no. P.R.O.M.P.T. is often used when a child cannot imitate speech. The P.R.O.M.P.T. technique uses touch and movement. Deborah Hayden's therapeutic technique was alluded to on page 117, so let's talk about it.

P.R.O.M.P.T. is an acronym that stands for "**P**rompts for **R**estructuring **O**ral **M**uscular **P**honetic **T**argets." P.R.O.M.P.T. uses "Dynamic Systems Theory" to shape, guide, and educate muscles for speech movements. The SLP will use tactile and kinesthetic prompts such as moving the child's lips or pressing her cheeks in a manner that elicits the correct sound. If you or your child is uncomfortable with the use of touch, then P.R.O.M.P.T may not be the therapy best suited for your family. To use this therapeutic technique, the SLP must be specially trained. Sometimes, SLPs can teach parents how to use some of these techniques at home with their child. For information on P.R.O.M.P.T. techniques, visit www.promptinstitute.com.

➤ **Actions with objects/toys:** rolling a ball back and forth or banging two blocks together
➤ **Subtle movements:** nodding head or wiggling fingers
➤ **Oral-facial movements:** blowing kisses, sticking out tongue, other facial expressions
➤ **Vocal play:** blowing raspberries

In her book *Becoming Verbal with Childhood Apraxia of Speech : New Insights on Piaget for Today's Therapy*, Pam Marshalla, CCC-SLP, devotes an entire chapter to the critical component of imitation in the ability to speak. Most humans can imitate facial expressions, words, sounds, intonation patterns, accents, gestures, actions, and emotions within the first year of life. However, Ms. Marshalla proposes that kids with CAS have a much more difficult time learning how to imitate than typically developing children. According to her book, children with CAS have the following problems with imitation:

➤ **Late Emergence:** Children with CAS begin the process of imitation development later than "typical" children.
➤ **Slow Maturation:** Most kids with CAS take longer to move from one stage of imitation to the next.
➤ **Stagnation:** Most kids with CAS will plateau at an early stage of imitation, making it more difficult to advance.
➤ **Inability:** Some children with severe to profound apraxia never do begin the imitation process at all.
➤ **Scatter:** Sometimes, kids with apraxia skip ahead to a more advanced stage of imitation, leaving the earlier stages incomplete

I remember these stages clearly with Kate—only she *wasn't* a baby when she was in them! Although I knew what was happening—she was experimenting with vocal play as a toddler—I found it exasperating and almost embarrassing. We might be at the grocery store or at a play date and Kate would make all of these "mouth noises" as though she were a six-month-old infant, but she was three and a half or four years old. There were times I would just cringe, or even tell her to be quiet. I look back on those days and wish I had reacted differently.

Kids with CAS *do* have the ability to acquire mature speech-imitation skills; it just may take longer than typical. Keep in mind that imitation is *the* building block to a fully functional communication system.

More Building Blocks: Approximations and Mean Length of Utterances

Once your child is able to imitate speech sounds, your child's SLP might begin to have her work on *approximations* of words—for example, "nana" for "banana." Of course, the goal will be for your child to say words with increasing accuracy, but this can be slow. If your child is only saying a couple of sounds, her SLP will choose words to approximate based on those sounds. This is a hierarchical approach.

After approximations comes *increasing the length of utterances*. A common speech pathology term is *mean length of utterance (MLU).* This refers to the number of language units (morphemes), on average, that the child says in one phrase.

Researchers have documented the average MLU for children of all ages, and these averages are one indicator that is often used to measure your child's progress or the amount of speech delay. The MLU is sometimes used in writing goals for speech therapy provided through EI or special education programs in the public schools. For example, you may see a goal like this: "Jack will increase his MLU from 3.5 morphemes to 5.0 morphemes in structured conversation by the end of the school year." If the goal has objectives, the objectives will involve teaching the various age-appropriate language structures that his speech is lacking (e.g., present progressive tense, plurals, possessives, or vocabulary).

Below-average MLUs may be used in justifying a child's need for speech therapy from the school/EI program. For more information on MLU, visit STIR (Speech Therapy Information Resources) at: www.speech-therapy-information-and-resources.com/mean-length-of-utterance.html. Here you will find an MLU/age-equivalent chart and a protocol for calculating MLU.

Once your child is able to say longer words and phrases, your speech pathologist will begin working on:

➤ *accuracy*—what percentage of the time your child says a word correctly. Often used in writing goals for speech therapy; e.g., "Jack will produce 20 one-syllable words with 90% accuracy by (date)"
➤ *clarity*—meaning how clearly—or intelligibly—your child is speaking those words.
➤ *increasing vocabulary*—understanding the *meanings* of words is not usually a problem for children with CAS, but getting them to branch out and *use* those words can be.
➤ *pragmatics*—the "social appropriateness" of conversation.

As you see, there are a lot of skills your therapist is working on. That's a big reason why kids with CAS need frequent and intense therapy.

Functional Expressions

A major piece of therapy in treating CAS is to provide the child with some functional expressions—words, phrases, or gestures that can assist in helping her get what she wants and needs. Examples of functional expressions might be:

➤ "More, please"
➤ "Help (me)"
➤ "I need..."
➤ "I want ..."
➤ "Please"
➤ "Thank you"

What You Can Do at Home: You can work on these phrases in real-life situations where the phrases would come in handy, particularly in motivating situations when your child actually wants a particular item or needs help with something she enjoys doing. For example, I used to have my daughter, Kate, place her order when we went out to eat. While it may seem like "mean ol' mom" here, I actually viewed our weekly lunch dates as therapeutic. Kate got to the point where she could order without a problem. (Of course, if she stumbled, I was there to help.)

How Can Parents Assist with Therapy?

➤ *Ask if you can observe sessions.* This may be the single most important thing you do for your child. It helps you understand what the SLP is doing with your child and it gives you some tricks for learning to communicate more effectively with your child. Plus, you will see that the techniques your SLP uses are not "rocket science." Once you see them, you can usually do them at home. This is crucial for home practice. If observing is not routinely done in your clinic, ask if there is a way to videotape a session.

➤ *Observe unobtrusively.* You may watch from a two-way mirror so that your child is not distracted by your presence. You could observe for just a brief period, say ten to twenty minutes of each session. You might just observe by listening—perhaps sitting in the hallway with the exam door propped open. Listen to the interactions between your child and the therapist. Some parents sit in the room for the entire session. When I did this, however, I became anxious waiting for those words to come. Sometimes it was boring; other times the SLP and I got to talking about something relevant to therapy, but then Kate got less therapy time. When I left those therapy sessions, however, I felt more motivated and eager to model good communication at home.

➤ *Know what your child's therapy goals are at all times.* If you don't know, ask. It's best to have them in writing so you can refer back to them. Plus, it makes you feel good when you can cross off an achieved goal. (Note that if your child is receiving speech therapy through an early intervention program or public school, the goals will be written in your child's IFSP or IEP.)

Margaret Fish, CCC-SLP, says this about a child's treatment goals:

> *"In addition to providing a warm and supportive environment for children, one of the best things that families can do for a child with CAS is to locate a therapist [SLP] who understands the unique needs of children with motor speech challenges. Request that your SLP explain the goals and methods, as well as the types of things you can be doing at home to support your child's communication skill development."*

➤ *Get to know your therapist.* Know a bit about her family and interests and ask about them periodically. Because of the intensity of CAS therapy, your SLP may become like a member of the family. We even invited ours to a birthday party! If the SLP doesn't mind sharing his or her email address, get it. Send therapy-related emails occasionally. Ask her opinion on something you read; update her on progress at home. But don't bombard her—remember your child is just one of many she treats. Developing a close working relationship with your child's SLP shows that you are interested and engaged and keeps your family on her radar.

Ronda Wojcicki, CCC-SLP, urges parents to get involved:

"Get involved with your child's teacher, speech therapist, local speech and hearing association. Participate with your child in therapy and learn how to take what they are doing in therapy and bring it to the home environment and elsewhere. This is a family journey, so treat it as such. And remember to celebrate each and every small victory along the way—this is how we ultimately get where we are going."

➤ *Ensure that therapy is an active process for you, as well as your child.* Bring reading material that directly relates to the technique your therapist is using. Read it in the waiting room and share it with your SLP. Use the waiting room time to review your child's progress. Create a timeline of improvements for you and your child to review or make a list of goals you'd like your child to achieve. It can really be motivating!

➤ *Make incentives for your child.* Perhaps you can take your child to the park after her session. Three sessions of speech therapy could result in a trip to the Dollar Store or an ice cream cone. Make it fun (and spontaneous) and you and your child will avoid burnout.

➤ *Track and celebrate progress.* Celebrate your child's small successes with CAS. Remember, every little word, phrase, or sentence is a result of much effort.

"The frequent and consistent speech therapy and the actual carry-over into [my son's] classroom created a big difference in his speech, language, articulation, reading, and fluency. Since then, we've seen incremental improvement each year, but not as great as the first year or two he was there: that was his 'burst.' But then, with our son, we are dealing with a lot more than apraxia (PDD-NOS, ADHD, anxiety issues, global sensory issues, etc.) so we are constantly changing gears and directions to solve the issue du jour. Progress is progress and baby steps are big steps in our world. We've climbed a mountain since he was originally diagnosed at 20 months old."

—Holly, mother of son with apraxia.

"Branded" Therapy Methods

In your CAS journey, you may come across some "branded" therapy styles—that is, methods that were developed by one or more individuals who have published materials or hold training sessions to teach others how to use their methods. I've received questions on them in my Small Talk: All About Apraxia sessions, so I will break them down for you here:

"Branded" Therapy Methods Sometimes Used for CAS

Method/Program	How It's Used	Where to Learn More
Language Is the Key: A Program for Building Language and Literacy (LIK) Kevin N. Cole, Mary Maddox, and Young Sook Lim (2006)	Uses constructive interactions between books and play (see below). The program uses "dialogic reading" and teaches parents to use open-ended questions (what, why, how) and make comments by responding to and adding more to the child's utterances. Best suited for a child who has delayed language development but normal cognitive function.	Washington Learning Systems, the company that creates and markets LIK, can be found at: www.walearning.com/products/language-is-the-key Parents can view the Language is the Key: Video Programs for Building Language & Literacy in Early Childhood, a video in the program *Talking and Books*, at above website.
It Takes Two to Talk: The Hanen Program for Parents Ayala Hanen Manolson, SLP (1985)	Teaches parents to use methods designed to facilitate speech development. Parents are taught to recognize their child's stage and style of communication, motivation, how to adjust daily routines and follow the child's lead in communication. Best for kids who are late-talkers and preschoolers with cognitive and developmental delays.	*It Takes Two to Talk: A Practical Guide for Parents of Children with Language Delays*, by Jan Pepper, Elaine Weitzman, and H. Ayala Hanen Manolson The Hanen Centre website: www.hanen.org

Picture Exchange Communication System (PECS) Lori Frost and Andy Bondy (1994)	A visually based communication method developed to help children with autism communicate. Children are taught to give pictures to others in order to express their needs, wants, and observations. Children work up from exchanging a single picture (e.g., cookie) to sentence strips expressing a complete thought (e.g., I want a big chocolate chip cookie, please). Does not inhibit children from developing speech, but serves as a bridge to speech. Best suited for kids with little or no verbal language and those with developmental delays.	*A Picture's Worth: PECS and Other Visual Communication Strategies in Autism*, 2nd edition, by Andy Bondy and Lori Frost (Woodbine House, 2011) Available from: www.woodbinehouse.com *Complete Visual Reinforcement System Set for PECS: Picture Exchange Communication System* PECS materials available from Pyramid Educational Systems: www.pecs.com

Criteria for choosing books and toys in the Language Is Key *program:*

Books—children will be more stimulated to talk with lively and colorful illustrations. Vary the content of the books. Children are *least likely* to converse with counting books, name-the-color books, or ABC books. Allow children to choose books; read them over and over if they insist (repetition helps them internalize the words). Allow children to flip pages until they come to one they like. Remember, the goal is not to read the book cover to cover, but to facilitate language development. (Teri Peterson, CCC-SLP, has written a book with this strategy in mind. Look for *The Big Book of Exclamations!*)

Toys—observe your child's interests and follow her lead in the types of toys she gravitates towards. What toys/items get her to vocalize most in "free play?" As your child plays, talk about what she is doing with the toy ("Oh, I see you are stacking the blocks").

I Am Not a Speech Pathologist

I am not a speech pathologist. If you have questions and concerns about the techniques presented in this chapter, I urge you to ask your child's SLP or to do some of your own research.

The strategies presented in this chapter are a general guide to working with kids with apraxia. As your child progresses in therapy—age and maturity—other areas of speech will need practice, such as correct sentence structure and grammar, as these are known to be problematic for kids with CAS.

Parents Ask...

What is Melodic Intonation Therapy (MIT)

Researchers have long realized that some adults who have lost the ability to speak due to strokes can still sing—or at least hum. Some of these adults have relearned to speak through use of MIT in combination with other approaches. Using this technique, the therapist sings (or *intones*) a word or phrase (generally using just two pitches) while using a visual cue (signing or tapping). Some speech-language pathologists and music therapists have also used the technique with varying success with children who have CAS. Kathleen Helfrich-Miller, an SLP with expertise in MIT, shares this, "[MIT] is a structured technique used to merge motor learning and sequencing sounds; skills that are difficult for children with CAS."

At some point in therapy, your child will need to work on intelligibility and speech precision. Intelligibility is the understandability of her speech, and depends on the correct sound production, including:

➤ Stressing certain words within sentences
➤ Pitch, volume, rate, and rhythm
➤ Phonological awareness (pre-literacy skills)
➤ Articulation

Your child will also need to practice these areas related to speech-language:

➤ Spelling, reading, decoding, comprehension (literacy skills)
➤ Listener awareness (repeating herself or making corrections if the listener doesn't understand her; adjusting how she speaks to others depending on their age, status, relationship—e.g., you speak differently to a little child than to a teacher or a friend
➤ Self-advocacy (learning communicative strengths and weaknesses and how to communicate with teachers, coaches, friends about these issues)

I am sure you are beginning to understand why experts recommend that therapy for kids with CAS be frequent and intense, and extend over the course of several years. There's a lot of stuff to sort out and a lot of coaching to get these kiddos to be effective communicators! Have faith and take it step by step. You and your child will get there.

Bridging Research and Practice

By now, I am sure you've realized: *there is no one method for treating CAS.* Why? Well, for starters there is not enough scientific evidence as to which method works best because researchers are still a little foggy as to what causes CAS, so we have several unanswered questions:

> Do kids with apraxia have problems talking because formulating motor routines and patterns is particularly difficult for them?

> Do kids with apraxia have problems storing verbal routines in their brain?

> Do kids with CAS have problems adequately retrieving the routines that have been stored?

See Chapter 6 for more information on what may cause symptoms of CAS.

Say That Again?! Chapter Summary

This chapter has been all about speech therapy—the types and subtypes that are available to help your child communicate. Your child's SLP will carefully map out a treatment plan designed to assist your child in producing intelligible speech based on attributes specific to your child (age, attention span, motivation, intelligence, etc.). However, a large piece to the therapeutic approaches used for CAS is *motor learning*, a process of gathering the skills necessary for producing a desired action (in this case—speech). Your child will get better with practice, self-confidence, intrinsic motivation, direct instruction, and modeling. Please discuss the best treatment approach with your child's SLP—that's what they're there for!

Finally, please remember: *The key to success with CAS is frequent, intense, long-term therapy, and plenty of practice at home!* Chapter 9 is entirely devoted to explaining how you can help your child at home. Practicing outside of therapy helps make speech skills automatic. Following through at home can help keep therapy on track, and maybe even speed up the process.

Read On! Recommended Resources

> *It Takes Two to Talk: A Practical Guide for Parents of Children with Language Delays* by Jan Pepper, Elaine Weitzman, and H. Ayala Manolson. If you are interested in learning more about this program, this is a must-read. Published by the Hanen Centre: www.hanen.org.

> *A Picture's Worth: PECS and Other Visual Communication Strategies in Autism* by Andy Bondy, Ph.D. and Lori Frost, CCC-SLP (Woodbine House, 2011). Although this communication strategy was originally developed for children on the autism spectrum, it can be applied to children with limited speech skills, such as those with CAS.

> You may also be interested in viewing the *PECS DVD,* which provides an overview of the potential benefits of the PECS program. It is available at www.pecs.

com, along with other PECS products, such as the activity binder, communication books, and the training manual with CD.

➤ *Talking Together: A Parent's Guide to the Development, and Problems of Speech and Language,* by Katherine T. Schetz and Stuart Kent, M.D., covers the basics of speech development, including charts of sound proficiency.

➤ *Teach Me How to Say It Right: Helping Your Child with Articulation Disorders* by Dorothy P. Dougherty, CCC-SLP. While this book is about articulation disorders (CAS is *not* a disorder of articulation), you may still find some helpful information on working with your child at home, as well as learning more about speech sound development.

➤ *Becoming Verbal with Childhood Apraxia: New Insights on Piaget for Today's Therapy* by Pam Marshalla, CCC-SLP. This is a great resource for SLPs treating CAS, but also accessible to parents.

➤ *Apraxia Uncovered: Seven Stages of Phoneme Development* by Pam Marshalla, CCC-SLP. Mainly developed for use by speech-language pathologists, this handbook is an appropriate reference for the motivated parent to use at home in conjunction with speech therapy.

➤ *Language Is the Key: Video Programs for Building Language and Literacy in Early Childhood.* This informational and instructional DVD is available from Washington Learning Systems, 2212 Queen Anne Ave. North, #726, Seattle, WA 98109 (www.walearning.com; 206-310-7401).

➤ Three instructional DVDs available through the Apraxia-KIDS store are *Kaufman Speech to Language Protocol, Taking it Home: Practicing Speech Where Kids Live and Play,* and *Overview of Dynamic Temporal and Tactile Cueing* (a DVD lecture presented by Edythe Strand, Ph.D., CCC-SLP). Order from www.apraxia-kids.org.

➤ *Just for Kids: Apraxia* by Martha Drake is a practical and effective treatment tool for SLPs working with CAS in individual and group therapy. There are lots of great suggestions for books, gross motor activities, and songs. You can find some used copies online, but new copies fall in the $80 range.

➤ *Easy Does It for Apraxia-Preschool* by Robin Strode and Catherine Chamberlin was developed for the preschool-aged child who has CAS. It is a systematic program designed to teach isolated sounds, syllable productions, sequencing, and closure as well as multisyllabic words, phrases and sentences, and consonant blend sounds. It is designed for SLPs to use in their practice, but parents may glean some examples of things to do at home.

➤ *Here's How to Treat Childhood Apraxia of Speech* by Margaret (Dee) Fish may be best suited for students in an SLP program, but it's written in such a way that motivated parents can glean valuable insight into their child's speech-language therapy.

Section Three

Helping Your Child

Chapter Eight

· · · · · · · · · · · · · · · ·

Fish Oil, Diet, Horses, Music, and More

· · · · · · · · · · · · · · · ·

Complementary and Alternative Medical (CAM) Approaches to Childhood Apraxia of Speech

"If there is something else out there that will help
my son, then I want to know about it!"
— Small Talk: All About Apraxia Participant

When I first learned of Kate's CAS diagnosis, I thought the only thing I could do was to schlep her to and from speech therapy a couple of times a week. Then I found out that we would need to do speech therapy homework, since much of her progress would be made at home.

When I started getting serious about learning about apraxia, a whole new world opened up to me. For better or worse, I was introduced to the idea of Complementary and Alternative Medicine (CAM). Well, maybe "reintroduced" is a better word. I am a nurse, after all, and I had heard patients praise such therapies. Heck, I've even tried some ideas on my own. Visualization, listening to relaxing music, and even yoga can all be classified as CAM. If you've ever lit a delicious-smelling candle and listened to classical music to relax after an exhausting day, then you, too, have experienced some form of CAM.

Just as with most things in life: you often have a choice. This chapter will outline some of the more mainstream alternative approaches to conventional therapy such as B-12 vitamins, Omega-3 Fatty Acids, dietary changes, and nutritional supplementa-

> **The Nuts and Bolts of This Chapter**

> ➤ An overview of Complementary Alternative Medicine (CAM), including who is qualified to treat individuals with these methods

> ➤ Nutritional modifications and how the food we put into our bodies affects the greater whole—including our ability to communicate

> ➤ Sensory-based therapies—including hippotherapy (horse riding), vision therapy, and therapeutic listening, among others

> ➤ Medically based therapies, including pranic healers, chiropractors, and others.

> ➤ Finally, a series of questions to get you asking the right questions to determine if a particular therapy is "right" for you and your child

tion—and some you may not have thought of or heard about before. The goal of this chapter is not to discount or offer substitutes for traditional therapy, but to offer a supplemental approach.

So What Is Complementary and Alternative Medicine?

Complementary and Alternative Medicine (CAM) is a constellation of medical and therapeutic practices and products not currently thought to be part of conventional medicine. Examples of CAM practitioners are chiropractors and acupuncturists; examples of CAM products, dietary supplements.

Integrative medicine (IM) combines mainstream medical therapies with CAM therapies. It treats the whole person, not just the disease. It's the best of both worlds—science and western medicine plus *evidenced-based* complementary therapy. Treating the individual through a dynamic team of partners, integrative medicine helps heal the mind, body, and spirit. Biofeedback, yoga instructors, massage therapists, and recreational therapists all fall under that umbrella we call integrative medicine.

We'll jump right in and start discussing the types of therapies that are available. Some of these ideas may just be too "out there" for you to consider. Have an open mind as you read through the next few pages, though. Something just may work for your child. As with anything, do your homework first. These techniques, ideas, and therapies should never replace traditional speech therapy. Also, bear in mind that there is no point in trying to treat symptoms your child does not have. For example, a gluten-free diet will not help your child if he does not have gluten intolerance. If you are concerned, or just curious, you can ask your pediatrician to consider a blood test to indicate whether your child might have an intolerance or allergy.

Nutritional Intervention: Gluten-free Diets, Fatty Acids, Supplements, and More

There are books upon books written on the subject of adding ingredients to or eliminating ingredients from one's diet to aid in the body's performance. I find that as a parent, you either want a general overview, or you already *know* your child has a food intolerance or allergy and have taken appropriate steps.

Let's assume you fall into the "just the facts, ma'am" category. The table on pages 140-42 offers a quick and easy guide to some of the benefits of diet modification. Please continue to seek out other resources—including your child's pediatrician—should you choose to travel along this nutritional journey.

Some Things to Keep in Mind about Supplements

➤ Supplements *are not* monitored by the FDA; prescription medications are.

➤ *Never, ever give your child supplements solely on the recommendation of a friend or something you've read!* I cannot stress this enough. This chapter is not intended to replace medical advice.

➤ Your child's pediatrician should *always* be consulted before giving your child any type of supplements.

➤ When you are selecting vitamins or any other supplements, be sure to look for companies that get their products tested by an outside source/third party. Look for US Pharmacopeia (USP), Consumer Lab, or NSF International on the label.

➤ Who will monitor the safety of dosages? A doctor typically does that, but if you are self-medicating your child, you'll need some professional guidance.

➤ If anyone claims that a particular product helps children with speech and communication concerns, ask for a source or a citation for that claim. If you do this in a tactful, diplomatic manner, they should be happy to oblige.

➤ If you are concerned that fish oil supplements could contain mercury, make sure the brand you are using has been tested for purity by a third party.

➤ A registered dietician (R.D.) may be helpful in making some dietary changes/modifications. Find one at www.eatright.org, website of the American Dietetic Association.

	Omega-Essential Fatty Acids (EFAs)	Gluten-Free Casein-Free Diet	B-12 (Cobalamin)
What it is:	Fatty acids that the body doesn't produce naturally, but are essential to the development & function of the brain, nerves, muscles, and organs.	A diet that eliminates wheat and dairy products. ***Please have your child tested for gluten and casein sensitivities before assuming there is a problem.*** Going this route takes a lot of time, commitment, and disruption to the child—and family's—eating routine.	Water-soluble vitamin.
Where it's found naturally:	***Omega-3 fatty acids*** (DHA) are found in flaxseed oil, walnuts, dark green leafy veggies (spinach, kale), and cold-water fish like salmon, trout, cod, and sardines (3-4 oz./week). ***Omega-6 fatty acids*** can be found in animal fats and linoleic acid (the primary oil added to processed food), and used in sunflower, safflower, and soybean oils.	***Gluten*** is a protein found in wheat, barley, and rye, as well as in oats that have been contaminated by wheat, barley, or rye. ***Casein*** is a protein in diary products such as milk, ice cream, cheese, and yogurt.	Often found in red meat, also in dairy and eggs; the body doesn't naturally make B-12.
What's the deal?	Some suggestions are that EFA's *may be able* to offer therapeutic benefits to depression, bipolar, ADHD, autism, heart disease, diabetes, autoimmune disease, and communication. It helps communication in the sense that it may improve attention and focus.	Typically, the body digests these proteins down into peptides. Some kids can't digest them well. They enter the bloodstream and *may* cause problems with brain development, as well as bloating, diarrhea, and other gastrointestinal problems.	B-12 works with folic acid to make DNA and red blood cells. It converts carbohydrates, fats, and proteins from food into energy. Also important in protecting nerve cells.

How it *Could* Help Kids with Apraxia:	One study from the Univ. of British Columbia found a positive correlation between amount of DHA in breast milk and the language development of children. Some folks feel EFAs help communication by improving focus.	*Nutritional Neuroscience* indicated a reduction in autistic behavior, increase in social and communication skills in kids who went on gluten-free, casein-free diets. These findings were determined after 12 years of studies on kids with autism. The Univ. of Sunderland in the UK found parents reported improvements in communication and concentration in kids with autism after a 3-month casein/gluten-free diet	Scientifically proven to target the communication center of the brain. However, it doesn't necessarily mean that children with CAS need more B-12 in their diets, but perhaps they are not metabolizing it as they should. Please check with your child's doctor to determine if your child has a B-12 deficiency.
Side Effects:	Mild tummy ache, fishy taste and/or smell; to avoid, use smaller doses throughout the day, mix with food (some say it's great when added to popcorn or smoothies). Another concern is that it could be contaminated with methyl mercury, especially over the long-term treatment in small kids. According to the CDC, mercury can be passed from mother to her fetus, and can cause brain damage, incoordination, blindness, seizures, and inability to speak.	It's a pain in the you-know-what! Constant monitoring of your food sources and intake can be exhausting. Lots of learning and meal planning involved. You have to stick with it—yes, that means bringing your own snacks to a birthday party.	Found to be a safe & nontoxic vitamin. Anything in excess can be bad—soon you're just nourishing your toilet bowl! May have some interactions with antibiotics; tell your doctor if you are giving your child B-12 supplements.
What You Can Do at Home:	Have your child eat more fish, give him a supplement; talk with your pediatrician before you do anything.	Read and learn about the diet. Try eliminating some of the above foods, one category at a time and keep track of effects on your child.	Incorporate more red meat. Find out if your child has a B-12 deficiency by having a blood test; proceed if your doctor recommends it.

(continued)	Omega-Essential Fatty Acids (EFAs)	Gluten-Free Casein-Free Diet	B-12 (Cobalamin)
Products to consider:	ProEFA, Nordic Naturals, Carlson Kids, & Dr. Sears Chewies	Nowadays there are a lot of products stocked on grocery store shelves that are labeled "gluten-free."	Sublingual (under the tongue) B-12 supplements that dissolve in your mouth are best because they go right into the bloodstream, bypassing the digestive system.
Resources	*The Omega-3 Connection* (Stoll) ***Children with Starving Brains*** (McCandless), ***The LCP Solution*** (Stordy), and ***What's Eating Your Child?*** (Dorfman)	***The Living Gluten Free Answer Book*** (Bowland), ***Getting Your Kid on a Gluten-Free Caesin-Free Diet*** (Lord), ***Special Diets for Special Kids*** (Lewis), ***Gluten-Free Kids*** (Korn), and ***What's Eating Your Child?*** (Dorfman)	***"Could It Be B-12: An Epidemic of Misdiagnosis"*** (Pacholock & Stuart)

Is There a Connection between Allergies, Apraxia, and Diet?"

Perhaps. A book recently published by nutritionist Kelly Dorfman, *What's Eating Your Child*, proposes that there is. In addition, a study published by Drs. Claudia Morris and Marilyn Agin in 2009 suggests that a link may exist between diet, gastrointestinal symptoms, allergies, and apraxia (CAS). Their article summarizes the literature supporting the idea that people with dyspraxia and apraxia (which they refer to as "verbal apraxia"), along with ADHD, dyslexia, and autism spectrum disorders (ASD), lack a sufficient amount of long-chain polyunsaturated fatty acids (PUFAs, aka fish oil). Dr. Morris also notes that many symptoms of "apraxia" are similar to those that develop in conditions resulting from a vitamin E deficiency. She asserts that apraxia is a syndrome that affects the whole child and is more than "just a speech disorder," even though the verbal apraxia component is often the most obvious symptom. According to the premise in their paper, if kids with these disorders were to have supplementation of PUFAs (fish oil), along with vitamin E, they *might* be more responsive to overcoming CAS. The article also supports traditional speech and occupational therapy *in conjunction* with nutrition supplementation.

Note that Dr. Morris's and Dr. Agin's study is an ***anecdotal case series*** based on data collected through an online apraxia support group in which parents shared their

Fishing for an Omega-3 Fatty Acid Product?

Here's a sampling of various Omega-3 Fatty Acids (a.k.a. fish oil, PUFAs) you may want to consider for your child with apraxia:

➤ **Cormega Kids Omega-3 Squeeze,** produced by European Reference Botanical Laboratories located in Carlsbad, CA. Coromega is a form of fish oil in a creamy, orange-flavored, pudding-like substance. Some come in portable, single-dose packets. Parents find it easy to add to juice or yogurt or blend in a smoothie; taking it "straight" generally not preferred. Kids don't usually mind the taste. You can order directly from the company: www.coromega.com, or www.lpcsolution.com.

➤ **Efalex** is a fish oil supplement rich in DHA. This is the very product that was used in clinical trials with ADHD, dyslexia, and apraxia in the U.S. and U.K. It is manufactured by Nutricia USA Inc. (Clearwater, FL). Check out their website at www.nutricia.com.

➤ **ProEFA (Ultimate Omega, Complete Omega)** is the Nordic Naturals version of Omega-3 fatty acids found in naturally occurring ratios. You can order directly through the company, www.nordicnaturals.com.

➤ **Dr. Sears Go Fish Brainy Kidz Children's Omega-3 DHA Soft Chews.** All-natural fruit-based supplement that supports brain development; no fishy taste or smell. This product is free of wheat, yeast, gluten, milk, and nut derivatives. From a "safe source," meaning that every batch of oil is third-party tested and certified for batch purity and to be free of detectable levels of over 250 environmental contaminants, including mercury, heavy metals, dioxins, PCBs, and pesticides.

➤ **Carlson for Kids** are vitamins and supplements designed with kids' nutritional needs in mind. All of their products are free of gluten, wheat, milk, casein, nuts, and eggs. They offer liquid fish oil, as well as cod liver oil, from fish caught in Norwegian waters and bottled at the site. Kids often prefer it mixed with a favorite food such as chocolate milk. Lemon flavor may be tasty in lemon yogurt. Visit www.carlsonlabs.com for more information.

experiences supplementing their children with vitamin E and PUFA treatment. Parents were encouraged to report their observations, both good and bad, and details of any perceived adverse effects were solicited along with perceived benefits. Families were also asked specifically whether their children had any additional symptoms beyond verbal apraxia, including the presence of an autism diagnosis, coordination difficulties (dyspraxia), sensory issues, abnormal pain sensation, low muscle tone (hypotonia), gastrointestinal symptoms, and/or food allergies.

Drs. Morris and Agin summarized characteristics of the largest group of children diagnosed with CAS to date, and found that verbal apraxia in this group of nearly 200 children rarely occurred in isolation. Boys were more often affected than girls, while coordination problems, low muscle tone, sensory issues, gastrointestinal complaints, malabsorption, and gluten sensitivity were common. In addition, the majority of children screened had evidence of a carnitine deficiency, a red flag for an underlying metabolic component to apraxia in some children that is rarely evaluated, and could be dangerous if not addressed properly by a specialist. Families in the study often had difficulties encouraging their medical provider to consider searching for an underlying medical cause of apraxia, even when symptoms of a systemic illness warranted a work-up. In addition, the majority of families exploring nutritional avenues reported benefits after using vitamin E and PUFA.

Dr. Morris recognizes that this 2009 study is not *the* answer, but it does generate some awareness of a potentially unrecognized syndrome. As she shared in an email, "[This study] was vastly criticized for its study design, as it was not a randomized control trial (RCT), meaning it was not a double-blind placebo controlled study, often the "gold-standard" for scientific studies. However, in my view, it's a *start*. It is hard to determine an ideal treatment, when the disorder you hope to treat has not yet been accurately characterized. All medical discoveries start with a simple anecdotal observation that initiates further investigation. Our case series justifies controlled trials for a group of children with a complex medical condition that includes verbal apraxia, whose medical needs are currently not being met." Furthermore, she acknowledges that not everyone will recognize CAS as a complex metabolic disorder, as she and her coauthor suggest it is—in at least a subgroup of children.

It is also important to note that this preliminary study had absolutely *no funding*—which limited the study design and methodology.

As with anything, interpret this study with caution. If you have questions, concerns, or would like further information on the particulars of this article, please consider bringing it to your child's pediatrician for advisement.

Sensory-based Therapies: Horseback Riding, Occupational Therapy, and Therapeutic Listening Programs

We all experience the world through our senses—including seeing, hearing, touching, smelling, and tasting (there's also the vestibular and proprioceptive senses, which are very important, but often less talked about). It is through our senses that we make *sense* of the sometimes overwhelming stimuli coming at us.

Most folks learn how to combine multiple senses in childhood so that they can effectively juggle them at one time. As a child, I used to say something along these lines,

"We are always using our brain even when we don't think we are!" I thought I was making an astute observation, but what I was probably trying to explain had something to do with the idea of sensory integration. For example, as you walk outdoors, you *see* the colorful fall foliage, you *feel* the warmth of the sun, you *hear* a school bus coming to a squeaky stop, you *taste* the gum you are chewing, and you *smell* the fire burning off in the distance. You are aware of these things, although you may not consciously be thinking about all of them.

But you *do* consciously think the bus is coming to a squeaky stop. Why? Your sense of hearing is alerting you that there is a possibility of danger. Questions run through your mind: "Where is my body in time and space?" "Could I—or my child(ren)—get hit by that bus?"

Some kids (and even adults) have a hard time sorting out sensory stimulation. They may have what is referred to as **Sensory Processing Disorder (SPD)** (the older term for the same phenomena was Sensory Integration Disorder (SID). You can find more information on SPD/SID in Appendix A.

Sensory Integration Therapy

Sensory Integration Therapy is the therapy that works with kids who have a hard time organizing their senses and their world. It's often recommended for children who have autism, but can be beneficial to any child who has trouble with regulating his senses.

Sensory Integration Therapy is done 1:1 with an occupational therapist (OT) and is generally fun, adaptive (working at correcting a deficit or problem), and child-directed. You might find kids in an OT session swinging in a hammock or other indoor swing (working on the *vestibular* sensation—movement in space). Or they may be dancing to music (*sound and movement*), playing at a table filled with water or dried beans (*touch*), crawling through tunnels (*touch/space*), doing *balance* beam work, tracking objects or lights with eyes (*vision*), and possibly doing spinning exercises (*balance* and *vision*). All of these ideas and activities are rooted in various disciplines: neuroscience, developmental psychology, occupational therapy, and education.

Kate participated in OT for help with a mild sensory integration concern and it worked wonders. She was better able to focus, attend in her classroom, and seek out opportunities to satisfy her need for sensory input. Will it work for your child? Possibly. That is, it wouldn't help with the CAS per se, but might help your child with underlying problems with tolerating sensations or focusing. The effectiveness is a bit controversial.

In *The Out of Sync Child* by Carol Stock Kranowitz, we learn that there have been just a few well-designed studies to support sensory integration therapy for kids. About half of the scientific literature suggests it's beneficial; the other half says there's no effect. Perhaps sensory integration therapy may be more useful in younger versus older kids (again, it's that idea that younger kids benefit from early intervention). Generally, the goal of sensory integration therapy is for kids to be better able to play, learn, and interact with peers—all of which are the *occupation* of a child.

Hippotherapy

What do *hippos* have to do with *anything*? Actually, *"hippos"* is a Greek word meaning horse, so hippotherapy is horse riding therapy.

Kids with abnormal muscle tone (high tone or low tone), poor posture, impaired communication, behavioral and cognitive disabilities, and some medical conditions (Down syndrome and cerebral palsy, especially) may benefit from the therapeutic effects of hippotherapy.

Physical therapists, occupational therapists, and speech-language pathologists *may* recommend hippotherapy, because they believe the rhythmic movement of a horse and the rider's need to constantly adjust to the horse's movements help improve muscle tone, balance, posture, coordination, strength, flexibility, and cognitive skills. Children who are motivated to ride a horse may also be motivated to try to speak to the horse in order to control its movements (e.g., you need to say "Walk on" or "giddy-up" to get it moving, "whoa," to stop, etc.).

Hippotherapy has been shown scientifically to help children with developmental disabilities including spina bifida, Down syndrome, cerebral palsy, multiple sclerosis, attention deficit, and autism spectrum disorders. Studies have yet to prove its effectiveness with CAS, but one can project similar results.

If you remember back to the discussion about stimulating your child's vestibular system (motor/sensory) to produce more speech, it's the same idea here. Your little one's motor and sensory systems are working hard to ride that horse, so he might as well practice speech sounds, too. Keep in mind, just as with traditional speech therapy, children will need repeated exposure to this therapeutic intervention. It is not a "quick fix." For example, if your child is working so very hard just to stay on that horse, he may not have the extra reserves to put forth vocalizing. But then again, he might.

Need more to convince you? Think back to Chapter 2 in which we talked about the underlying mechanics of speech: postural control, respiration, motor control, timing, and rhythm. Since riding a horse helps in all of those areas, it stands to reason that it could also be helpful in speech production.

You may also consider the therapeutic use of an exercise ball in speech therapy. Your SLP may place your child on top of the ball, hold him there, and gently bounce him up and down. The hope here is that your child is better able to make more vocalizations than when he is sitting still.

Sandi Foreman, COTA/L, Pediatric Occupational Therapist, says this about riding horses as a therapeutic intervention: "Hippotherapy is such a great tool for a variety of diagnoses! It provides great sensory input, is good for strength, balance, and motor planning [of limbs and body]. It is so motivational for the kids. The best part is that it is fun and rewarding for both the client and the therapist!"

The American Hippotherapy Association indicates physical gains in the form of "balance, posture, mobility, and function; as well as psychological gains in cognitive, behavioral, and communication functions of clients of all ages." The AHS further asserts that a variety of diagnoses may benefit from hippotherapy, including language disabilities.

According to "Friends for Therapeutic Equine Activities," in Winfield, Illinois, the therapeutic results include such things as improved motivation, self-confidence, self-esteem, balance and coordination, cardio-respiratory function, sensory motor-organization, language and cognitive skills, and increased confidence and self-control.

Parents Share...

Experiences with Hippotherapy

➤ *"My four-year-old daughter [with CAS] went once a week and loved it! She worked with an occupational therapist who had her reaching for different objects, throwing balls into hoops as she rode. Since kids with apraxia [CAS] have trouble with planning movements of the muscles of the mouth to make the proper sounds, I thought it helped her with motor planning, as well as coordinating all of the muscles in her entire body. Overall, hippotherapy helped her mouth muscles, overall coordination, and balance."*

➤ Another mother thought her child was able to "open up" more with the horse than with people. *"[There was] something about not feeling any pressure to talk to people...he could just talk to the horse!"*

➤ Other parents who used hippotherapy as part of their child's treatment program have indicated improvements in mood, happiness, exercise, confidence, and animal bonding.

Is Hippotherapy Right for Your Child?

You may be asking yourself, "how do I know if hippotherapy is right for my child/family?" Here's a step-by-step list of questions that may help you decide:

1. First and foremost, you will want to *assess whether your child has a fear of large animals.* This sounds relatively easy, but you may be surprised at your child's reaction.

2. Is there a *suitable therapeutic riding facility in your area?* You can start by asking others or at your school, Googling it, or posting a question on a listserv.

3. *Is therapeutic riding covered by your insurance company?* If so, talk with your child's pediatrician. To receive insurance coverage, hippotherapy may require a doctor's prescription

4. *What are your other time commitments,* and how much time can you commit to hippotherapy? (The drive to and from the facility should factor into this equation.) Most kids have the best benefits when they have at least 1 hour a week of therapeutic riding.

5. *What qualifications do staff have?* You'll want involved, educated, specially trained and professional staff working with your child. In some cases, there are three staff members to one child!

Jill, mom of Finley with CAS and other developmental disabilities, points out one thing to keep in mind if you are hoping for insurance coverage: "Be aware of how you inquire about riding programs. Hippotherapy is not the same as therapeutic riding, according to some facilities. In our experience, 'therapeutic riding' was not covered by insurance, but 'hippotherapy' was."

Therapeutic riding lessons range in price, depending on where you are located in the U.S. (larger cities tend to charge more, as do those on either coast). In my research, I came across a range of prices, from as high as $175 per class to a low of $25 per half-hour. Some insurance companies may cover a portion of the expense. Check to see if yours does.

Therapeutic Listening/Auditory Integration Therapy

Because children are generally not great listeners, I would wager that most parents would gladly enroll their child(ren) in a therapeutic listening course without really knowing what it is!

While therapeutic listening (sometimes called Auditory Integration Therapy) may be able to help regulate a child's listening skills, it's not a cure-all. What Therapeutic listening really aims to accomplish is to train a child's ears to attend to and discriminate among sounds.

Children listen—through specially designed, costly earphones—to music that has been carefully engineered so that certain sound frequencies are modulated or distorted. They listen for a prescribed amount of time each day while going about their regular business.

The theory behind therapeutic listening programs is that the electronically altered music stimulates neural pathways in the brain. The brain is then supposed to be better able to tune in to higher frequencies that make up human speech.

Does it help? Some folks contend that therapeutic listening *does* help with organizing thoughts, attention, behavior, and speech-language difficulties, while plenty of others suggest it *doesn't*. Some scientists will tell you it is not effective or that it is still experimental. For example, some doctors say that patients responded negatively. And studies completed at MIT and Northeastern University indicate that the frequencies in the music could be harmful to one's ears. The American Speech-Language-Hearing Association (ASHA) studied the Berard Auditory Integration Therapy (the most commonly used program in the U.S.) and then published a technical report in 2003. They found that these particular programs did not meet scientific standards for safety and effectiveness. You can read this technical report on the ASHA website at: www.asha.org/docs/html/TR2004-00260.html.

Vision Therapy

We've got another sense that helps us see the big picture, literally. Our eyes bring a wealth of knowledge and stimulation to our minds. Together, occupational thera-

Our Experience with Therapeutic Listening

Our OT tried therapeutic listening with our daughter, Kate, during 1:1 therapy. Kate liked it and *was* better able to attend to other OT exercises while wearing the headphones. But I felt that the earphones were too expensive for her "mild" diagnosis of sensory processing disorder. We opted not to go for it.

Instead, we created our own homemade version: listening to white noise on regular headphones while Kate was going about her regular routine. The idea was to screen out distracting sounds rather than retraining her ears. While it's not exactly the same idea, it worked for us in the sense that Kate was less interested in extraneous noises and more likely to focus on a task.

Kate *still* doesn't hear me when I suggest she clean up her room or set the table, though! Bottom line: kids are *always* going to have selective hearing, and there is no evidence that I am aware of that indicates that therapeutic listening tasks improve the speech of children with CAS.

pists and developmental optometrists have developed vision therapy to hone in on visual discrimination and hand-eye coordination. Trained providers use fun, educational activities to strengthen eye musculature. It helps children tune out environmental distractions by integrating various inputs from other senses. Let me explain.

When we began seeing an OT for Kate's attention-control issues, the therapist told me that Kate was frequently distracted with visual stimulation. *Everything* was interesting and exciting for Kate to look at. It's like when you are vacationing in a new place—you look around, flashing lights and attractions catch your eye. You can't get enough. Or maybe you do, and you become overwhelmed. That may be how your child feels, too.

Our OT said that Kate had difficulty focusing her eyes on something for a significant (or even normal) amount of time. She was darting from activity to activity, losing interest quickly, and getting distracted. Most kids have a tendency to do this anyway—they *are* kids, after all!

But there is a difference between being a "typical kid" and being a child with a visual tracking problem. **There is no reason to believe that a child with CAS will have a visual tracking problem.** A child can have both, CAS *and* visual tracking concerns, but they are independent problems.

Kids with tracking problems have weaker musculature around their eyeball(s). Vision therapy presents exercises to do at home to strengthen them. For example, your child may be asked to track a light source with his eyes only (without moving his head or body to follow the light). Or he might look at two objects at the same time, but focus on one first (in the foreground), then the other (in the background), which helps with visual discrimination.

Of course, you want to know if vision therapy will help *your* child with CAS. It *might*. Remember, though: while vision therapy may help improve focus and decrease distractibility, it does not directly improve motor speech issues such as CAS. However, if you think the reason your child is not progressing in speech therapy is because of a suspected visual tracking problem, then you may want to mention it to your SLP or OT.

It's also worth noting that there is not much awareness of vision therapy. Therefore, there is not much scientific evidence to prove its effectiveness. It's typically not covered by insurance.

Other suggestions that may help your child if he has a visual tracking problem:
➤ De-clutter work and play spaces your child frequents (more on this in Chapter 10).
➤ Ask your child's teacher to make accommodations in worksheets; for example, removing unnecessary graphics or increasing the text size.
➤ Talk about a toy, game, or activity to help your child understand what is expected before presenting him with the new (visually stimulating) item. This helped my daughter Kate.

To get a full list of what vision therapy can do to help your child, please visit the websites listed in the resource section of this chapter.

Medically Based Approaches

Some folks you'll encounter on your apraxia journey will tell you that there are some medically based approaches that may help your child's apraxia. For most of these approaches—including cord blood/stem cell transplant and hyperbaric O_2 chamber therapy—there have not been any scientific studies of their effectiveness in treating CAS, so I feel it would be irresponsible to delve into them here. I feel it is worth discussing chiropractic treatment, however, because many insurance plans will pay for this, and there have been some case studies published in the literature that shows it *may* be effective for children with CAS.

Chiropractors

Some folks strongly believe in the healing touch of a chiropractor. If you are interested in having a chiropractor help your child with CAS, make sure he or she is familiar with kids and their issues. Doctors of Chiropractic (D.C.) medicine do not treat disease, but instead remove spinal nerve stress. That is really a fancy term for a "pinched nerve." Spinal nerve stress interferes with the proper function of the nervous system, according to chiropractors.

According to Dr. Tony Ebel, a chiropractor in Crystal Lake, IL, the reason that chiropractic treatment can help children with CAS is that there are "kinks" in the up-

Parents Ask...

Can the style/difficulty of birth cause CAS?

I am not aware of any major studies linking communication delays—specifically CAS—and style of birth (C-section vs. vaginal) or difficult birth. Many of the birth histories reviewed at speech clinics, however, indicate *some* concerns perinatally (around the time of birth), such as cords wrapped around the child's neck, loss of oxygen at birth, and emergency C-sections.

There is really no reason to believe that C-sections "cause" CAS. But note that a child born via C-section does not experience that tight "squeeze" through the birth canal that usually activates the lungs and accessory muscles associated with breath control. *If* the C-section was in response to an emergent situation (loss of oxygen), that *may* have affected speech development.

Be honest when your SLP asks you about your child's birth. Don't beat yourself up over the possibility that the style of your child's birth *caused* CAS. Chances are, nothing could have prevented this.

per neck and occiput region that prevent messages from flowing normally between the brain, nervous system, and muscular/motor system. Chiropractors are trained to find and detect this misalignment (subluxation) through touch (palpation) and examination. A chiropractic exam looks for the three components of the subluxation—misalignment, fixation, and nerve interference.

A chiropractor then uses specific, gentle adjustments to correct and remove the misalignment, allowing proper neurological function to return.

So, is there any research to support using chiropractic adjustments for children with CAS? There are some case studies, but nothing that I am aware of that is a randomized control study (RCT). A recent *case study* (Cuthbert and Barras, 2009) followed 157 children with developmental delay syndromes, including dyspraxia (CAS), dyslexia, attention-deficit hyperactivity disorder, and learning disabilities, who received chiropractic care. Individual and group data showed that at the end of treatment, the 157 children showed improvements in several areas, including in ability to concentrate, maintain focus and attention, and control impulsivity, as well as in their performance at home and school. However, the researchers did not say specifically whether the children with CAS improved, or if the children with CAS also had other concerns such as ADHD (a co-morbid condition).

Please consider talking with your child's pediatrician or others for recommendations of a chiropractor who works well with children. The "best of the best" have received either a Certification and/or Diplomate in pediatrics through the International Chiropractic Pediatric Association (ICPA). The "Find a Doctor" portion of the website would likely be the best place to start (www.icpa4kids.org). You may want to bear in mind, however, that there are many articles about specific aspects of chiropractic care (as well as other types of complementary and alternative treatments) on the Quack-watch website: www.quackwatch.com.

Music Therapy

Anthropologists may call music the "universal language," and they just may be right. Think of an opera singer singing in Italian. You may not know any Italian, yet you know that he is very emotional about something. You can sense his hurt, passion, love, etc. without really knowing what words he is using.

Music therapy is an established healthcare profession that uses music and music experiences to attain *nonmusical goals*—motor, cognitive, social, emotional, and speech communication. Kimberly Sena-Moore, a board-certified neurologic music therapist in private practice, gives several examples of how children with CAS may benefit from music therapy:

"Music therapists (MT) can use rhythm to help organize the oral-motor mechanisms (e.g., speaking in a steady rate where each syllable equals one beat), or they may use singing to help practice speech production. MTs may also select—or compose—specific songs in order to practice specific issues in speech production." For example, the song "The Witch Doctor" by Ross Bagdasarian (a.k.a. David Seville) is especially helpful for practicing vowels, as it repeats "Oo ee oo ah ah ting tang walla walla bing bang" several times throughout the chorus. Finally, a music therapist may use musical improvisation to learn and practice back-and-forth "dialogue," between speaker and listener, which is an important component of communication.

Another music therapist, Emily Sevcik (MT-BC), is a strong proponent of singing and its connection to the oral-motor piece of apraxia. She explains: "[Singing] is something that can address many important aspects of speaking, such as breath support, tongue movement, and lip movement. Singing can also be used to teach new vocabulary concepts. Songs can range from singing simple nursery rhymes or current songs on the radio to highly structured songs that focus on one particular letter sound or other language concept."

Why Does Music Work as a Therapeutic Intervention?

According to "Music, Rhythm, and Their Potential Benefits for Childhood Apraxia of Speech," an article by board-certified music therapist Kimberly Sena Moore, music therapy works for these reasons:

➤ *Music is a core function of the brain.* Our brains are wired to respond to music, as proven in various studies on babies as young as one day old.
➤ *Our bodies naturally move to music.* That is, we move to a rhythm without thinking much about it. Tapping our toes to the beat, for example, is usually an unconscious movement.
➤ *Children generally respond well to music.*

➤ *Music shares neural circuits with speech.*

➤ *Music can make learning easier.* For example, the ABC song helps kids memorize the letters in the alphabet. Try it with other things your kids are expected to know/remember such as their phone number, address, or spelling words!

➤ *Music is predictable, structured, and organized.* Think of a favorite song. There is a verse with one melody that is followed by a chorus with a different melody, which is usually the same every time it is sung. As we know, kids with apraxia need lots of repetition, so go ahead and belt out those tunes!

➤ *Music can help improve attention skills.* Listening to and reciting music takes concentration and that, in turn, improves attention.

➤ *Music is a noninvasive, safe, and motivating intervention—plus, it's FUN!*

Ms. Sena Moore ends with this observation: "Music therapy is a natural fit when targeting speech, language, and communication goals. From using singing to help re-wire the brain for speech to using rhythm to coordinate oral motor skills, music therapy works because of the unique way music engages and changes our brains." For more information about Ms. Sena Moore and how music therapy can help your child, visit her blog at www.MusicTherapyMaven.com.

On top of the benefits mentioned above, music therapy can help with managing stress, promoting wellness, and enhancing memory. It can also help children to improve communication and express feelings. Hmmm…now, that might be something to sing about!

What Can You Do to Encourage Speech through Music?

➤ Encourage your child to dance to the beat and clap his hands when the song mentions a certain word or phrase.

➤ Try fill-in-the-blank singing: "Old McDonald had a ____." (This fill-in-the-blank style of eliciting a response is called the Cloze task in speech-language pathology.)

Does Research Support Music Therapy for Kids with CAS?

Perhaps. One clinical case study of a three-year-old girl with CAS found that she was able to produce many syllables, combination sounds, and words by the end of therapy (she was nearly nonverbal when she started therapy). She received twenty-four therapy sessions over a period of nine months.

A critical look at this study makes it difficult to say whether this little girl's improvement had anything to do with her developmental age, or if she was receiving speech therapy in addition to music therapy. More randomized controlled studies (RCT) need to be done to determine the effectiveness of music therapy on kids with CAS.

➤ You can also practice repeat-after-me style of singing.

➤ Try to sing a scale with your child by going really high and then really low with your voice. Can your child imitate you?

➤ Have your child imitate musical instrument sounds. You play the kazoo and then have your child play the kazoo in the same manner you did, likewise for other instruments like drums, cymbals, and maracas. (We will talk more about incorporating music at home in the next chapter.)

Ask your SLP about incorporating more music into therapy sessions if you think this is something your child may respond to.

To make your case, you may want to refer to these possible benefits of using music in treatment noted in *Here's How to Treat Childhood Apraxia of Speech*, by Margaret (Dee) Fish, CCC-SLP: "Incorporating music into treatment facilitates opportunities to repeat target utterances multiple times, practice producing varied intonation patterns, and model and produce target utterances at a reduced rate by prolonging the vowels."

If you want to pursue formal music therapy, you can ask the American Music Therapy Association for help finding a therapist at www.musictherapy.org.

Does Any of This Nontraditional Therapy Do Any Good?!

Sometimes you will find scientific research that supports the treatment claims you hear or read about regarding CAM products, but sometimes you won't. Many folks will ask, "So, if it's not scientific, why bother?"

It's been my experience that parents want to know what else may help their child. Since we live in a society in which "more" sometimes equates to "better," why stop at "just" speech therapy?

Knowing about—even trying—additional therapies or remedies gives hope to parents whose kids are struggling. ***For children with CAS alone, it is just as beneficial to work with them on a frequent, intense basis to remediate symptoms associated with CAS.*** If your child has additional concerns, Complementary and Alternative Medicine (CAM) provides options to augment more traditional therapy.

For instance, one parent in my Small Talk: All About Apraxia group noted:

> *"We had really hit a plateau in speech therapy. Once we started occupational therapy [OT], my daughter really took off in terms of speech and language. We still continued with speech therapy, but I firmly believe it was the addition of OT that did the trick."*

While many "claims to cure" are anecdotal success stories, it never hurts to be a smart consumer. Ask questions, be critical, and then go with your gut. I'll show you how in the next section.

Assessing Alternative Treatments

When you go online, it's likely you will find hundreds of websites, listservs, blogs, and message boards that will tell you "ABC Wonder Remedy" will cure or dramatically improve CAS.

That's why you need to get really good at *assessing* alternative treatments. Here are a few tips to keep in mind:

➤ *Consider the source.* You don't believe just anything you see, hear, or read, right? I hope not. Sites you can generally trust include: websites of a government agency, national organization for a specific disorder, nonprofit organizations, or a medical school, or a speech pathology department page within a university website. *Buyer Beware:* if you're on a website with success articles and products for sale, be extra cautious before whipping out that credit card.

➤ *Sounds like an empirical question.* Want to know if a study is valid? Find out if there have been any scientific studies done using the scientific procedure you learned about in school. Think hypothesis, data collection, results, conclusions…then go beyond that and think "controlled studies," "peer review," "reputable journal," and "randomized control trial." A good study needs all of those elements. Sometimes you will run across studies that *sound* good, but they are limited by sample size (too small to make generalizations) or are testimonials—sometimes called anecdotal—from just one doctor, or just one SLP or only one patient. It could very well still "work," but for the results to really be valid and conclusive, it should be tested using the scientific method, which involves having a control group as well as an experimental group, and sometimes a "blind" study in which researchers are not told which group has had which treatment, so as not influence their conclusions.

➤ *Really? Or are you just saying that?* Fads come and go. The evening news will report something is "breakthrough," and it's not yet ready for the public market. You need confirmation and not just speculation on a new claim. Always go to the primary source—a journal article in an academic publication or the reputable website associated with the claim.

➤ *Says who? Is there an expert in the house?* Expert opinion should be objective, meaning the expert has nothing to gain personally or professionally from the product or claim. What does your SLP have to say about something you are willing to try? What does the ASHA have to say about it? Check it out at www.ASHA.org.

➤ *Go with your gut.* You know when something feels "off." Listen to that little voice and then sleep on it, ask around, make a pro and con list, whatever you need to do to feel better about things. If the treatment could cause a problem, especially to your kid—but even to your bank account, be conservative. Quackwatch.com is a good place to check out dubious sounding therapies or even therapies that just sound "too good to be true."

Say That Again?! Chapter Summary

I don't mean to suggest that any of the approaches covered above are cures. They may not even help. But then again, you may have just found *your* magic bullet. Kids are individuals and just as they do not all like the same toys or colors, they also don't respond to the same CAM approach in the same way.

Whatever approach you decide to try, do your homework. Take a close look at the resources in the following section to further your knowledge on the subject. Make certain there is no risk to your child. It's best to try one approach at a time. Take careful notes and be systematic about it. Trying several at a time to increase the likelihood of progress can be confusing, and you may have a hard time determining just what was helpful—was it the gluten-free diet or the fish oil that helped your little pumpkin talk? Pick and choose a few approaches, but don't knock yourself out, or you could be trying them until your kid is thirty!

Read On! Recommended Resources

➤ If you want to know more about hippotherapy (therapeutic horseback riding), look into *Special Needs, Special Horses: A Guide to the Benefits of Therapeutic Horseback Riding,* by Naomi Scott and J. Warren Evans. In addition, you may want to visit Horsefeathers Center in Lake Forest, IL at www.horsefeatherscenter.org for additional information on benefits of hippotherapy.

➤ *The Out-of-Sync Child: Recognizing and Coping with Sensory Processing Disorder* by Carol Stock Kranowitz and Lucy Jane Miller is a great resource for parents who are looking for ways to understand a child who has different modes of interpreting vision, hearing, motor skills, and nutrition, among others.

➤ If you liked *The Out-of-Sync Child* (above), then try this one next: *Growing an In-Sync Child: Simple, Fun Activities to Help Every Child Develop,* by perceptual-motor therapist Joye Newman.

➤ *Raising a Sensory Smart Child: The Definitive Handbook,* by Lindsey Biel (a mom with a child with sensory concerns) and pediatric occupational therapist

Nancy Peske, will give you some hints, tips, and understanding of sensory issues from a practical view.

➤ Two additional resources for information on sensory processing difficulties: *Sensational Kids: Hope and Help for Kids with Sensory Processing Disorder* by Lucy Jane Miller and *The Sensory Processing Disorder Answer Book: Practical Answers to the Top 25 Questions Parents Ask* by Tara Delaney, MS, OTR/L.

➤ For information on **chiropractic treatment,** try the websites of Anthony J. Ebel, DC, CACCP, *Certified Pediatric Chiropractor* (www.PremierWellnessChiro.com) or Katie Stull, D.C. (www.stullchiropractic.com), both of whom provided me with information helpful in writing this chapter.

➤ *The International Chiropractic Pediatric Association* is a nice online resource if you are interested in looking at chiropractic care for your child: www.icpa4kids.com. You may also appreciate the *Intersect4Kids program,* a very advanced certification for chiropractors in the area of Neuro-Developmental Disorders, Spectrum/Sensory Challenges. Their website is www.intersect4kids.com.

➤ *Gluten-Free Kids: Raising Happy, Healthy Children with Celiac Disease, Autism, and Other Conditions,* by Danna Korn (Woodbine House, 2010), the mother of a son with celiac disease can help you understand the pros and cons of going gluten-free.

➤ *What's Eating Your Child?* by Kelly Dorfman (Workman Press, 2011) presents a parent-friendly explanation of theories about the hidden connections between nutrition and chronic childhood ailments such as ear infections, allergies, and ADHD. You may also gain valuable information from Ms. Dorfman's website: www.whatseatingyourchild.com.

➤ *Healing the New Childhood Epidemics: Groundbreaking Program for the 4-A Disorders: Autism, ADHD, Asthma & Allergies,* by Kenneth Bock and Cameron Stauth (Ballantine Books, 2007).

➤ **The American Hippotherapy Association** can provide you with guidance and information on hippotherapy/therapeutic riding: www.americanhippotherapyassociation.org, or 877-851-4592.

➤ The Listening Program (TLP) is one of the main companies that specialize in *auditory integration therapy.* Look to their website for an overview of the program or to find a provider: www.thelisteningprogram.com. You may also like Vital Links, www.vitallinks.net, which has a similar product.

➤ For more information on *vision therapy,* refer to The Optometrists Network: www.visiontherapy.org.

➤ *Seeing Through New Eyes: Changing the Lives of Children with Autism, Asperger's Syndrome and Other Developmental Disabilities through Vision Therapy,* by Melvin Kaplan (Jessica Kingsley Publishers, 2008).

➤ *The Holistic Pediatric Association* at www.hpakids.org is a good source for information on treating kids in a holistic manner.

➤ Timothy Culbert and Karen Olness have written a book called *Integrative Pediatrics* (Oxford University Press, 2009) with guidelines on Complementary Medicine in an easy-to-read, evidence-based manner.

➤ For more information on music therapy, check out the *American Music Therapy Association:* www.musictherapy.org or 301-589-3300.

➤ *Music, Language, and the Brain,* by Aniruddah D. Patel (Oxford University Press, 2010), is a comprehensive volume of the neuroscience behind language and music.

➤ You may find these various *music therapy websites* helpful to you and your children:
  ➤ Milestone Music Therapy: www.milestonemusictherapy.com
  ➤ Listen and Learn Music: www.listenlearnmusic.com
  ➤ Kimberly Sena Moore's website: www.neurosong.com
  ➤ Music Therapy Round Table: www.musictherapyroundtable.com

➤ You can read Kimberly Sena Moore's original article, "Music, Rhythm, and Their Potential Benefits for Childhood Apraxia of Speech," on PediaStaff at www.pediastaff.com/blog/music-rhythm-and-their-potential-benefits-for-childhood-apraxia-of-speech-647 (originally published online, May 28, 2010).

Chapter Nine

. . . .

What You Can Do at Home

. . . . .

Tapping into Your Inner Speech-Language Pathologist

*"I learned the most from the sessions on what I can do
at home to help my son. I didn't know there was so much I could actually do.
I had thought only the SLP could do some of this stuff. Don't get me wrong; they do a lot.
But I can do some pretty cool things to help my son, too."*
—Small Talk: All About Apraxia parent participant

This may very well be the chapter we have all been waiting for. It's the one I am the most eager to write. You may have turned to this chapter first, for it is the one thing you can actually feel good about doing—making a difference in your child's struggles with Childhood Apraxia of Speech.

Here you will find tips and ideas for helping your child make progress in a fun and nurturing speech-rich environment at home and on the go. Simple toys and books can become therapeutic; music and games can promote speech development. This chapter combines all aspects of your parenting brain: teaching, nurturing, creating, role-playing, and limit-setting. So get ready!

Even adults remember new information best when they are having fun. If you had a traditional education, you grew up with desks, blackboards, and the teacher at the front of the class. You were taught that this is how people learned. It might be time to shift your view and throw out the flashcards! This chapter does not take place in a classroom. It does not even suggest you turn your dining room into a speech clinic (al-

---

The Nuts and Bolts of This Chapter

➤ Your "toolbox" with a host of fun ideas to get your child talking, playing, and learning

➤ How to have fun with speech and language each day in a variety of settings, as you move through your family's daily routines

➤ Gross motor, musical, and multimedia avenues to get your child's speech system warmed up and ready to go, and to actually facilitate speech

➤ How to identify your child's learning style and preferences and how you can best tap into these

---

though that's not necessarily a bad idea). But it *is* about learning how to help your child overcome apraxia of speech in a natural environment: your home and community.

Here are a few ideas to get you started:

➤ *Have a family game night.* Traditional favorites will do the trick. The speech payoffs here: turn-taking, counting, requesting, being a good sport, and other communication opportunities.

➤ *Visit your public library.* Let your child find some books of interest and then read them to her. Speech payoff: child-directed learning, introduction to new vocabulary, 1:1 time with you in which you are modeling pronunciation and articulation. You might even hear some sounds or word approximations from your child!

➤ *Experience and connect with nature.* Speech payoff: identify and describe what you see, hear, and smell. Think holistically—this is more than *just* a walk in the park.

➤ *Exercise* by biking or sledding, walking, or swinging. Speech payoff: vocalizations and words are often heard with movement. Exercise also increases self-confidence, which these kiddos need more than anything. Children with CAS often crave movement.

➤ *Do some art.* Speech payoff: Besides the 1:1 time all kids need, it also unleashes creative potential and gives you something to talk about: "What color should we make the banana?" Practice saying "banana" or "yellow" while you're at it.

➤ *Listen to music.* Speech payoff: Kids need physical movement, and what better way to get them moving than with some rockin' tunes? Even if they can't get the lyrics out, they can hum along. Plus, music has a positive effect on mood—even yours!

➤ *Bake cookies or cupcakes.* Speech payoff: identify ingredients as you toss them into the bowl, have your child repeat the words (flour, sugar, butter, etc.) if she is able, and talk about shapes as you roll out sugar cookies. Share your cookies with friends and neighbors and let your child do *some* of the talking—if possible—when the two of you deliver the goodies. It can be as simple as saying, "cookie" or "bake"—even an approximation will do.

Learning Styles

Before we have a deeper discussion about what you can do at home, it's important to talk about different styles of learning. We all learn best in different and unique ways. Sure, we can learn in a classroom by reading books and sitting at desks in neat, straight lines. But is this the *best* way for everyone to learn? How do you learn best? How does your child learn best? Don't be discouraged if the two of you learn in different ways. We'll touch on melding those differences later in this chapter.

When I sat down to write this chapter (at a coffee shop, where I tend to do my best writing and learning), it came as no surprise that I had several piles of information corresponding to different learning styles. The biggest pile was about gross motor/sensory/whole-body/kinesthetic learning. By now, you know why: *CAS is a disorder of the motor-speech system.* Many children with CAS may also have other motor programming problems such oral and/or limb apraxia. Adequate sensory processing is necessary for good motor programming.

But there are lots of other learning styles and preferences. Without getting into too much of the psychology of learning and different educational theories, let's review them in brief. Be sure to note the traits that sound most like your child.

Howard Gardner, a developmental psychologist and professor of education, suggests that humans have multiple intelligences. Individuals tend to be more skilled in some areas than others, which leads to a preferred or certain style of learning. Gardner has identified eight different types of intelligences, shown in the table on pages 162-163, all of which work together to create a whole.

Did you see yourself in any of these categories? Your child? Perhaps you saw attributes in more than one category that describe you and/or your child.

Despite the many strengths identified by Gardner, schools, teachers, and even parents tend to expect children to have just one of three learning styles: auditory, visual, and/or kinesthetic.

How do you like to learn new material? By *seeing* it done (demonstration), *reading* about new information, *hearing* someone else describe what to do, or *doing* the new task until you feel you've "got it?"

Of course, your little one with CAS likely can't tell which learning style she prefers. It takes time and introspection to figure out one's best learning style, and most children have no idea what theirs is. It's up to you to observe and see how your child responds to different approaches. Particularly good teaching instruction will employ *seeing, doing, hearing,* and *reading.*

Before we can help our children at home with speech and language, it is helpful to have some idea of how they best learn, so we can best help. The bottom line with this information on learning styles and intelligences:

Multiple Intelligences

Area	Description	Strengths
LINGUISTIC	Strong awareness of: ➤ Sounds ➤ Rhythms ➤ Words	May be adept at: ➤ Organizational abilities ➤ Logical deduction ➤ Good memory of spoken words & written language ➤ Structured & sequenced instruction
LOGICAL-MATHEMATICAL	Proficient in: ➤ Logic ➤ Patterning ➤ Conceptualization ➤ Abstraction	Likely enjoys: ➤ Problem-solving ➤ Patterns ➤ How and why things work
MUSICAL-RHYTHMIC	Easily discriminates: ➤ Auditory tone ➤ Pitch ➤ Rhythm	Generally good at: ➤ Auditory patterning ➤ Remembering things that he or she hears
VISUAL-SPATIAL	Naturally: ➤ Understands the relation-ships between objects, concepts, or images ➤ Looks at events from different viewpoints.	These learners: ➤ Can mentally create and visualize very well ➤ Good at drawing maps and diagrams ➤ Looks at big picture first then fills in details
BODILY-KINESTHETIC	Loves to: ➤ Move body through time and space ➤ Perform sequential movements	Generally: ➤ Has a good sense of time ➤ Understands proportion ➤ Predicts sequences well ➤ Can visualize movements before they occur
INTERPERSONAL	Highly proficient at: ➤ Perceiving moods ➤ Empathizes well with others' feelings	Typically: ➤ Interacts well with others ➤ Natural leader ➤ Can do the above well because they can sense emotions, needs, desires, and intentions of others

INTRAPERSONAL	Confident in: ➤ Knowing self well ➤ Believing strongly in one's values and goals	These individuals: ➤ Can reflect well on one's own thoughts and feelings ➤ Introspective ➤ Analyzes own behavior through reflection
NATURALISTIC	Highly Perceptive of: ➤ Things in the natural world ➤ Plants ➤ Animals	Generally, it is easy to: ➤ Organize things into categories ➤ Make detailed observations ➤ Recognize patterns

➤ Your child will not fall neatly into one camp.
➤ You will see bits and pieces of your child's traits in each category, but there will be one category that seems to be the "best fit."
➤ Kids with apraxia are individuals, just like other children. It is your job to find out how you can best help *your child with CAS.*
➤ Hopefully this information will help you hone your skills so you can best help your child.

Parenting Primer

There are a few things you need to keep in mind as your "golden rules" in working with your child with CAS:

➤ *Have your child repeat, repeat, repeat!* Movement repetitions build strong motor planning/programming/gestures. *Can you say that again?*
➤ *Provide lots of opportunities throughout the day to get your child to talk or vocalize—about* **anything.** Your child will begin to see that communication is indeed a fun part of life.
➤ *Be goofy and funny.* If you are relaxed and your kiddo is relaxed, words will come easier.
➤ *Make talking and speech practice more about your lifestyle and less about "sit and speak" time.*
➤ *Team up with your SLP.* Have her give you ideas for homework and report back to her. Let her know what your kid does well at home and see if it works as well in the clinic. Think of your SLP-parent-kid connection as a circle with no beginning and no end; make it appear as if you are driving a fancy automatic car—smooth and effortless, even if it's really a jumpy 5-speed jeep.
➤ *The more talking feels like work, the less willing your kid will be to do it.*

➤ *Imitation is huge, too.* "Can you say what I say?" Try it. If imitation is too hard, try doing it in unison. Even singing the ABC song is a form of imitation in the form of chanting memorization.

➤ *You are mom or dad first.* You do not need to become your child's SLP. Kids are smart. They will know what you're up to and won't participate if you act too much like their SLP.

➤ *Your goal is to complement your SLP's efforts in your own home.* Talk to your SLP about a reasonable amount of home practice. This will also depend on the age of your child. As one apraxia parent named Mike says, "An SLP is like a personal trainer at the gym. You go, your trainer works with you for an hour and teaches you things to do on your own, but it's up to you to do the rest."

Home-made Speech and Language Lessons by Category

Feeling ready to kick it up to high gear? I hope you have a notebook or a highlighter handy. You'll want to make a list of your favorite activities—ones you think your child will respond to best, based on personality, interests, personal motivators, and age. Your willingness and ability are other factors to contribute—time, effort, support, and sometimes money. Remember, your goal here is not to get your child to say things perfectly, but to encourage speech communication.

GET YOUR MOTOR RUNNIN': Gross Motor and Whole Body Activities

1. Bounce Your Way to Words!
What you need: Get a trampoline appropriate for your space and budget. You can find small basic trampolines in the sporting goods department of your favorite retailer for about $30. Bigger (outdoor) ones come with a higher price tag and other concerns like space, insurance, and neighbor kids. Look for one made just for kids; a stabilizer bar is helpful. Keep it in a place in your home where your child will see it and use it.

What you do: Bounce on it, of course! Use it for at least 15 minutes a day over a period of several months and you're bound to see a jump in words. You can also have your child jump and practice saying target sounds and words.

Speech payoff: It's fun! The underlying issue in CAS is neurological motor planning. Jumping requires motor programming. Movement helps your child's mind and body work together more effectively.

2. Box It Up, Please

What you need: Boxes—big, little, and in-between sizes—plus imagination. Make sure there are no sharp brads or corners and then let the kids have at it!

What you do: Create toys, forts, stages, and playhouses. Probe your child to describe—using words, of course—what she is doing. Is she making a robot? Ask her to identify and describe body parts. "Building" a dollhouse or castle can focus on words like window, door, inside, outside, and the many other descriptions that can go with building.

Speech payoff: Kids use their imaginations and creativity to paint, cut, tape, fold, and construct. It builds problem-solving skills and a larger vocabulary.

3. Freeze Frame

What you need: Music (CD player, radio) and kids.

What you do: Put on some tunes and have the kids dance, wiggle, jump, and move to the music. When the music stops, everyone freezes and says a word, phrase, or approximation of a word, either related to how they're posing, or some other target word or phrase you determine ahead of time. The key is they have to say *something*!

Speech payoff: Besides providing fun and exercise, it works the vestibular system and helps those words come out.

4. Rollin, Rollin'— Keep Those Kids Rollin'

What you need: Kid(s), adult(s), and a flat, open, safe place to roll around.

What you do: Lie down, grab your kid, and gather her to your chest with your arms. Roll back and forth saying, "I've got...mommy/daddy/baby brother/teacher/friend/neighbor/grandparent." You and your child take turns saying who they've "got." If your child can't say the entire phrase, "I've got Papa," just have her say "papa." You can even use fill-in-the-blank to help your child: "I've got _____."

Speech payoff: You can practice names of family members in a nonthreatening, on-the-spot manner. Aunt Shannon isn't really there when you are practicing this activity, but the next time you see her, your child will be more comfortable with saying her name. It also encourages parent-child bonding and stimulates the all-important vestibular system.

5. Get in the Swing of It!

What you need: Swings at the park, in your backyard, or even hanging from the rafters in your basement.

What you do: Push your child as long as she will allow, and you have energy for. As you push, think of target sounds, words, or phrases to work on with your child. Practice the ABCs, work on perfecting her name, count to ten, etc. Do this at least once a day for 15 to 20 minutes over the course of a few months, and you just may see a surge in talking.

Speech payoff: Can we say, "vestibular system?!"

Parents Ask...

What's the big deal about motion, again?

In the first couple of chapters, we talked about CAS being a disorder of the neuromotor system. In fact, physical and occupational therapists who have worked with children with speech disorders have commented that children become much more vocal when engaged in movement such as rocking, swinging, bouncing, sliding, or even rock climbing. These activities are often referred to as *vestibular stimulation activities.*

We found that Kate did much better in her speech therapy sessions when we complemented them with occupational therapy. I would go as far as to say that it was the combination of speech and occupational therapies that was the "key" that unlocked Kate's voice.

6. Do a Little Dance, Make a Little Word

What you need: Adult and child.

What you do: The adult calls out different kinds of movements: "Touch the sky way up high—touch your toes way down low—wiggle your hips—rub your tummy." Child plays along and can repeat words as she feels ready. Add in other body parts like nose, ears, hair, mouth, tongue, knees, etc.

Speech payoff: Whole body movements can help get your little pumpkin talking; they also encourage listening to directions and enhance receptive language and identification of body parts.

7. If We Could Talk Like the Animals

What you need: Nothing but you and a child with CAS.

What you do: Can you make a great pig noise? Do it—but really act like a pig by rolling around (as if in the mud). After you are done oinking, say the name of the animal. Bark like a dog, jump like one, pant and lick like one. Meow like a cat, rub your head on a loved one, purr, and curl up like a cat.

Variation: As your child gets better at this, she has to identify the animal by name ("Dog") before moving on to the next one.

Speech pay-off: Besides the fun and giggles you're sure to get, it helps your child learn about different animals and their sounds. Plus, making animal sounds may be less intimidating than saying actual words. In fact, the Kaufman Speech Praxis Treatment Kit: Basic level begins with the animal sounds. These are often some of the first words children say.

8. Roll It to Me, Baby

What you need: Kid(s) and a ball.

What you do: Sit on the floor, with legs apart and take turns rolling the ball back and forth (or tossing the ball in the air as your child's skills improve). Practice saying target words or telling about a favorite something (food, color, season, friend, etc.) while you roll/toss the ball. Do this until you (or she) tires of it, but aim for at least six passes.

If your child is nonverbal, you roll the ball and say, "Mommy's turn." When it is your child's turn, say, "Kate's turn" for her.

Speech payoff: This is a wonderful way to encourage conversational turn-taking: speaker + listener = conversation. Teach this concept early.

9. Hullabaloo (Cranium Games)

What you need: Get yourself to the toy store and put Hullabaloo in your cart. You'll be glad you made the investment. This game is best for kids ages 3-8.

What you do: The game comes with a machine that calls out directions to players: "Hop to a mat with an animal"; "Slither to a blue." It's sort of like Twister meets charades.

Speech payoff: Kids have to pay attention, because if you miss something, you miss the whole thing. The game works on colors, categories, and shapes and is great for building receptive language. Step it up by adding in a word or a phrase (a target speech sound) your child must say (or attempt) on each turn.

10. Take a Hike

What you need: Yourself and a fun/interesting place to walk.

What you do: Walk around your park, neighborhood, or local arboretum with your family. Using the letters of the alphabet as a guide, find items along your path that begin with the letter, sound, or word your little child is working on in therapy. First choose words and sounds your child already knows and build upon that base.

Variation: Label every tree (or other item) you see as you pass by (a form of concentrated practice; auditory bombardment).

Speech payoff: Repetition, whole-body learning, develops a love of nature, plus it's a fun way to sneak in those speech drills.

11. Stage a Scavenger Hunt

What you need: 4 to 5 items that interest your child and that target a sound/word/phrase you are working on.

What you do: Show the items to your child and then hide them around your house. Set a timer for an appropriate amount of time and have her look for the items. When she finds the item, have her identify what it is, three times. After three attempts at saying the target sound, reward her with something of value (a sticker, a food treat, more play, a video game, or movie).

Variation: Make it a mobile scavenger hunt by doing it in the car. First, list items you might spot on the route you choose. Sneaky parents will think of the target sounds that are challenging (e.g., /ST/ blends in the words "stop sign, store, stone," for the child who has advanced to this level). You could even draw pictures of a stop sign, store, stone, etc. or cut them out of magazines. When you drive by that spot, your child shouts out what she found.

Speech payoff: Kids, like adults, get bored with the same ol' routine. This activity shakes it up a bit, plus it encourages memory and works on repetition.

12. Create an Obstacle Course

What you need: Whatever you have on hand and don't mind your kids crawling through, jumping in, bouncing on, or climbing on top of—chairs, blankets, trampolines, etc. Throw in some directives, too. "Do two somersaults and now three jumping jacks!"

What you do: Design the course and then have your child complete the activities. You can make it more challenging by having your child say key words/phrases/sounds at each station. Encourage verbalization at the end, such as, "I'm a winner," "Hooray," or another similar phrase. Afterwards, you can pull out the speech flashcards. You may be amazed at how much faster and easier they are once the body (and brain) have been "warmed up" with a vestibular/movement activity.

Speech payoff: Fun, silly play beats boredom any day, and it just might be what your rough-and-tumble kid needs to stimulate the verbal part of her brain.

13. Switch It Up

What you need: Flashcards (make your own or buy some), speech exercises/worksheets from your therapist, objects from around the house that correspond to sounds, words, or phrases you are currently targeting, even coloring books will do! You'll need access to music and your kid(s).

What you do: Arrange the items you gathered on the floor. Then start the music and the dancing. When the music stops, have your child pick an item from the floor to talk about, or practice. Do several rounds.

Speech payoff: Again, it's work disguised as fun involving movement, rhythm, and vestibular activation.

14. Target Toss

What you need: Hula hoop and bean bags, foam balls, or other soft toys.

What you do: Set the hula hoop on the floor (or grass). Invite your child to stand a certain distance away from the hula hoop and toss or drop bean bags, foam balls, or other soft toys into it. Each time she tosses something into the target, have your child say "toss/throw/in" or a target sound/word/phrase.

Speech payoff: Fun for little ones, especially when targets are large and accuracy is not important. Plus, it's active fun for little minds.

15. Fall Fun

What you need: Rake (child-sized is best), kid, and lots of fall leaves.

What you do: Help your child rake leaves in the yard. Talk about the sounds the leaves make as you rake them. You can stress the words "in" and "out" as you put leaves into bags.

Speech payoff: Working together promotes bonding and teamwork, respect for nature, and, again, it's a whole-body movement that not only exercises the body, but the mind as well.

16. Touch & Talk

What you need: Container, rice or beans, and various small objects.

What you do: Fill the container with uncooked rice or beans, add small objects, shake it up, and then have your child reach in and find an object (look for objects that contain target sounds or words). Talk about what the object does, looks like, and what other things can go with it. Description is a powerful language development activity.

Speech payoff: This activity is great for those touchy-feely kids who learn best by doing. It encourages problem-solving, language development, and critical thinking skills (what can we do with it? what else goes with that?).

17. Be a Superhero

What you need: Something your child can use as a cape or crown.

What you do: Pretend your little one is a superhero—"Super Word Boy/Girl" or the like. Let her run—but not aggressively—in a safe place, with her cape or crown. Encourage neat words that superheroes often use: "Kaboom, bam, boink, and pow" and let your child have fun saving the day with verbal power!

Speech payoff: This activity is a great outlet for kids' super-charged energy. Those silly action words are a lot of fun to say. Plus, when speech drills and therapy wear them down, this feels like play, yet you know it's secretly work.

18. Block Head

What you need: Table blocks, colored stacking blocks, cardboard brick blocks, even empty food boxes.

What you do: Have your child build with blocks. Encourage her to talk about what she is building. For example, "I see you are building a tall tower….How do you get to the top?" Or, "Who lives in the house?" If your child is reluctant to answer questions, make statements and give her time to respond. Some children with speech concerns are sensitive to too many questions.

Speech payoff: Again, it's active play that ties together gross and fine motor work (speech is fine motor work). Your child is actively playing with something that already interests her and may not notice that you are getting her to talk about what she is doing. Words just might "pop" out.

Books/Words

We all know that books can open a whole new world of imagination, but they can also help open a whole new world of speech. Here are some ideas for using books, magazines, and catalogs to get some word practice in for your child.

1. Vacation Time

What you need: Nothing!

What you do: Pretend you are going on a trip to the beach. Ask your child to help you "pack." Have her make suggestions by giving prompts: "We wear this when we go swimming," or "So we don't get sunburned, we will need to bring ____." Fill-in-the-blank is a *great* way to encourage speech production. Suggest a couple of silly items that your child knows won't be going in your suitcase to the beach. Try a pretend vacation to the mountains next.

Speech payoff: It's a fun way to pass the time if you are waiting. It also develops vocabulary, word associations, and critical thinking skills. You can focus on target sounds/words/phrases.

Other resources to consider: *Smart Kids* makes a double-sided flipchart entitled *"Where are you going? What would you take?"* On it are colorful pictures of various vacation destinations—beach, jungle, camping, skiing, airport, etc. It's a great tool to stimulate early speaking, listening, and language development. Look for it at www.janellepublications.com.

2. Art Appreciation

What you need: Picture books or real artwork at home or around town **Try these books:** *Can You Find It Inside?* and *Can You Find It Outside?* by Jessica Schulte. They're great hardcover art appreciation books for kids in which you search and discover famous pieces of art based on rhyme-style clues.

What you do: Study the pictures/illustrations/art. Ask your child questions about what's happening. Together, you can create a story. "Who lives here?" "Why do you think she's sad?" For less verbal kids, just identifying what you—the adult—see in the picture can encourage your child to vocalize. The more you talk, the more she learns. Just be sure to give your child time to respond. Some adults are uncomfortable with silence, especially when their communication partner is struggling. You will get better at this!

Speech payoff: Exposure to new media and styles of art increases observational skills/attention to detail and encourages story-telling.

3. A Picture Is Worth 1000 Words

What you need: Magazine, scissors, and glue.

What you do: Cut out magazine pictures of things that interest your child—people, places, and things like toys and food. Try to make the picture of a single object, say pizza, grandma, etc. Then glue the images to a note card or construction paper. When you have a sizeable amount (it will vary based on your child's age, attention span, and verbal ability), arrange the cards on the floor and use the pictures to create a story. You can target specific speech sounds/words/phrases.

Variation: Rip an action picture/photo from the magazine. Ask your child to tell you about it. Where are the people going, what are they eating, are they happy or sad, etc.? Can your child ask *you* about the picture? This can help your child develop question-asking skills.

Speech payoff: This can target sequencing (see below), and stirs the creative juices to develop story-telling. It can get your child talking about things that interest her.

4. Folding Fun

What you need: Kumon *Fold and Cut* workbook for preschool (ages 2 - 5 years), available from most places that carry books.

What you do: Pick a few activities from the book and do them together with your child. Ask her about what you are doing. For example, one activity is a picture of a little boy smiling. When you open the folded part, he's crying. You could ask your child to say "smile" (working on an "s" blend and/or ask her to say "cry."). Ask other questions such as "Why is she happy?" Even if your child answers with "I don't know" (or some variation of it—as long as it's verbal), it still counts!

Variation: If your child is reluctant to answer questions, try comments or fill-in-the-blank.

Speech payoff: Fun, engaging, and 1:1 time with a parent. The activities are varied and can be used just about anywhere. Keep a Kumon workbook in your car or bag and see where it takes you.

5. The Big Book of Exclamations

What you need: *The Big Book of Exclamations* (Chatterbox Books, 2008), written by SLP Teri K. Peterson.

What you do: *Look* at it with your child. This book is not a traditional storybook. The captivating illustrations give your child lots of opportunity to practice speech words and sounds in a fun, nonthreatening way. It helps parents learn to talk about the illustrations in books. Teri's technique is useful for other illustrated books as well. (See "Literacy Is Key" in Chapter 7 and dialogic reading later in this chapter as well as in Chapter 12 for more tips on this style of looking at books with your child.)

Speech payoff: If you're a bookworm, you'll find this is a fun way to bond with your child while sneaking in speech practice. Check out Ms. Peterson's website for more information: www.TheBigBookofExclamations.com.

6. Auditory Bombardment

What you need: List of words beginning with the same sound (a target sound for your child). For example, 16 words beginning with a "k" or hard "c" such as coat, cane, cage, kick, camp, kite, court, cup, cut, cab, card, cone, king, kid, kiss, and key.

What you do: While your kiddo is sitting at the table, playing quietly in the sandbox, or any another quiet moment, read the list aloud several times slowly and clearly. Read the list a couple of times a day. It will only take you a minute or two to get through the words.

Variation: Have your child search through magazines and catalogs looking for items on the list. Make a collage. On a silly note, I used to make up stories about the words on the page: "The kid kicked the cat's cage and then kissed the king."

Speech payoff: Your child will hear that beginning letter sound over and over and begin to internalize it. Speech requires auditory recognition and discrimination of sounds on which your child is working.

7. Magic Words

What you need: Good manners.

What you do: Model those "magic words" wherever you go (e.g., "Thank you," "please," etc.). The more often you do this in the presence of your children, the more likely they will do the same. Thank your kids for the small things, too: "*Thank* you for playing so nicely with your sister. *Thank* you for taking your plate to the sink. *Thank* you for getting buckled up so quickly in the car." After you have modeled polite words for awhile, see if your child can imitate you or say the words in unison with you. Unison can be easier than imitation. This is sort of like the auditory bombardment idea above. Your child hears it so many times she'll eventually "get it." You'll need to exaggerate the words and get your child to look in the person's eyes and say it (even an approximation) with you or right after you say it.

Speech payoff: Children with CAS may not be able to say much, but it's no excuse for not being polite. Explain that a "thank you" or "please" makes people feel good and when people feel good, they may help you again in the future. Watch folks smile when your child uses manners, even if it is just an approximation.

8. Act It Out

What you need: Nothing.

What you do: Think charades with a therapy twist. Bring therapy ideas home, and get creative. For instance, the "j" sound is typically very tricky. You can turn that into a jump-a-thon at home in a sort of "say it, do it" fashion. Act out the word "push"; exaggerate the "p" sound as you push open doors, or push a toy ride-on around the room. Have your child bring in a grocery bag. Say, "It's *heavy*. So *heavy*. Can you say *heavy*?" Exaggerate the "h" sound. "Can you say *ha-ha*?" (Keep in mind, some SLPs may not want you to work with hard/tricky words at home with your child at first. They want to see you and your child be successful at home with easier sounds/words/phrases before making "homework" more challenging. Check with your SLP first.)

Speech payoff: It's a fun way to entertain and engage (whole-body) kids with their speech practice. It shows them you are serious about their interests/activities and that you have "found" a way to incorporate them at home. Plus, it might help you get some household chores done!

9. Book Talk (Dialogic Reading)

What you need: Picture books your child likes.

What you do: Read with your child and *let* him interrupt. Allow lots of time for a reading session. Remember, you don't have to read everything on the page. Study the pictures together and ask wh- questions (who-what-when-where-why), and see what your child can come up with. You might just start by pointing out the items in the picture. Give choices if your child has a hard time spontaneously identifying objects: "Is this an umbrella or a boot?" When you ask *what* a character is doing in the book, you'll get an answer that works on action words and the –ing word ending (running, walking, jumping, washing). You can expand on this and say, "Show me running," and allow your child to run around the room once or twice and finish the exercise by saying, "Run!"

Speech payoff: Besides facilitating language development and introducing new vocabulary words, you are engaging in what experts call *dialogic reading*. It's reading as though you were having a conversation—stopping to discuss pictures and new words, and identifying feelings and emotions of the characters. The key with dialogic reading is to read with expression and enthusiasm.

10. Show and Tell for Mom and Dad

What you need: A nifty little item you want to talk about (e.g., your new iPhone/iPad, a cool new cooking gadget) with your kids, perhaps at the dinner table.

What you do: Instead of your child being the center of attention with their favorite item, it's *your turn* to "show and tell." You can expose your child to new words like "[app]lication," "download," "garlic press," "nutcracker."

Speech payoff: Your child is likely familiar with the game from school, so you are expanding on that experience by introducing her to new vocabulary. This helps our see-it-touch-it-learn-it learners.

Rhythm/Music

The jury's still out on the role music plays in the learning process. Scientists are continuing to look at whether music supports verbal and math skills. In the meantime, it is fun and what could it hurt? Music can help kids express themselves, relax, and release tension, and it may even help with attention, focus, and creativity. Here are some products designed with speech improvement in mind, some specifically for CAS:

Time to Sing! CD

The tempo of the songs on this CD has been slowed from the originals to encourage kids with apraxia to sing along (the original pace of these songs may be too fast for young apraxics to keep up). Includes traditional favorites such as "Wheels on the Bus," "Itsy Bitsy Spider," and "Old MacDonald Had a Farm." Look for it at CASANA/Apraxia-KIDS, www.apraxia-kids.org.

SPEECHercise CDs

These CDs were created by SLPs to help kids (ages 3 - 6) with speech disabilities at home, at school, and in the car. They combine silly songs, mouth activities, and speech drills. Plus, there's a parent guide, worksheets, and lyrics if you order the "enhanced music CD." Available at www.twinsisters.com.

Marvelous Mouth Music: Songs for Therapy and Beyond

It's a little pricey for the book and CD but those who use this set like it. Suzanne Evans Morris, Ph.D., created this product along with the performers. It gets kids working on speech breathing and voicing in fun ways. Morris's website is New Visions (www.new-vis.com) where you can also locate articles about music and learning.

Sing Out! & Ta-Da! Music to Enhance Language Development

Written and performed by Katie Eshelman, an "apraxia mom" who is also a music therapist, this CD has been helpful to many who need a little nudge where language development is concerned. For more information, visit www.singoutonline.com.

Kids' Express Train (CD)

This company helps kids with speech and language difficulties sing simple songs through fun, transportation-themed albums such as "Drills on Wheels" and "Conversation Station." Check them out at: www.expresstrain.org.

Make a Sound and Move Around

An SLP and musician created this program consisting of a CD and booklet. The program works on basic communication, socialization, and movement skills. It is best suited for kids aged 18 months to 3 years. Available at www.pediatrictherapynetwork. org.

Dr. Jean Feldman's Albums

Dr. Feldman has lots of albums under her belt—all with fun titles sure to get a giggle (*Kiss Your Brain, Going Green,* and *Totally Math*). An educator for over 35 years, Dr. Feldman has a way with kids from preschool through the elementary years. Look for her website at www.drjean.org.

Silly Mom Jingles

Even though I can't carry a tune in a bucket, I still sing songs to my kids. After a few poor attempts at singing lullabies, I quickly learned that the better form of song for me is the jingle. I challenge you to think of ways to turn everyday comments or directives into a song. Before you know it, your little ones may just join in on the chorus. Here are a few examples of things I sang/chanted around the house during our daily routines:

➤ "Yummy to my tummy, yummy to my tummy, yum, yum yum!"
➤ "Pee pee in the potty, pee pee in the potty, pee pee pee!" (Or substitute poo poo.) This jingle worked wonders when we were potty-training.
➤ "This is the way we dry your hair, dry your hair, dry your hair. This is the way we dry your hair so early in the evening."
➤ "Go with the green light; go with the green light; go with the green light. Go!" or "Stop with the red light, stop with the red light; stop."

Traditional Songs to Sing with and to Your Kids

➤ ABC song,
➤ "I'm a Little Teapot,"

- ➤ "Rain, Rain Go Away,"
- ➤ "Head, Shoulders, Knees and Toes,"
- ➤ "Twinkle, Twinkle Little Star,"
- ➤ "Pat a Cake,"
- ➤ "This Little Piggy,"
- ➤ "Wheels on the Bus,"
- ➤ "Pop Goes the Weasel,"
- ➤ "Itsy Bitsy Spider,"
- ➤ "Five Little Monkeys Jumping on the Bed."

I like these songs because many of them have an action component. Since we know that CAS is a motor-based disorder, these motions go hand-in-hand with the lyrics.

You may also want to try the "call and response" style of singing with your child(ren) in which you say something and they repeat or "answer" your "call"—as in "Who Stole the Cookies from the Cookie Jar?"

Props
Consider investing in some of these to have on hand for a music experience:
- ➤ Kazoos to encourage vocal intonation used in singing and speech,
- ➤ Harmonicas to encourage breath control and direction of air through the mouth,
- ➤ Toy microphone that amplifies the voice and increases auditory feedback,
- ➤ Echo microphone (Rapper Snapper) to provide auditory feedback via reverberation.

Look for these items at party supply stores and dollar stores.

Sequencing

Sometimes kids with CAS have difficulty following directions or following an orderly sequence of events. They may need extra time to absorb what is being said/asked of them, and they may need directions repeated during the middle of a task. Help them out by offering to strengthen those skills through some fun games. Just remember to vary the activities to keep your child interested and engaged.

1. Follow the Leader and Simon Says
What you need: Child(ren) and a little bit of time (5 - 20 minutes).

What you do: You're probably already familiar with these classic childhood games, so start small—simple actions and concepts go a long way in these "do as I do" games. Make them more challenging by giving two or three commands at each turn as your child's skills increase: "Stomp your feet, turn around, touch the ground." It is important that your child have successful listening experiences.

Speech payoff: Attention to detail and memory are stressed, as well as receptive language and sequencing skills.

2. Memory Take-Away

What you need: A Memory game, or objects from around the house.

What you do: Instead of playing Memory in the traditional sense, pull out just a few cards with target speech sounds/words/phrases (from 2 to 5, depending on your child's ability, tolerance, and attention span). Talk about what's on the cards. Place them face up on the table or floor. Take away one of the cards while your child covers her eyes. Her job is to tell you which card you took away.

Variation: Let you child be the teacher and quiz *you*. Many kids are much more engaged when they're in charge. Switch it around so you're the teacher again. As your child gets better at this, try taking 2 cards away and then 3 from a set of 5 or 6. Some children do better with objects than with pictures. Try it both ways and see what works for your child. My daughter did so much better at this activity when we used actual objects that she could touch and relate to.

Speech payoff: Develops memory skills, attention, and focus—which may be a struggle for kids with CAS. It also helps with vocabulary and targeted speech sounds/words/phrases.

3. Photographic Memory

What you need: Camera and child.

What you do: Take pictures of your child completing activities around the house: washing hands, setting the table, getting ready for bed, heading out the door. Keep the steps in the routine manageable—say, no more than 5 photographs (steps) of the same routine. Print them out and laminate, or stick them to note cards. Have your child arrange them in order from start to finish. Have her tell you her own story about these sequences to the best of her ability. If she struggles with this, you can tell *her* the story. For a challenge, have her arrange them in *reverse* order!

Variation: Take photos of an item that changes over time—seeds to sprouts to flower (or trees in and out of bloom), seasons, or baby to child to mom to grandmother. If your child is really interested in cameras, consider giving her one of her own. You may appreciate this book: *Picture This: Photography Activities for Early Childhood Learning* by Susan G. Entz (Corwin Press, 2009).

Speech payoff: Kids respond best when they are center stage. So, taking actual photographs of your child doing everyday things will be a motivator to remember steps in an important household routine. Talking about these routines can make your child "the star of the show."

4. First...Then

What you need: Not much of anything...unless you'd like to create a picture board, in which case you'll need an 8½ x 11 piece of construction paper, two half-sheets of construction paper, a marker, and a laminator (if you really want to get fancy).

What you do: Use simple directions to get your kid to do two-step commands. For example, "*First* wash your hands. *Then* we'll eat." Don't over-talk a request: "I need you to go to the bathroom and wash your hands—they're really dirty and we're eating soon. Gosh, you look like you've been playing in mud all day." See how confusing this could be to your child when all you really want her to do is wash her hands?

Variation: Make a picture board in which you show activities of "first" and "then." You can use clipart to show pictures of things your child does around the house—hand washing, teeth brushing, TV watching. Tape a picture of "clean your room" in the "first" category and a picture of a TV in the "then" category. Visually it gets your kid thinking and remembering what to do.

Speech payoff: If your child is a visual learner, she'll love the picture board. You'll find that life is easier and you are less frustrated when your child cooperates with your requests. Think of how you use visual reminders like Post-It notes to remind yourself of something you need to do—it's the same idea for your child.

5. Movin' On: Songs for Transition Times

What you need: This CD (order from a special needs catalog; see resources at the end of this chapter) and a CD player.

What you do: Let your children listen to appropriate songs at transition times as a cue to get moving. Songs on the CD are "Hello Hi," "Clean-Up," "Wash Your Hands," "Please and Thank You," etc. If you don't have the CD handy, *you* can sing the transition song and your child can sing along.

Speech payoff: For kids who respond to music, but not always to your voice, this CD is a useful resource. It may also prepare and help strengthen transition skills needed in school, even if it is "just preschool," as children make many transitions in a school day.

Household and Family Routines

Kids thrive on routine. One of the best things you can do as a parent is to establish your own daily routine. Remember, there is a difference between a routine and a schedule. A *routine* is a typical pattern of events that happen roughly about the same time each day. For example, after we eat lunch (between 11:30-12:30), we have quiet time (for two hours), followed by some activity or outing (usually around 3:00). A *schedule* is precise, as in every day at 9:30 we have to be at preschool.

1. Visual Routine Sequences

What you need: Pictures (photographs, clipart, or Boardmaker) of daily activities.

What you do: Choose the daily routine you would like to visually depict (getting dressed, eating a meal, getting out the door, packing a backpack). Draw, print, or find clear, simple pictures showing the specific steps involved. Aim for about four steps in each routine; more could be too complex. Post it in an area where you and your child will see it. Point to the steps and repeat them aloud together.

Speech payoff: Not only does this exercise help with sequencing, it also helps with time management and vocabulary development.

2. Speech and Language Star Charts

What you need: A simple chart that shows the days of the week. You can make your own on the computer or with old-fashioned poster board and a marker. Also get some gold stars or other small stickers.

What you do: Tell your child that for every day of the week she completes a speech/language activity (see end of chapter *Read On!* for hints), she gets a star. She can receive a small prize at the end of the day as a reward for her hard work or she can "bank" the stars for a bigger prize at the end of the week: "If you earn 5 stars by the end of the week, you can earn a new ____." Make sure the prize is something your child is invested in. Keep in mind that rewards don't have to be monetary. Most kids love earning special 1:1 time with Mom or Dad or a trip to the park.

Speech payoff: You can get your child to do just about anything for the right motivator. Just make sure you are targeting a *positive* behavior—one you want her to do most of the time. Some parents may target negative behaviors. For example, when a parent says, "No booger picking," the child just hears, "Pick my boogers—okay!" and the "no" is ignored. Bringing attention to negative behaviors often reinforces them. If you want a bad habit to end, mention an appropriate alternative.

3. Create a Speech Star Chart

What you need: Poster board, computer print-out on which you have created a daily or weekly grid, or a store-bought chart designed for good behavior or chores (Board Dudes Magnetic Dry Erase Rewards Chore Chart, for example). You can even make a list of speech exercises (suggestions below) and use stickers or tally marks to mark off those your child completes.

What you do: Come up with lots of questions that will get your child to answer with words. For example, "name a color in the rainbow," "tell me two things you wear in the winter (summer, fall, spring)," "a glove goes on your hand, a shoe goes on your ____," "name five animals that belong in the zoo," "tell me the name of our neighbor's dog," "ice is cold, fire is ____," "tell me what you know about a cat (other animals)." Once you think of a few, you'll be amazed how many more you can come up with! You'll likely just do one or two of these star speech tasks a day, too many may overwhelm your child. When your child completes one, give her a sticker or other incentive. Remember, these are only suggestions. If these examples seem too difficult, tailor them for your child.

Speech pay-off: It's a fun way to practice words/sounds/phrases with your child. It's also another opportunity to engage your child in conversation, work on critical thinking skills, and memory skills.

4. Schedule Play Dates with Typically-speaking Peers

What you need: A child and parent you and your little one enjoy spending time with.

What you do: Find a time each week or month you all can get together to talk and play. Play dates don't have to be confined to your family room. Branch out and have them at the park, a bounce place, or a fast food restaurant with kiddie play area.

Speech payoff: It's amazing how peer interactions can work in a positive way. Repeated interactions with kids who speak at developmentally appropriate levels may encourage your child's communication as well. Plus, it gives *you* a chance to catch up with other parents. Try not to make your child's speech issue the main topic of your adult conversation, though.

More information: Here are a couple of resources you may find helpful when planning a play date—

> ➤ *What to Expect at a Play Date* (a children's book) by Heidi Murkoff (Harper Festival, 2001)
> ➤ *How to Be a Friend* by Laurie Krasny Brown and Marc Brown, the husband-wife team of the "Arthur" series (Little, Brown & Co., 1998)
> ➤ *Let's Talk about Playing with Others* by Joy Berry (Gold Star Publishers, 1999).

5. Remember Me Always

What you need: Photos of loved ones, neighbors, friends, babysitters, and even pets. Cut and laminate into smaller, say, 2 x 2 inch cards. You'll also need a key ring or binder ring.

What you do: Place the cards on a key ring and toss them in your bag for use in waiting rooms, in the car, or at home. Have your child flip through them while you tell her who's in the picture. Next quiz your child; approximations will do just fine. Then get silly and point to the dog and ask, "Is that Grandpa?" You can also use fill-in-the-blank sentences such as, "This is ____." Wait for your child to respond with a word, sound, approximation, or phrase.

Variation: Take photos of your child *doing* things she enjoys—playing at the park, digging in the sand, jumping through the sprinkler. This activity focuses on action words and the suffix *–ing*. Ask, "What are you doing here?" "Riding [my bike]." Work on expanding those responses as your child's skills grow.

Speech payoff: This is a fun way of encouraging language development and getting your kiddo to say the names of key people in her life. Repetition and repeated exposure doesn't hurt, either.

6. D is for Describe

What you need: An object to talk about.

What you do: Talk about an object—how it looks, sounds, feels, tastes, smells, or makes you feel. Name its parts or talk about what it's made from. For example, talk about an orange—it's heavy, it's orange, it smells sweet, and it feels a little bumpy, maybe even cold. After touching and hearing you talk about it, ask your child to say "orange." She just might surprise you. Again, try the fill-in-the-blank approach here. For example, "The orange feels ____?"

Speech payoff: Quite possibly one of the most powerful speech development activities we can do for our kids is to describe things. Touch-feely learning in a real-life environment is much more effective for kids with apraxia than your run-of-the-mill sit and speak approach.

7. S Is for Stretch It Out

What you need: A child who can follow simple directions and say about 50 words.

What you do: Help your child put those 50 or so words into two-word phrases like "more juice," "go bye-bye." For example, if your child says, "go," *stretch* it out by saying, "Yes, Mommy go."

Speech payoff: Kids hear appropriate language models. Show delight, pay attention, and respond when she tries to put words together. This way she knows you're listening and understanding her.

Multimedia

In today's tech-crazy world, there's got to be an app for apraxia right? Well, yes and no. Read on to determine if there is some bit of technology that might apply to your family.

1. Tune In!

What you need: Television, DVD player, and access to programs such as those listed below. Check local listings on www.pbskids.org. Ask your librarian for DVDs, or consider purchasing them.

What you do: Find time to watch the shows or videos with your child. Talk about what you see and learn during commercial breaks, or when you pause or hit "stop."

Speech payoff: Watching TV is a time to rest. Your child isn't likely to become any smarter or overcome CAS by sitting in front of the TV. However, it *will* provide some reinforcement from the ideas and activities you have provided for your child in a more active, hands-on setting.

➤ *WordWorld* (PBS Kids): Everyday words are spelled out in the shape of the actual item, helping your visual learner see the words she hears all day.

➤ *WordGirl* (PBS Kids): She might be small and she might be a cartoon, but this girl knows her words!

➤ *Emma's Extravagant Expedition* (DVD): An elephant dresses up and introduces your child to advanced vocabulary such as embellish and magnificent.

➤ *Signing Times* (DVD): These videos teach beginning American Sign Language (ASL) through the help of Leah, a deaf four-year-old, and lots of catchy songs. It's geared for kids between the ages of one and eight, and teaches many first words. Don't be deterred by sign language. It can encourage more verbalization and help you understand those sounds your child is using to communicate.

➤ *Baby Bumblebee* (DVD). According to the website and many parents, these products—with their real-world images—have helped many kids with autism spectrum disorders, speech and language delays, and general developmental delays. Check it out at www.babybumblebee.com.

➤ *Baby Chatterbox* (DVD): Teaches cognitive skills and helps little ones form sounds and words and establish early speech patterns. Plus, they are funny!

➤ *Preschool Prep Series* (DVD). Geared toward kids aged fifteen months to six years, this DVD series has won many national awards. It teaches words, shapes, numbers, letters, colors, and words. Look for the DVDs at www.preschoolprepco.com.

Parents Ask...

How much TV is OK for my child to watch?

Not much, at least according to the American Academy of Pediatrics (www.aap. org). If your child is under two years old, the recommendation from AAP is *no* television. If your child is over the age of two years, the AAP recommends no more than two hours a day. Television may provide *some* supplement to hands-on teaching with your child, but it is not a substitute for education or speech-language therapy. Choose television programs wisely. See also the section in Chapter 14 on "Exercise and Extracurricular Activities to Help Your Child Thrive."

---

2. Software for Your Brain

What you need:

➤ *School Zone Preschool-Kindergarten Super Scholar.* This computer program is designed for kids aged 3 to 6 years old. It builds language skills through word searches, crosswords, mazes, pictures, and imaginative puzzles, plus early math skills. You may also appreciate **On Track: Beginning Sounds** software, which helps your child work at recognizing sounds and associating them with words and objects. Check it out on www.schoolzone.com.

➤ *Dr. Seuss Preschool Learning System.* Classic and loved for his rhyming, Dr. Seuss does it again taking kids through the alphabet. It is a little less than conventional—but what would you expect from Dr. Seuss? Check it out at The Learning Company: www.learningservicesus.com.

➤ *Flash Pro 2 (CD-ROM).* With over 10,000 photographic images in 65 categories, you can select, preview, and print flashcards to teach and quiz your kids on certain words. The price may be worth it if you think of ways you can use it in the future—for school projects and homework, as well as with younger siblings. Available from Spectronics: www. spectronicsinoz.com/product/flash-pro-2.

➤ *Boardmaker (CD-ROM).* Boardmaker is a software program that allows you to make materials using the Picture Exchange Communication Symbols (PECS)—line drawings widely used by speech-language pathologists. You may be surprised at all of the uses for this program. From valuable printed materials to communication boards, to home-made sequencing games to developing a schedule or creating flash-cards, this program is very versatile. Many schools and speech clinics have access to Boardmaker programs, so this makes a nice extension for home use. For more information, visit: www.mayer-johnson.com.

What you do: Work with your child on the computer to see those brain connec-tions grow and words a-coming.

Speech payoff: Introduction to computers is a great way to practice speech exer-cises. It just might help shake the boredom off the traditional approaches you've been trying, plus it feels delightfully "grown-up."

3. Log On

What you need: Child-safe access to the Internet.

What you do: Go online with your children and discover various sites. Consider:

> *Starfall* (www.starfall.com): a great resource for kids in preschool through early elementary years, including those with special needs. The goal of the site is to make learning to read with phonics fun.

> *Bemboszoo* (www.bemboszoo.com): Just click on the letters of the alphabet and you will see letters spelling out your favorite zoo ani-mals—which pop up and morph into a picture of one and make silly animal noises.

> *Speaking of Speech* (www.speakingofspeech.com): This interactive web-site is really intended for parents, teachers, and SLPs and provides a host of advice, information on products, resources, and web/Internet links.

4. Gaming for Words

What you need: Wii or Nintendo DS plus games that interest your child. Or con-sider less expensive and "younger" products by Fisher-Price (Smart Fit Park) or V-Tech.

What you do: Allow your child to play certain games that she is interested in and that you find appropriate.

Speech payoff: The Wii provides gross motor activities that involve movement. Engage the vestibular systems to encourage vocal play. Plus, it can give your kids in-creased speech practice opportunities—ones they may not even notice doing!

Toys & Games

Kids play. It's their job and they see it as serious business, just as you see your job as a parent. What are they really getting out of play, you ask? It's an opportunity to learn about the world and how they fit in it. It's through play that kids can rehearse scary or worrisome situations (like going to the doctor or dentist), experiment with a new object or idea, and learn what they are good at doing—and not so good at doing. Here are some ideas to slip in speech practice while your little one is hard at play.

Choosing Toys for Your Child

I could give you lots of suggestions for types of toys to purchase or how to play with the ones you already have cluttering your living room. Instead, I'd like to emphasize that *anything and everything can become a therapy tool/prop!* Please, don't rush out and purchase expensive "therapy" toys, unless you just want to (and have an abundant supply of "toy cash").

The next time you decide it's time for a new toy, keep these tips in mind, from the National Lekotek Center, a division of Anixter Center—a nonprofit organization with a national network of affiliates dedicated to making play and learning accessible to children with disabilities:

1. **Multisensory Appeal.** Does the toy respond with lights, sounds, movement to engage the child? Does it have scent, texture, or contrasting colors? Will these aspects of the toy irritate or intrigue your child (or you)?

2. **Method of Activation.** Will the toy provide a challenge, but not to the point of frustration? What is the force required to activate? What are the number and complexity of steps required to activate the toy? Some children with CAS also have limb apraxia and may find some toys too complicated to activate.

3. **Places the Toy will be Used.** Will the toy be easy to store? Is there a special place in the home for playing and storing the toy? Can the toy be used in a variety of ways?

4. **Opportunities for Success.** Can play be open-ended with no definite right or wrong way of using the toy?

5. **Current Popularity.** Is this a toy that will make your child feel like *any other kid*? That is, she will like it because it's considered a "cool" toy, and not another "tool" to help with her speech.

6. **Self-expression.** Does the toy allow for creativity, uniqueness, and making choices? Does it provide experiences with a variety of media?

7. **Adjustability.** Does it have adjustable height, sound volume, speed, and level of difficulty?

8. **Child's Individual Abilities.** Does the toy provide activities that reflect both developmental and chronological ages? Does it reflect *your* child's interest?

9. **Safety and Durability.** Is the toy appropriate for kids of your child's strength and size? Does it have moisture resistance? Are the toy and its parts sized appropriately (i.e., not a choking hazard)? Can it be washed and cleaned?

10. **Potential for Interaction.** Will the child be an active participant during use? Will the toy encourage social interaction and engagement with others?

The National Lekotek Center also provides supportive family services. For more information, visit www.lekotek.org or www.ableplay.org.

If you are just an ordinary parent like me, you might have fewer criteria than what's on this big, official list. Choose the most important points to you.

Managing Toy Chaos

At our house, we manage toy chaos with "Toy Trade Tuesday." It may well be the very best thing we've done as parents—in terms of managing all of the "kid clutter." Here's how it works: First I organized our toys by "family"—farm, zoo, dress up/role play, cars and trucks, building and constructing things, baby dolls, cooking and baking items, and pets and vets.

Then, everything that somehow related to a particular group of toys—puzzles, books, art supplies, stickers, and placemats—went into a large plastic storage bin. I slapped a label on each box and stored eight of them in the basement, leaving one out in the family room where the children spent most of their time playing. The girls were able to keep several special toys out at all times: their favorite stuffed dog, for example, never got packed away, nor did the miniature dollhouses. When Tuesday rolled around each week, it was time to trade the toys the girls had been playing with for one of the bins downstairs. I'd ask the girls, "What should we do for Toy Trade Tuesday?" They almost always had a request. Sometimes I'd try to tie the week at home in with a unit of study at school. (If you decide to try this with your kids, you can have them help you with categorizing your toys—it's a great language categorization activity.)

When we went to the library on Wednesdays, I'd look for books that connected with our theme. On Friday, we had "fieldtrips" and headed to the zoo, visited a working farm, set up the tent in the backyard, or popped into the pet store for a visit. We could almost always relate these activities to the toy theme we chose on Tuesday. The field trips were a fun way to end the week.

Managing your toys like this helps with clutter control. It also helps you concentrate on specific vocabulary and target speech sounds/words/phrases. It gives you and your kids something to look forward to. Plus, it's exciting to see how much your children have grown and progressed when you pull out a group of toys they haven't seen in awhile.

You will also want to regularly add to and update the boxes so that the toys offer a bit of a challenge and change.

Since "Toy Trade Tuesday" has made its way into our life, I have several questions I ask myself before allowing a new toy into our home:

1. Does it match with one of our existing toy themes? Which one?
2. Is this something the girls will get some challenge and pleasure out of for awhile (a year or more)?
3. In what way can I make it educational?
4. Will it fit—physically—into my box?

Try "Toy Trade Tuesday" or "Swap-it-out-Saturday" or "Mix-it-up-Monday" today! You'll be amazed how your child(ren) respond to this.

If Toy Trade Tuesday sounds too organized for your style, then try this variation: get a tote, basket, or box that you can call your Speech Box. Fill it with special toys, treats, and crafts that only make an appearance at home speech time. Periodically update the box (as a surprise, perhaps, or as a "job well done," with things you know will excite your child.

Toy Trade Tuesday Themes

Think you may want to adapt Toy Trade Tuesday at your house? You can create as many themed weeks as you have space and toys for. Generally, you'll need about 5 to 10 objects per theme. Look at what you already have and build on it, based on your child's interests. Here's a list to get you started:

- Zoo/Safari/Wild Animals
- Food/Baking/Nutrition
- Seasons/weather
- Dinosaurs
- Tools, Machines, & Measurement
- Family and Homes
- Cultures of the World
- Ocean and Beach
- Shapes/Alphabet/Colors/School
- Transportation
- Community and Careers + Role-Play
- Farm (we combined farm with weather)
- Pets
- Earth/Environment/Camping (we added space exploration to this one)
- Exercise
- Folk Tales and Nursery Rhymes + Dress-Up

Toys to Encourage Communication

Here are some more qualities you can look for in toys that encourage speech/vocal communication:

1. **Amplification and Reverberation.** These toys have the ability to change or make your child's voice louder. Think: megaphones, microphones, and echo-phones. Why: they motivate your child to use her voice in a fun—and sometimes—goofy way. Plus, they provide the auditory feedback some children need to hear the details of targeted speech.
2. **Speech.** These toys encourage the development of spoken words. Look for: toys or dolls that speak, flashcards that use phonics, etc.
3. **Verbal Talk-Back Response.** These toys respond to your kids and help develop receptive and expressive language. Be sure to look for toys that have clear, simple voices.
4. **Words and Pictures.** These toys use words and pictures that can be pointed to and talked about. Look for: books, puzzles, games, and electronic toys that use the alphabet (e.g., Leap Frog products have a lot of options).
5. **Communication.** Remember walkie talkies from your childhood? It may be fun to introduce them to your child. Old telephones work well, too.

6. **Pretend Play.** Dressing up and pretending to be someone or something you dream about may help with communication. Hand puppets work in this way, too. Kids can talk "through" the puppet so they tend to feel less self-conscious. Children can use different voices and play with speech sounds. You might be surprised at the speech you hear from your child when she pretends to be someone else.

Parents Share...

Puppets Are a Handful—and May Help with Speech!

"My daughter must have been about 20 months old. She wasn't diagnosed with CAS yet, but we were concerned about her lack of speech. I remember telling my husband that I thought this would help her use her words. While she didn't love the puppet like I thought she would, she did enjoy watching me have conversations with her and the puppet and even made some new sounds during puppet play."

—mother of a girl with CAS

A Few Personal Favorites

I know I said I wouldn't tell you what to run out and buy, but I just have to share the merits of:

Legos. Whether you have a son or a daughter, you most certainly have a set of Legos. They have the utmost power to bring to life a child's imagination, and perhaps her verbal skills as well.

Deb Tomarakos, CCC-SLP, elaborates on the uses of plastic building blocks: "Legos or Duplos can be used to work on: receptive and expressive vocabulary skills related to people, places, and animals; following directions; articulation of target sounds that are pictured in the scene; identifying and producing animal and environmental sounds; direction/location concepts (up/down, left/right, beside/front/behind); community workers (policeman, pilot); categories (farm animals, zoo animals, vehicles); color labels and identification."

"For the older crowd," she shares, "I love the **Lego City Comic Builder.** [It's] a great way to work on story narratives; story sequencing; story elements including setting and characters; main idea formulation; problems and resolutions; sentence formulation; humor; social skills stories." Visit Deb's blog, "Speech Gadget," at www.speechgadget.com. Visit the Lego website (www.lego.com) to find other ways to target speech/language practice.

Zingo! It's like Bingo with a zing—think word lessons and picture matching instead of letters on the bingo card. Each player gets a Zingo board; all of the chips are stored in a kid-friendly slider case. Each player takes a turn sliding the device to reveal what chips are doled out. The chips have both a picture *and* spelling of a common object (house, shoe, bird, sun). We started using this with our daughter when she was about three and a half. We'd have her practice saying the words as they appeared on the chips. As she got older, we'd have her string together more words, "I have a ____(sun)," or "Here's a sun!" "Does anyone have a ____ house, bird, sun, etc.)?" The game teaches turn-taking, patience, listening, sight words, and target word practice.

There Was an Old Lady Who Swallowed a Fly Doll and CD Set. This award-winning toy works on language development and learning through rhyming and repetition and silliness that will surely get some giggles—if not words out of your little sweetie. Look for it at Young Explorers: www.YoungExplorers.com.

What's in Ned's Head. This toy from Fat Brain Toys may appease your sensory-seeker or the child who enjoys "gross stuff." Basically, Ned's head is a large plush "head," with an assortment of gross stuff inside (a large tooth, a frog, a lab rat, Ned's lost lunch—rubber vomit, an alien, a worm, moldy cheese, among others). The players are dealt one card each with a picture of an item in the head. They all then reach into Ned's head through his mouth or ear holes—to try to find their item. You can practice having your child say these "gross things"; they may be icky enough to illicit some chatter.

Play with Your Food

1. Table Talk and Toss

What you need: Just you and your family members at the dinner table, plus any school papers and artwork your child created that day.

What you do: Whatever kid-created pieces of paper come out of your child's backpack go directly on the table as though they were placemats. At dinner, ask your child to tell you about what she created. Ask open-ended question, such as, "How did you come up with this idea?" or "Tell me about this" (and point to what you want more information on). Be sure to show positive interest.

Speech payoff: It gives your child a chance to share something meaningful about her day and it gives yet another opportunity to practice new words. Plus, when dinner's over, you either save the paper or toss it in the recycling bin, reducing the mounds of paper that are sure to make their home on your kitchen counter.

2. Favorite Part of the Day

What you need: Family members talking.

What you do: This activity was best done at our dinner table. Bedtime also works. Go from person to person and ask about their favorite part of the day. You may need to give choices—even silly ones—to prompt your child, depending on her verbal skills. "Was your favorite part of the day getting in trouble for coloring on the wall?" "Was your favorite part of the day going to the donut shop?" "What color donut did you get?"

Speech payoff: It's a great way to hear the highlights of everyone's day, and it encourages communication.

3. This or That

What you need: A couple of food or beverage options at meal or snack time (this also works with just about anything at just about any time).

What you do: Offer your child a choice between two items: "Would you like milk or juice?" As you say milk, hold the milk jug up and clearly enunciate. Do the same for juice. "Would you like hot dogs or chicken nuggets?" Then wait for a response from your child. Any response besides a grunt or a point will do (unless that is all your child can do at the time). After a speech attempt, clearly say, "Okay! Chicken nuggets it is! Can you say chicken?"

Speech payoff: It can be grueling to wait for a response when it would be easier to fill the glass with chocolate milk and present it to your kid, but giving her some say in the matter will make her feel empowered. Choice-making is a basic part of communication; young children are eager to make their own choices.

4. Meal Time Prayers

What you need: Mealtime prayer and child(ren).

What you do: If your family says a mealtime prayer, see if you can modify your traditional prayer to make it more fun and kid-friendly. Can you add gestures? (We give everyone a high five at the end of ours.) Ask your child to lead the prayer and coach her along, or use fill-in-the-blank if you say a routine prayer.

Speech payoff: Having a family tradition at the table can be a fun way to bond and connect. Saying words in unison (almost like a chant) can be easier than having your child say it on her own.

5. Handful of Goodies

What you need: M&Ms, a small bowl, and a child who likes candy.

What you do: Have the bowl of M&Ms on the dinner table. When everyone is finished with the meal, have them reach in and grab a few. Each family member is to say something for *each* M&M they grabbed. It can be as simple as a sound your child is learning in therapy (like the st-blend), a target word (me), first name, etc. Eat the M&Ms one at a time as a special treat.

Speech payoff: The M&M serves as an incentive. "If you can say ____, then you can eat the M&M." The whole family is doing it, too—safety in numbers and good role modeling, right?

Dinner Games & Activity Cards

You may want to invest in this deck of 51 cards designed for dinner time conversations. It comes in a handy container with lid so you can take it with you on the go (restaurants, camping, picnics). The cards provide great prompts for conversations, thought-provoking questions, memory games, and more. This product even comes in a beginner series (ages 3+). The regular series is best for kids 5 to 12 years. Look for them in various catalogs, bookstores, and online.

Arts & Crafts

Art is not just about the outcome—the final masterpiece. The process is equally important. Kids can express their originality and feelings through art, while improving their coordination (fine/hand motor), learning colors and textures, and developing pride in their artistic accomplishments. Take time to talk with your child about the art she is creating. Encourage confidence and satisfaction in creativity by asking questions like:

➤ "Tell me about your picture!"
➤ "How did you decide what to draw?"
➤ "I like the colors you used. How did you decide which ones you wanted in your picture?"
➤ "Where would you like us to hang it?"
➤ "Should we send it to Grandma?"

If your child does not respond well to questions, comment about her work and wait for her response. For example, "Oh, I see you drew a big, bright sun." Stop and wait. It may take a moment for your kid to come up with a response.

1. Draw & Label

What you need: A child at the table with markers, crayons, a blank sheet of paper, and imagination.

What you do: Let her work for as long as she wants. Listen and make observations. When she's finished, say, "I like your picture. Tell me about it." Point to items on the page. Ask her to describe it for you. Any little word will do. Write down what she says in quotations right next to the image. Put her name on it and date it. You can save these in a binder so that you can go back and look at her progress—not just artistically—but verbally, too.

Speech payoff: It's fun and interesting to see what our kids are drawing; consider it a little window to their world. Plus, it helps catalog where she's been—in terms of ability.

2. Sketch Book

What you need: Find a notebook with plain paper—one that's spiral-bound works best. Add crayons, markers, colored pencils—whatever media you feel most comfortable with.

What you do: Allow your child to make several entries daily (maybe during quiet time)—label and date them. What's really fun is to make the sketch book into a sort of scrapbook. Collect pictures, articles, ticket stubs, leaves, feathers—whatever fascinates your child. Have her describe the item, the scents, colors, and textures and capture that in the book.

Speech payoff: In many ways, this activity combines the elements of learning—collecting, identifying, researching, and talking. It introduces new experiences and vocabulary. Again, it's a good way to measure progress.

3. Pen Pals

What you need: A friend or family member (cousin or grandparent) who lives in another zip code.

What you do: Provide your child with envelopes, stamps, pens, paper, stickers. Your child can draw or write a biography of herself as well as including artwork and other tidbits about her life. The pen pal will hopefully respond with similar items. When letters arrive in the mail, talk about what you've received.

Speech payoff: While this activity is fun, it may actually be better suited for older kids. It gives kids the message that communication—even if written—is very important.

Parents As Partners in CAS Treatment

No pressure here, but you are very much a partner in your child's speech-language treatment. Don't let your child know that, though, or she'll be less likely to go along with your ideas! You need to be clever. Here are some suggestions for tapping into your inner speech-language pathologist.

1. Car Schooling

What you need: A vehicle and an adult willing to go for a drive.

What you do: While you are running errands with the kids, quiz them on some of the words and sounds you know they know. For example, "Where do Nana and Papa live?" Or, "Who lives in St. Louis?" (Papa and Nana). Other ideas: "What does a dog say? (woof, woof)," "Who's at work? (dada)," "Who's driving the van? (mama)," etc. Then throw in a new word your child is working on, or one you'd like her to say. Practice it.

Speech payoff: The backseat is a safe place for your little ones to practice those new words and sounds. There's less performance anxiety. Plus, they are a captive audience. One time when I was doing this activity, Kate said—"No more talking!" I considered that a success—her first three-word phrase!

Please keep safety in mind. I found this type of activity was best done as we were traveling roads I was familiar with. Speech work shouldn't cause you to become a distracted driver!

2. Teach and Drive

What you need: Vehicle and parent running errands.

What you do: Tape a kid-friendly lesson to the back of the headrest in your vehicle—right in front of your child's eyes. These lessons could be as simple as a worksheet from your SLP's office on a target sound or a picture of a family pet. Make sure your lesson includes pictures/drawings if your child isn't reading yet. Your child will see the "lesson" each time she's in the car and eventually will learn things such as her ABCs, phone number, and what sound the letter "l" makes.

Speech payoff: Repeated exposure, repetition, and something on which to focus on while you are driving.

Keep safety in mind. Speech work shouldn't cause you to become a distracted driver!

3. From Sounds to Words

What you need: A little person who has a few sounds such as "da" and "ba" in her repertoire.

What you do: Encourage your child to build on sounds she already has by introducing words that begin with that same sound. For example, she can say, "ba" so build on that by encouraging her to imitate you when you say, "bottle," "ball," "book," "baby," and "bath." Emphasize and exaggerate these words throughout the day whenever you get the chance. For example say, *"ba-ba — bottle."*

Speech payoff: It exposes kiddos to new words containing sounds they can already say.

4. Expand-o-matic

What you need: A child who can say about 10 to 15 words spontaneously.

What you do: When your child says a one-word sentence with clear intent she wants you to *do* something, expand on the gesture/sound/word. For example, she's at the kitchen table and offers you her cup, saying "more?" You can expand by saying, "Oh, you want more milk? Okay! More milk coming right up. More milk."

Speech payoff: In a brief interaction, you have repeated the request three times and have modeled more words while completing a simple task for your child. She will surprise you in the future by saying more than "more!"

5. Parallel Talk

What you need: A happy child engaged in play.

What you do: Describe what your child is doing with her play. "Oh I see you are playing with your cars. It looks like they are driving really fast. Vroom, vroom. Beep, beep. I like the blue car best. Do you like the blue car, too?"

Speech payoff: This sort of parallel talk (talking about what your child is doing in short phrases and sentences) helps your child attach words to the actions and objects she is experiencing. It really takes the pressure off of speech production, and can give your child the freedom to comment.

6. Make a Speech Sounds Practice Book

What you need: All of those worksheets your SLP hands you after a session with your child, plus a small three-ring binder or folder with brads and some sheet protectors.

What you do: Let your child decorate and color the "pages" so she feels a bit of ownership. Give her free rein on the cover, too. Review the items in the book several times a day at your convenience with your child. We often looked over ours at breakfast and lunch and as a part of our regular reading routine.

Speech payoff: Putting worksheets from your child's speech sessions into a binder is a great way to make an individualized study guide. It directly strengthens the skills that your SLP is working on with your child. You can look back and see the progress your child has made. Date the pages and put the new ones on top. This helps manage the paper clutter you are sure to accumulate from weekly worksheets!

7. Who's in Your Family?

What you need: Various objects from around the house that represent a hobby or interest of each family member.

What you do: It's fun if you can make this a family activity. Gather at least one object per family member (e.g., Mom's favorite magazine or book, Dad's remote control or newspaper, baby sister's rattle, big brother's videogame). Put the items in a pile in the middle of the room. Ask your child to match the item with the "right" person. Practice saying that person's name and the name of the object. Combine them into two-word phrases such as "Daddy's remote."

Variation: Hide the objects (tell or show your child what they are first); take turns having different family members select objects for the game. Name the objects as they are found, as in "Mom's book."

Speech payoff: An exercise like this involves the whole family, can be fun, and helps your child make connections, develop critical thinking skills, and improve vocabulary.

8. "Play" Speech Therapy

What you need: You, your child, and a pile of stuffed animals or dolls.

What you do: Set up a pretend speech therapy session with your child's favorite little critters. Let your child be the SLP, or you can pretend to be the SLP. Teach the toys while your child watches.

Speech payoff: If your child loves her animals or dolls and likes playing teacher, this type of activity will be right up her alley. Your child is doing a couple of important things—role playing, processing what she's learned in therapy, and spending time with a caring adult. You just may be surprised to hear what your child can say when she takes on the teaching role. It's sort of like a tea party with a twist!

OK—that's a big list of things to try. Don't feel as if you have to try them all. None of them are designed to be *the* magic bullet, either. The ideas presented are just a fun way to get that much-needed speech practice in.

Encourage, Encourage, Encourage!

Once your child starts talking more, you'll need to give her lots of praise and encouragement. Here are some tips to keep in mind as you work with your child:

➤ *Your child will do her best communicating when she's not under pressure.* How well do you communicate when you are in that important meeting or on a stage? For this reason, don't insist that your child demonstrate her speech skills in front of an audience (even if it's just grandma and grandpa). Instead, let your child's speech come out more naturally, particularly with folks she is unfamiliar with.

➤ *Let (and encourage) your child to use whatever props she needs to communicate to her very best ability.* That means letting her use gestures, sign, show you pictures, or act it out.

➤ *Validate your child's desire to communicate with you.* When I couldn't understand what our daughter was trying to tell us, I would say, "Kate, I know you are trying to tell us something really important, but we're having a hard time understanding." Depending on the situation, I might add, "Show us [what you are trying to explain, do, desire]." It worked 99 percent of the time.

➤ *If you can understand some of what your child is trying to say, let her know.* "I see...you are talking about George and the Man with the Yellow Hat, but I didn't understand what you said after that. Tell me again." She's going to feel a lot better knowing that something got through and will do her best to revise what she just said so you can "get" the rest.

➤ *Our SLP often said to give choices with small parts of the day.* It's all about having some control in the choices they make. For example, you might say something like, "Do you want milk or juice?" An approximation of the word such as "Ju" is good enough, but a grunt is not. Finish the word yourself by saying, "*Juice!* OK, you want *juice.* I'll get you some *juice.*" Then, if you're as goofy as I am, you might break into a song about juice. "Juicy, juicy juice...yum, I love juice. Juice helps me grow strong and gives me important vitamins. I love juice, don't you?!"

➤ *Do not demand that your child use speech to make requests.* (For example, "Tell me what you want to drink. You won't get anything unless you can tell me what you want." Yikes!) Your child may never feel ready to talk if she's under that kind of pressure.

Parents Ask...

What is an approximation?

When you are working hard to help your child talk, you just might accept *anything* as an attempt to say the word correctly. That's an "approximation." **But, you must not respond to grunts, squeals, crying, and fussing as an appropriate approximation.** Set the record straight beforehand by saying something like, "I need you to try and use your words. It's OK if it's not perfect. Just try to say ____." When your child feels confident and not so pressured, she'll try it. It might take a minute; be patient.

At first, it's OK to accept practically anything that pops out of her mouth that sounds like speech. Give her *lots* of praise when that happens—a smile, a hug, and victory jump have worked wonders with us! Your child will quickly learn that in order to get what she wants, she is going to have to try to say *something.* One day, a true breakthrough will happen and she will attempt to talk with you *without* your prompting!

Where's the Research?

Many of the suggestions in this book are rooted in the research world. An October 2008 article in the *American Journal of Speech and Language Pathology*, "When 'Simon Says' Doesn't Work: Alternatives to Imitation for Facilitating Early Speech Development," discusses ways clinicians can provide evidence-based strategies to facilitate kids who are not readily imitating sounds. The suggestions in the article are:

> ➤ *Provide access to AAC.* There is evidence to suggest an augmentative and alternative communication (AAC) device *does* facilitate speech development.
> ➤ *Minimize the pressure to speak.* High pressure requests are direct requests to speak, whereas a low pressure technique would be modeling what you want to hear.
> ➤ *Imitate the child.* You've likely heard certain sounds from this child before. Remember what they are and pick targets that get the child to produce words based on those sounds.
> ➤ *Use exaggerated intonation and a slowed tempo.* This helps with intelligibility.
> ➤ *Augment auditory, visual, tactile, and proprioceptive feedback.* Children with CAS need appropriate sensory input to progress. This is a different approach than traditional articulation treatment.
> ➤ *Avoid emphasis on nonspeech-like articulation movements.* We learn to talk better when we practice talking! Work on tasks in context so children are better able to generalize in different environments.

What's AAC? Does My Child with CAS Need It?

The American Speech-Language-Hearing Association (ASHA) defines **A**ugmentative and **A**lternative **C**ommunication (AAC) as the means to "temporarily or permanently compensate for the impairments, activity limitations, and participation restrictions of individuals with severe disorders of speech-language production and/or comprehension."

ASHA proposes a continuum of AAC. That is, there are multiple ways in which communication can be assisted. For example, *unaided communication* involves using one's body to convey a message—through gestures, showing, even word approximations. *Aided communication* requires the use of an *external tool* to communicate a thought, feeling, message, need, or want. For example, a child may find it easier to communicate using a picture/symbol such as one produced with Boardmaker, or writing down a request in a notebook. Higher-tech ideas may include using an iPhone or iPad, a voice output communication aid (VOCA) such as a Dynovox, or something of similar ilk.

Not all children with CAS need AAC. But if a child has very limited expressive speech or reduced intelligibility, AAC can be very helpful. Talk to your child's SLP to determine if this would be appropriate for your child.

According to Dee Fish, CCC-SLP, and author of *Here's How to Treat Childhood Apraxia of Speech*, kids with CAS can benefit from AAC in the following ways:

Benefits of AAC

Increased effectiveness of communication	Decreased reliance on familiar adults to serve as interpreters
Increased *quality* and *quantity* of the child's language	Reduced challenging behaviors caused by limited ability to express ideas
Increased opportunities for social interaction across a wider variety of setting, with a wider variety of individuals, and for a wider range of communication functions	Decreased communicative passivity

Adapted from Fish, Margaret, *Here's How to Treat Childhood Apraxia of Speech* (San Diego: Plural Publishing, 2010), 197. Used with permission of the author.

Let's Get Tech-y

There is no doubt our children will be exposed to technology from a young age. You may find that introducing your child with apraxia to an iPad early on actually helps her communication skills. In fact, many organizations these days are advocating that children with special needs have access to an iPad or similar tablet. For example, Apps for Children with Special Needs (www.a4cwsn.com) offers tips and videos that demonstrate how products work so that parents and educators can make sensible buying decisions about electronic devices and apps.

Not only are iPads and other tablets less expensive than most devices used in speech-language therapy (which can run well over $1,000), but they are sleek and trendy. Children with an iPad at their fingertips are less likely to be stigmatized for being "different." Plus, it's lightweight and can be customized for each child's communication needs. Still, the expense of an iPad may simply be out of reach for some families.

As Mirla G. Raz, CCC-SLP, a private practice speech-language pathologist in Arizona and author of the *Help Me Talk Books* shares, "[The iPad] is an extremely motivating device [for children].... It is a wonderful gadget with a multitude of uses." But she points out that parents must really weigh whether the initial cost of the iPad plus the sometimes steep prices of apps is worth it.

If you decide that you'd like an iPad for your child with CAS, don't give up hope that it is "too expensive." Many companies and foundations are developing programs that award iPads to deserving families. You can start by asking your school, your speech clinic, or EI coordinator if they know of anything along those lines.

For more information on the benefits of using an iPad to supplement your child's speech at school, talk to your school/child's teacher first and then do a bit of your own homework. You may want to refer to "How Schools can Successfully Implement iPod touch and iPad for Children with Special Needs" by Eric Sailers, an SLP and assistive technology specialist. The article can be found at Closing the Gap: www.closingthegap.com.

Say That Again?! Chapter Summary

Holy cow! That was quite a list. Did you take note of the activities you want to try with your child? The key to success with kids with CAS is to give them plenty of opportunities throughout the day to practice their speech and language skills. Better yet, disguise this "work" as fun. Keep your environment and approach healthy and supportive by remembering to be goofy and funny and not always a serious teach-and-talk type of parent. Make sure to keep your SLP in the loop, and let her keep you in the loop, too. You are partners in this process, after all!

Parents Share...

We love our iPad!

In a Small Talk: All About Apraxia meeting, a parent participant pulled out a shiny new iPad2 purchased for a three-and-a-half-year-old boy with CAS. "We love this thing," he crooned. This dad couldn't be happier with the results and functionality the iPad brings for his son's speech. "It's cool, it's portable, and it's fun. He will ask for his iPad so he can communicate something more complex. It's great!" Yet there is a cost to all of this.

Courtney, the mother of a child with CAS in Coloma, Michigan, offers advice on affordable apps: "I won't spend huge amounts of money on an app when there are so many good low-cost or free ones available. We really like *Phonics Word Family*, *Word Wagon*, *Parents Magazine* apps, *Tic-Tac-Talk*, and *Talking Memory*. *Talking Memory* is cool, because it says a word to you, and you repeat it. It's good practice for my son, who needs a lot of repetition." She mentioned several apps that she wouldn't bother spending the money on, however: "We didn't particularly like *Speech Tutor*. While the idea behind it is good, it just doesn't seem to connect with kids; plus, it's pricey." However, Courtney *did* positively endorse the more pricey *Artik Pix*: "It's probably the most functional app we've purchased." She also points out that many book apps are free—such as the popular BOB series for learning to read and Sandra Boynton books for children.

An iPad may be useful for your child at school, as well. The mother of a six-year-old who has CAS and cri du chat syndrome says that her daughter "uses her iPad at school daily to help with her communication. She can press a button and the iPad will talk for her. Not only can Finley participate, but it helps cut down on behavior problems due to being nonverbal. It's empowering."

Finally, I want to reiterate that *kids with CAS are unique individuals. It is your job to find out how you can best help your child with CAS!*

Read On!

● ● ● ● ● ●

➤ *Easy Does It for Apraxia-Preschool* by Robin Strode and Catherine Chamberlin (LinguiSystems, 1994) has been developed for SLPs to use with the preschool-aged child who has CAS. A systematic program designed to teach isolated sounds, syllable productions, sequencing, and closure as well as multisyllabic words, phrases and sentences, and consonant blend sounds.

➤ Interested in your child's *temperament and goodness-of-fit?* Try the child temperament profiler at www.childtemperament.org, a free assessment for kids aged 2 - 8 years. It provides a graphical display of the goodness of fit between your expectations and your child's "real" behavior. The test takes about 15 – 20 minutes, is anonymous and confidential. It's run by the Department of Psychology at the University of Geneva-Switzerland.

➤ *Lekotek* (source of the list provided earlier in this chapter on selecting toys) also provides supportive family services. For more information, check them out at www.lekotek.org.

➤ *AblePlay* has independent ratings and product reviews on play products in four disability categories including: physical, sensory, communicative, and cognitive. See www.ableplay.org.

➤ *PlanToys* markets toys created with the help of developmental specialists and design experts. They are also the world's first and foremost manufacturer of wooden toys—very sustainable and eco-friendly. Visit their website at www.plantoys.com.

➤ *Toys R Us* makes a mini-catalog of toys for kids with special needs. Icons indicate toys that aid in auditory discrimination, creativity, fine and gross motor skills, language, communication development, tactile, critical thinking, and visual discrimination tasks. Available at www.Toysrus.com/DifferentlyAbled or at your local store.

➤ *Mindfull Games* is a company founded by Kristin Edmonds, a former speech-language pathologist. The company focuses on improving literacy and standardized scores, along with speech development: www.mindfullgames.com.

➤ For more *educationally-based toys,* as well as *balance boards, exercise balls, foam mats and blocks, and trampolines,* check out these catalog/Internet companies:
  ➤ Beyond Play: www.beyondplay.com
  ➤ Great Ideas for Teaching: www.greatideasforteaching.com
  ➤ Therapy Shoppe: www.therapyshoppe.com
  ➤ Toys to Grow On: www.toystogrowon.com
  ➤ Super Duper, Inc.: www.superduperinc.com
  ➤ Weplay: www.weplay.com

➤ Titles of interest to stock your *recreation resource* shelf: *The Secret of Play* (DK Publishers, 2008) by Ann Pleshette Murphy, former editor-in-chief of Parenting magazine, as well as *Unplugged Play* by Bobbi Conner—700 kid-tested activities to keep your 1-10 year old active and engaged (Workman Publishing Group, 2007), and *Get Out!: 150 Easy Ways for Kids & Grown-Ups to Get Into Nature and Build a Greener Future* (Free Spirit Press, 2009) by Judy Molland and *Last Child in the Woods: Saving our Children from Nature Deficit Disorder* by Richard Louv (Algonquin Books, 2008) are great books for parents concerned about too much "screen time" (TV, computers, etc.).

➤ *Let's Talk Together: 55 Home Activities for Early Speech Language Development* by Cory Poland and Amy Chouinard (Talking Child Press, 2008) offers many ideas for stimulating speech and language in every room of the house.

➤ *Picture This: Photography Activities for Early Childhood Learning* by Susan G. Entz (Corwin Press, 2009). Plenty of activities with sound development practice in this easy-to-read book for the shutterbug parent and child.

➤ *The Kaufman Speech Praxis Treatment Approach* by Nancy Kaufman, M.A., CCC-SLP. Many parents find the *Kaufman Speech Praxis Workout Book* colorful, engaging, and reproducible. It's designed to help kids develop expressive language after mastering some basic sounds. See www.treatapraxia.com or www.kidspeech.com.

➤ Websites you may want to look into:
  ➤ The Discovery Center in the UK: www.boxofideas.org
  ➤ Kiz Club: www.kizclub.com (you may especially like the flannel board pictures for familiar books)
  ➤ PreschoolRock.com (parenting articles and fun ideas for home and school)
  ➤ Dr. Jean Feldman's website: www.drjean.com (great resources for early childhood education through elementary school).
  ➤ Mirla G. Kaz, CCC-SLP, blogs about apps for iPads: www. appsforspeechtherapy.blogspot.com

Chapter Ten

. . . .

An Eye for Design

. . . .

Creating a
Language-Rich Environment at Home
& Encouraging Sound Sleep

Do you pore over the kids' decorating catalogs that clog your mailbox? Do you wish to create a "learning lab" in your basement that the preschool envies? What if you just want to get organized? Then this is the chapter for you! As a self-proclaimed "Mini-Martha," I'll help you discover the joy of designing a special niche for your child with apraxia to flourish in. This chapter will focus on becoming very familiar with your child's interests, passions, and strengths and making them become a reality in your own home—all with a financially friendly approach.

The Nuts and Bolts of This Chapter

➤ How to turn your home into a speech-rich environment, even if you don't care about decorating

➤ The indirect relationship between one's environment and the individual benefits gained from a well-planned space

➤ Transforming rooms in your home into more kid-friendly areas

➤ Research to back this all up and thoughts from parents who have been there

➤ Hints and tips for working with your child as you decorate and design

➤ A discussion on sleep and the connection to apraxia

For some of you, decorating and organizing is a no-brainer. You love it and are good at it. Your kids benefit by having age-appropriate toys at their fingertips and you love the clutter-free lifestyle. Plus, you relish the fact that your living environment reflects what is most near and dear to you.

But I know not everyone has a knack or even an interest in interior design. *You don't have to!* Many of the ideas presented here don't require much decorating talent, just a little know-how and some awareness. You may be surprised by the hints and tips within this chapter that just may help your child with speech and language.

Your Home—A Walk-Through

When you walk into a home, you nearly always get an immediate sense of personality, values, and priorities. Let's take a critical look at your space. Answer these questions as honestly as you can, without giving much thought as to how you *should* answer.

1. Imagine walking inside your home. Do you get an immediate sense of welcome?
2. Does your home smell good?
3. Do you see personality in the form of photos, drawings, objects with personal meaning?
4. Do you feel relaxed and comfortable in your surroundings?
5. Is your home well-organized?
6. Can you find most items effortlessly?
7. Is there a designated place for toys and play?
8. Do the colors in your home uplift you?
9. Is there anything about your home that bothers you?

Once you have completed the simple yes and no portion of this exercise, go back and think about ideas for improvement. Try not to censor your thoughts based on time, money, space, or creativity...just jot down what first comes to mind. These ideas will serve as your inspiration for creating a better place for you and your child to grow and learn.

You are probably wondering why this is important: "Decorating is so not my thing!" you say, "and how does this relate to CAS anyway?"

➤ In a nutshell: *You have better access to materials.* Having to spend less time looking for items means you are more efficient and relaxed and inspired.
➤ *When kids (and parents) work and live in a well-planned environment, it helps keep the focus on learning and living.* The focus is *less* on cleaning up, locating, and managing chaos.
➤ *You'll feel empowered to do your work as a "speech assistant."* As parents we have lots to worry about. Why not make this aspect of your job a little easier?
➤ *Your child benefits from a sense of welcome and belonging.* Enhancing your child's emotional and communicative security is a wonderful result you'll be proud to claim.

Before you get started, you must remember two things:
➤ No environment is perfect.
➤ You'll probably never be able to create the most perfect room or house, but you can *enhance* what you already have.

Your Dream House/Room

Imagine walking into the most inviting, well-planned room you've ever laid eyes on. Go ahead, close your eyes and put yourself there. What catches your eye as you first walk in? What does it smell like? What colors are prominent? Is it cold, warm, just right? What sounds do you hear? Trickling water, crashing waves, soothing music, upbeat music, sounds of nature, screaming kids, silence? What is in the room? How is the room arranged? How do you use the room? How does the room use you?

That last question is a bit of a trick question. When a space is well planned, it should be serving you, *not you serving the room.* So, if something just isn't working, make it work. That might mean being a bit unconventional.

For example, my kitchen pantry was not conveniently located near the place where I stored the kids' plastic snack cups. I kept going back and forth from cabinet to pantry filling snack cups. Not only was it annoying, but it was inefficient. Then it dawned on me: *why not just keep these two items together?* So, I purchased an inexpensive plastic tote to store snack cups *in the pantry*. Genius? No, but now my kitchen was serving me, not me serving my kitchen.

Your 5-mile Radius

Your home and your child's space(s) should be powerful, inviting places to grow and learn. Think about the world of a child—it's pretty small when you get right down to it! Now, think of your world as an adult. You have a home where you sleep, eat, bathe, rest, work (this is a loaded task—could mean chasing after kids, home office, cleaning, maintenance), and entertain. In addition, you may be employed outside the home, and probably have a handful of places you go to regularly: the grocery store, child's school, health club, place of worship, favorite eateries, and the local park.

Chances are you don't venture too far out of your "comfort zone." In fact, most everything you do regularly is probably within a 5 to 10 mile radius of your home. Using this example of "the world ain't so big," I will show just how important your home is to your child's growth.

Really? Yes. Behavior, thoughts, and feelings are shaped by lots of things, including genes, neurochemistry, history, and relationships, but also surroundings.

Think of a cluttered kitchen counter. Dishes to be done, mail to sort, bills to pay, bulging backpacks, a flashing light indicating new voice mail, a lost sock, a novel to finish. Agh! Your *behavior* may be to ignore or tackle the mess, your *thoughts* may be,

"Who cares?" or "Yikes, I've got to do something about this!" Your *feelings* may be, "I'm such a slob," or "I love the abstract pattern of clutter on my counter. I feel so artistic."

Now those genes and the way your neurochemistry handles it is a little more complex. Let's just say that it's the genes that shape your personality that determine your immediate reaction to a cluttered kitchen counter.

History and relationships come in the picture in two ways. For example, maybe your mom always kept a spotless kitchen and you will, too. See how history (past kitchen neatness) and relationships (your mom) come together? History could also mean "personal history," as well: "Before I had kids, my house was a wreck; what's the point now that these little tornados have arrived?"

Your cluttered kitchen counter is screaming, "Do something with me—take care of this, take care of that!" If your home is cluttered, your children's thoughts, behaviors, and feelings might be too.

Creating a Great Space

The very best spaces are a result of thought, inspiration, knowledge, and information. When approaching a room to be decorated, it helps to keep these things in mind:

➤ Overall vision for the space. Go back to that first exercise on page 200.
➤ How the space will be used and by whom
➤ The room's inspiration piece (often becomes the theme)
➤ Your "splurge" item
➤ What you can create yourself
➤ Showcasing a collection of your child's interests, passions, and personality
➤ Matching sets aren't always a "good thing"
➤ Combining and blending accessories, colors, and pieces often creates the best look
➤ Decorating is a process that takes time, planning, coordination, and an eye to tie it all together—And it should be fun!

With those ideas in mind, let's get started with your child's bedroom.

Your Child's Bedroom

Most parents may assume that their kids don't really care about how their room looks or the stuff they keep in it. That's actually a poor assumption—many kids really *do* have a clear preference for how their space looks. Please ask your child if it's okay to decorate or redecorate before you dive in. Young kids become quite attached to belongings and personal spaces, even if you think less of them.

A child's bedroom is more than just a place to sleep. It's a little sanctuary from the world—a place to escape from the stresses of everyday life, to relax, to read, to daydream, and to just be.

A child's room should be filled with things that matter and interest him. Make a list of those things now. Be honest. It doesn't matter if *you* like Thomas the Train or Tinker Bell, just get the ideas down; you can always pare it down later. Here are some ideas to get you started:

➤ (Your child's) favorite colors (see textbox on color)

➤ Favorite TV shows

➤ Favorite type of music

➤ Favorite books

➤ Collections

➤ Sports (spectator or participant)

➤ Fascinations (bugs, space, nature, princesses)

Does Your Child Have a Favorite Color?

If your child has a favorite color, help him understand how the color can be used in the room. As a parent, you may not want bright orange paint splashed on the walls, but perhaps you *could* deal with a warm terra cotta accented with brighter orange accessories?

If your child isn't sure what his favorite color is, make a game out of it to determine if there is a clear theme to color preference. Sort objects and toys around the house together. Crayons, markers, blocks, Play-Doh that he gravitates towards could indicate a preference for a color. What colors are in some of his favorite clothes? What colors does he regularly use in his artwork?

Do Colors Influence Mood?

Yes! Warmer colors (orange, brown, red) tend to stimulate activity, whereas cooler colors (blues, greens) can produce feelings of calm.

➤ *RED*—Increases restlessness and attention. Use sparingly.

➤ *ORANGE*—Similar to red, but friendly. Use to increase feelings of friendship.

➤ *YELLOW*—Sharp focus, cheerful, use to draw attention to achievement and/or themes in the room.

➤ *GREEN*—Decreases muscular tension; good for concentration

➤ *BLUE*—Does not attract attention; can be too calming (decreases focus)

➤ *PURPLE*—Combination of active red and passive blue; neutral and pleasing.

➤ *BLACK, WHITE, & GRAY*—Emotionally neutral, unless used in large areas.

Plan Before You Decorate

Decorating your child's room should be fun! As parents, it gives us an opportunity to recreate some of our own childhood dreams. Think back to what you were passionate about as a child. Chances are, you and your kid have similar ideas.

Your goal at this stage should be to design a room that matches your child's individuality and grows with him. He won't love Sponge Bob forever, so avoid a costly under-the-sea mural or pineapple wallpaper!

Start by evaluating the space. Walk around the room at various times of day. Make notes. Too big, too small? Too hot, too cold? Too dark, too bright? What storage/closets already exist? Sketch out a floor plan of the room, including doors, windows, built-ins, and closets. Rough-in furnishings and rugs. Involve your child by showing him a more detailed plan with colors and specific objects.

Next, think about what your child needs. It's easy to get caught up in *"wants,"* but try to be as objective about this part of the exercise as possible. Think about how your child uses (or will use) his or her bedroom. Will homework be done in the room? Arts and crafts projects? Reading together or alone? Getting dressed? Listening to music? Playing with friends or siblings?

A child's room is his sanctuary. A child's room ought to reflect nearly every aspect of his life. Consider having these elements in his room:

➤ **Sanctuary**—a place to get away from the stress of everyday life. Develop a place to read, relax, daydream, and feel an overall sense of welcome.

➤ **Knowledge**—You may want to include a desk, books, computer, puzzle, globe, or maps.

➤ **Family**—Casual photos of your child with beloved family members work especially well. Consider enlarging and framing favorite candid shots for wall décor. Use matching frames, or matching mats, or make all photos black and white, sepia, or color for a cohesive look. You can have different frames if you keep some other element (such as the mat color) the same.

➤ **Possessions**—collections of any kind—display neatly and artistically, bank, dresser, closet (keep it well organized).

➤ **Recognition**—Highlight awards, trophies, and other accomplishments.

➤ **Friendship**—Photos with friends, games, and a table with two to four chairs encourage friendship.

➤ **Creativity**—Blocks, creative playthings, art supplies, computer, materials, and items that are shiny or catch your eye work well.

➤ **Diversity**—Computers, CD player, posters, dollhouses, books that depict various cultures.

➤ **Careers**—Mobiles, aquarium, comfy chair, floor lamp, books about careers.

➤ **Pride and Ownership**—Add something that is uniquely your child's. Consider special artwork (frame some he has created), a growth chart, his name spelled out in wooden letters, frame a favorite item from babyhood (birth certificate, blankie, or booties).

Bedroom Considerations Specific to Apraxia

Aside from not being able to communicate as effectively as typically developing kiddos, your child with CAS presents his own unique challenges. Think of *your* child in this exercise and jot down your answers as you go along. This will help you in planning a speech-rich environment for him.

➤ What motivates him? Excites him?
➤ How does he respond to external stimuli?
➤ How does he respond to internal stimuli?
➤ Is he active?
➤ Is he quiet and reserved?
➤ Is music calming or distracting?
➤ Are too many objects/toys/decorations overwhelming?
➤ Does your child have difficulty settling down after a long day?
➤ How does your child self-soothe?

With those ideas in mind, consider these decorating and design tips:

If your child needs a calming influence, consider:
➤ Using soft lighting such as table lamps
➤ Painting the room in muted colors
➤ Wall-to-wall carpeting
➤ Soft, smooth textures
➤ Rounded corners on furniture

If your child could benefit from gentle stimulation, consider:
➤ Overhead and table lighting, or a task lamp over a desk
➤ Brighter colors
➤ Hardwood flooring with area rugs to determine "stations" for certain tasks
➤ Glossy finishes on furniture
➤ Square corners on furniture
➤ Interesting textures, such as corduroy or ruffles

Keep in mind that just because your child has some communication (and possibly sensory issues) doesn't mean his room should be void of the "fun stuff." Get creative, use your parenting intuition, and let him know that his room is a safe, fun, and inviting place.

More Inspiration Needed?

At four years old, Kate was a friendly, outgoing girl with high energy needs. She loved gross motor activity, art, the color purple, flowers, dogs, and books. She had a difficult time unwinding at the end of the day and needed much sensory stimulation.

Quick Plan: Initially, we thought the theme for the room could be a garden/flower or dog theme. Keeping in mind that we wanted the room to grow with her, we involved her in the decision. We actually went for a "doggies and daisies" theme for Kate. It reflected her interest in gardening and her love for animals. Together, we selected items that we could both agree on that went along with the overall theme. We chose items that could easily be replaced, should she grow bored with them. For example, the peel-and-stick wildflowers on her wall are not permanent, the stuffed dogs can easily be relocated.

➤ Kate's **high energy** meant she needed a wide open space to play, jump, twirl, and stretch out without feeling restricted. I scooted furniture to the edges of the room in hopes it would prevent bumps and bruises (it did, mostly).

➤ Since Kate loved (and still loves) **art,** I involved her in selecting pieces of wall art. I also had her create her own with finger paint on a blank canvas. I even framed some of her favorite drawings and artwork from preschool that coordinated with her room.

➤ **Books** are a big deal to Kate (and her family), so I made sure they were prominently displayed. You might consider turning books into art by installing a book ledge along the wall and purchasing beautifully illustrated hardcover children's books that coordinate with the overall theme of the room.

Your Child with CAS Doesn't Talk Much...Yet

In reading through this chapter, you no doubt noticed me saying, "Get their input," over and over. Don't despair if your child isn't saying, "Well, Mom, what I'd really like is a sanctuary I can call my own. I'd like the walls painted quaking grass and the bedspread to be handcrafted by the best quilter in town with all of my favorite colors and coordinating art work." No kid will ever say that unless he is destined to be an interior designer!

What's a parent to do?
➤ Clip photos or pages from a catalog or magazine for your child to cull through with you.
➤ Take him with you to look at paint chips. "Which color would you like to paint your room?"
➤ Ask if he'd like to go along to shop for accessories for his train-themed bedroom. You can even "shop" from toys/items in his toy chest, selecting models or toys that fit into the dinosaur-themed bedroom or the space-and-rocket playroom.
➤ Try asking questions like, "Where do you like to play/have a playroom? Can you show me?"

Get creative and find ways you can ask for your child's input. Most kids can indicate "yes or no." And finally, don't just assume that because your little one can't articulate much doesn't mean he doesn't care.

➤ Achieving Kate's high need for **sensory stimulation** was done by incorporating various textures and surfaces. Beanbag chairs provided that cocoon-like feel she so desired (consider also floppy pillows or floor cushions). We even kept fidget toys and oral stimulation pieces in her room for those times she needed extra input.

➤ Kate's day concluded with a **bath, calming lotion** (lavender, vanilla, chamomile scents work well), relaxing music, and quiet reflection time.

I am not suggesting that your child with apraxia is "just like" Kate. The key with apraxia is it is as unique as your child. Apraxia does not present itself the same way every time.

Designing a Playroom for Your Child with Apraxia

Sure, we spend about a third of our life sleeping, but that means that two-thirds of our life is spent awake, doing things, learning things, and enjoying things. Children may spend some of that awake time in their own room, but chances are, they are going to be playing near you, their parents. This section will focus on developing a playroom just right for *your* child.

Again, you'll have to assess your space. Where do you tend to spend most of your day when you're at home? Are you in the kitchen, a home office, the family room, a basement rec room? Young kids will want Mom and Dad in eyesight and you might require it, too.

An ideal playroom will be devoted to your child(ren) and will make learning fun and safe.

➤ *Determine where you will set up shop.* Think of your basement, a loft, the corner of a family room; maybe you can convert a rarely used dining room, living room, or guest bedroom into "kid central?"

➤ *Try to keep all toys in a designated space.* That way your entire home won't feel like the dumping ground for the local toy store.

➤ *What kinds of toys do you already have?* Make a list.

➤ *Which toys do your child(ren) play with the most?*

➤ *What kinds of playroom furnishings do you own?* Toy box, bookshelves, kiddie table and chairs, easel, storage containers, etc.

➤ *What are the major traffic ways in and out of the room?*

➤ *Draw a floor plan.* Include windows, doors, closets, and any built-ins (bookshelves, fireplaces, window seats).

Think of your newly minted play space as a rival to your child's classroom. In classroom speak, the usefulness of a classroom is referred to as "vitality." It's all influenced by the amount of stuff—furniture, decorations, and materials. You may think that more is better. You may feel your kid(s) will be smarter if he has more. Actually, the opposite is true. Clutter depletes energy.

An ideal playroom will incorporate areas for play and work. And remember, in your child's world, it really *is* work to color in the lines or learn to use scissors. It requires skill and concentration to assemble a puzzle, even if it only has five pieces.

Playroom Considerations Specific to Apraxia

When you think of a child's classroom at the preschool level, you may envision work stations or "centers"—a kitchen area, a craft and color table, building and constructing, pretend play, and so forth. For your home play space, consider replicating that preschool vibe.

Preschools are also cognizant of allowing the environment to "grow with the child." Teachers are constantly assessing their students to see what they can do, what they are about to do, and what challenges them. You'll want your child's play area at home to grow with him, also. For example, once the alphabet is mastered, you may want to replace the ABC wall strip with sight words he is learning to read, such as "and," "the," and "see."

> *Other things you can do at home:*
> ➤ Periodically *review* the toys/items in your child's play space/room for skill level, ease of use, child's interest, etc.
> ➤ *Remove* toys/items that seem too "babyish."
> ➤ *Replenish* the room with items your child may see as a "reach," or challenge. (We found that introducing items that were slightly beyond Kate's current level gave her renewed interest and motivation to communicate.)

Please, ***don't*** take this advice as "you need to go out and purchase new toys for your child." You can very well store items your child receives as gifts in a closet and pull them out when he is ready for them. You can arrange a toy-swap in your neighborhood in which you trade toys on a rotating basis. Some communities even have a toy lending program. Garage sales are often good places to get "new" things that may interest your child.

> Here are some more ideas for creating a playroom that grows with your child:
> ➤ *Have a special section on phonological awareness.* Stock it with magnetic letters, alphabet stamps, letter flashcards, books on letters, workbooks, letter manipulatives (foam-shaped letters, blocks), etc.
> ➤ *Label everything.* Use big, bold letters and put signs on furnishings: "CHAIR," "TABLE," "EASEL." Lisa Circelli, M.Ed., an early childhood teacher at The Brokaw Early Learning Center in Oswego, IL, recommends using upper and lower case letters in your signage. "Kids need to see the correct way of writing words so they can begin to internalize it."

- ➤ *Prominently display alphabet cards at eye level.* Many folks place them at the top of the wall around the perimeter of the room, but children won't see them there.
- ➤ *Have a "letter of the day."* Work on that sound for the entire day (even if it is *just* you saying it), point out objects that begin with that sound, look for the letter when you are out and about in the community.
- ➤ *Encourage gross motor work.* Engage the vestibular system with a swing or trampoline. Quiz and drill your child on that speech homework from your therapist while he moves his body.
- ➤ *Create a safe and easily-accessible art center.* Stock it with child-safe scissors, glue, construction paper, coloring books, markers, crayons, etc.

I love this idea from Joy, the mother of twins with global apraxia and fine motor delays:

*"One whole end of our family room has a padded floor with table and chairs and our old toy bin, which we stock with all kinds of supplies (including recyclable items like tissue rolls and egg cartons). Both my kids love doing art, but my ulterior motive is to give them as many opportunities as possible to manipulate materials (from tape to a stapler to scissors) and also hold a writing utensil so they can sign all their work and/or write about it. Nobody wants to work on writing letters since it is so frustrating, but [they] will do artistic challenges that include the basic elements. I am even thinking of doing art challenges and tying it with verbal cues from **Handwriting without Tears** and then moving to working on letters if I can sneak it in."*

Robbin, mom of Kennedy (3.6 years with CAS) and Jack (2 years), says her art room has become the therapy room at their house:

"My kids love [our art room]…they have no idea we are working on speech. My daughter's SLP comes to the house and works with her with all the things I have in there. It's great!"

Parents Share...

Mirror, Mirror, on the Wall

Rita in Ohio shares this experience: "Our six-year-old daughter *loves* to have mirrors around wherever she is. It's a place where she can go touch base with where her mouth is (proprioception). She spends almost an hour sometimes looking at her mouth, inside [her mouth], sticking out her tongue, and touching her teeth. When she was younger, she did this even more. Eye-level mirrors have been key for us in all living areas."

In fact, speech clinics often use mirrors as a therapy tool—there just may be something to it!

Sensory Stimulation and Apraxia

By now, you should be aware that motion affects the speech and language center nestled deep within your child's brain. But did you know you can create cool features at home that foster good times and social development while allowing your child with apraxia to feel comfortable and increase his vestibular stimulation?

➤ *Got an exposed beam in your basement or attic?* Hang a swing from it, or a hammock (some even come with stands, so no need to have an exposed beam).

  "Thinking back, if we had the means, we could have put a swing in our basement and a trampoline out back: two very sensory-friendly things for Jack that stimulated his speech. We compromised on two large yoga kind of balls, jumping on the bed, and a Jim Gill CD featuring the "Washing Machine Song," where he'd run himself in circles each night before bed (seriously). Those less expensive, unobtrusive yet very typically kid-friendly items still stimulated the speech and sounds we were looking for, plus fed the vestibular and proprioceptive systems[stimulation]. Sometimes it isn't about what, but more about how."

  —Holly, mother of a son with CAS

➤ *Develop an indoor sports spot.* What you need: space (unfinished basement?), small trampoline, kid-sized basketball goal, exercise balls, jump ropes, maybe even a slide, tunnel system, or climbing wall. Add some music and you've got the recipe for burning energy. Kids into gymnastics? Get some mats, make or buy a beam, and voila—a gymnastics studio.

➤ *Some kids love to perform.* Consider developing a stage for theatrical productions and allowing him to sing his heart out. It doesn't have to be elaborate—just a slightly raised platform and a toy microphone will do. Who knows, it may even get him to try new words!

➤ *Some kids with apraxia crave sensory stimulation.* Consider converting an old sandbox or large under-bed storage box into a messy table. Fill it with popcorn kernels, dried beans (if your child is over three and won't swallow small items), feathers, or ribbon, or make your own slime. Add old measuring devices, bowls and spoons, a kid or two, and bake for hours of play.

Keep in mind: *any* individual—young, old, with or without apraxia—learns best when actively engaged in the learning process.

Creating a Book Nook

In our busy lives, it's hard to find the time and place to practice speech "homework" given to us by our SLP. One thing that can help: a book nook at home with comfy furnishings for you and your child (beanbags or floor pillows) to snuggle down and look at books together. Pull in a crate or bookshelf to store your materials, and you've got a wonderful area to practice speech in an inviting environment.

If you're short on space, there is no reason not to have your art center in the corner of the family room or kitchen, just as you can also have a quiet reading area in the dining room. It may work well to have "reservations" to use the space: "Dining room closed for speech practice from 2:00 - 2:30 pm," or something along those lines.

➤ *Consider making a "book" from the handouts and flashcards your speech pathologist gives you.* Use a folder with brads, or a ½"-1" binder and slip the worksheets into sheet protectors. We kept our notebook in Kate's room and reviewed that week's lesson every night and at naptime. I mixed it in with the other reading we did, so it didn't seem like such a chore.

➤ *Make a habit out of practicing speech with your child by pointing out pictures in children's books.* This worked wonderfully with Kate when she had difficulties with /s/ blends. "What's this?" I'd say as I pointed to a snail, a snake, a smokestack. I'd look for an /s/ blend on every page. A sigh and a few attempts later, Kate would produce the right blend. This worked because she loves books. If your child isn't the bookish type, don't despair.

What about Homework? Creating a Study Center

We can't get away with this idea that play is work forever. Don't be surprised if your preschooler brings home an assignment or two. By kindergarten, you'll likely see something every night.

➤ *Please have a regular place for your child(ren) to study.* Even if you're just working on the ABC's and 123's, practicing handwriting, or drawing shapes, establish a consistent place and keep it sacred. It can be a part of the playroom, in the bedroom, or elsewhere in the home (like the kitchen, a loft, even a wide hallway). The key is that homework is done in this area.

➤ *Stock your child's study center with school supplies.* Hit the before-school sales and buy double of what your school wants your child to bring. Keep an extra set of supplies at home. Consider purchasing other items like poster board and display boards, binders, report covers, pens, markers, and highlighters. You never know when that last-minute project may crop up.

➤ *Make it comfortable with well-appointed desks and chairs that are child-sized.* Add a cushion to the seat if sitting for prolonged time. Hang a bulletin board or dry-erase board to post assignments, ideas, task lists, and notes.

➤ *A filing cabinet for each child is handy, too.* It teaches filing and organizational skills and develops a sense of accountability. Stuff it full of progress reports, IEP information, and report cards, along with special projects and interests specific to your child(ren).

➤ *Keep some reference materials handy.* Consider dictionaries, thesauruses, atlases, and encyclopedias; nowadays, you can find it all on the computer.

➤ *Assess when and if you want your child using a computer.* At what age do you think having a computer is reasonable? Expected? How will you monitor your child's activity on the computer?

➤ *Keep your child's personality and work style in mind when setting up the study area.* Ask for his input. If it's an area that's naturally pleasing to your child, he's more likely to use it and succeed there. Let the area grow with your child. Homework is going to be a big part of his life for many years to come. *Last but not least, let it reflect his fun and unique style.*

Music Influences the Environment, Too

Music and moods go together like milk and cookies. Songs can make us feel good, evoke happy memories, or help us focus. Kids like music and having some playing in the background just adds to the space. You know your child best, so think about how he responds to music. Would classical music help him focus? Would some funky kid music get him up and moving?

Use different types of music at different times of the day and you may be surprised how it affects your child (and your parenting). You can use different music to signal transitions between activities—between play time and clean-up, for example. Or between awake time and calm-down-and-get-ready-for-bed-time. Gross motor time on the indoor trampoline makes for some great speech practice. Put on some rockin' tunes, get him jumping, and pull out the flashcards—he may forget he's even "working!"

Why Sleep May Be a Challenge for Kids with CAS

• • • • • • • • • • • •

I have heard from many parents with kids who have CAS that sleep can be a problem. Before we jump to conclusions, it's not always apraxia that is *the* cause for sleep issues. Just be aware that there is a *correlation* between apraxia and poor sleep. Your child, however, may be a terrific sleeper and still have apraxia. Again, not all children with CAS present exactly the same.

On that note, you'll want to be aware of any potential sensory or medical issues your child may have. See Appendix A for more information on sensory processing.

"My four-year-old [with apraxia] usually wakes during the night for three or four hours. We've tried melatonin, dietary changes, probiotics, sensory input before bed, strict schedule, white noise machine, black-out curtains, weighted blanket, homeopathy, Epsom salt baths….Short of prescription drugs—you name it, we've tried it. Not one thing has helped. The pediatrician and neurologist shrug their shoulders with a 'yep, nature of the beast with these disorders' attitude."

—Amanda, mom to twins with CAS, ADHD, SPD

Sensory Concerns Affecting Your Child's Ability to Relax

While it's easy, in some regards, to call CAS "the bad guy," identifying it as *the* source of all concerns for your child, it isn't true *all* of the time. However, if you are truly concerned about the possibility of sensory issues with your child, please seek the services of a pediatric occupational therapist or consider a comprehensive neuropsychological evaluation/assessment.

Here are a few ideas you can try if you suspect sensory issues *along with* CAS (but really, these ideas would work with just about any child, regardless of CAS):

➤ *Try kid yoga.* Your child may be very receptive to this idea, especially if he can "share" it with a parent or teenaged sibling as special bonding time. Yoga has powerful, yet soothing effects on the body and mind. For more information, look to the *YogaKids* DVD series (2010) and *Yoga for Families: Connect with Your Kids* (2009). You may also like the book *The ABCs of Yoga for Kids* by Theresa Anne Power, which shows how to teach the formations of letters (and their sounds) through yoga poses (Stafford House, 2009).

➤ *Explore visualization/meditation.* Along with, or in lieu of yoga, you and your child may appreciate a little guided visualization just before going to bed. Sit with your child in a comfortable spot for awhile, taking deep refreshing breaths. Using words, you can create a visual escape to your "destination" of choice…an ocean, wooded forest, mountain top. Use vibrant descriptions and encourage him to use all of his senses as you describe this location—smell the salty sea air, feel the warm breezes. I love this book: *Angel Bear Yoga Adventure Stories: Children's Stories Perfect for Relaxation, Sleeptime, or Kid's Yoga* by Christi Eley (2007).

➤ *Relax with a stress-relieving neck wrap.* They come filled with rice or beans, sometimes flax seed or buckwheat; some may be scented. You can warm them in the microwave. The weight (just a couple of pounds) can be very soothing for kids who have difficulty slowing down. Beanbags can produce a similar result.

➤ *Make a pig-in-a-blanket.* Try wrapping your child tightly in a heavy quilt, with his head poking out during bedtime stories. The tight feeling can be quite soothing and comforting to some kids (think of swaddling a baby). Unwrap him before tucking him in bed.

➤ *Try a bedtime snack.* Some folks swear that certain foods have magical powers that lull one to sleep (turkey, anyone?). Consider these wonder foods:

- *Cherries* (fresh and dried) are one of the only natural sources for melatonin, the chemical that controls the body's internal clock. Researchers recommend eating them about an hour before you want to fall asleep.
- *Bananas* are chock-full of potassium and magnesium, which are natural muscle relaxants. Also, bananas contain L-tryptophan (an amino acid), which is converted by the body to serotonin (5-HTP, a neurotransmitter which is a natural relaxant) and melatonin.
- *Toast* is one of those carbohydrate-dense foods triggering insulin production, making one drowsy by releasing tryptophan and serotonin. That's why you often feel tired after eating a muffin for breakfast without a source of protein.
- *Oatmeal* also triggers a rise in blood sugar, just like toast will. Oats also have melatonin.
- *Warm milk* may sound a bit old-fashioned, but there's science behind the magic. Again, the amino acid L-tryptophan is at work here, converting to 5-HTG, releasing serotonin. Milk is high in calcium, too which promotes that drowsy feeling. (Add a teaspoon of vanilla extract for a little added flavor.)

➤ *Consider heavy blankets and quilts.* You may want to turn down the thermostat at night (best sleeping temperatures range from 65 to 72 degrees Fahrenheit). The cooler temperatures are actually more conducive to sleep, and heavy blankets often produce a soothing effect for the sleeper.

Medical Concerns Regarding Sleep

Some of the parents I spoke with during the writing of this book indicated that their children with CAS also have medical concerns such as sleep apnea, swallowing problems, or overly large tonsils.

One mother of a child with global apraxia mentioned that her child had obstructive sleep apnea up until the time her tonsils and adenoids were removed. Another parent indicated that her son's speech/swallowing/apraxia/motor planning concerns were tied very closely to his overly large tonsils. Her explanation went something like this:

1. Initially her son relied on his large tonsils to help close his airway when he was speaking and swallowing.
2. After his tonsils were removed, his speech sounds were more nasal.
3. This led to the need for speech therapy and swallowing therapy.

After a little digging, I found a study published in *Pediatric Neurology* and found that there is, indeed, something to this. The article discusses a case study of a young boy, Max, who had CAS and a seizure disorder, who was also found to have obstructive sleep apnea. After a life-changing surgery, little Max was cured of sleep apnea and made considerable gains in speech.

Jodi Mindell, a clinical psychologist specializing in pediatric sleep medicine and coauthor of *Take Charge of your Child's Sleep,* shares that: "[Overall], children with any medical/psychiatric issue seem to be at higher risk for sleep disturbances, and parents should definitely consider the possibility of any underlying sleep disrupter, such as obstructive sleep apnea and restless legs syndrome/periodic limb movement disorder. Any sleep disruption will definitely exacerbate other daytime issues."

Back to Sleep

If you're pretty certain that your child doesn't have any additional sensory or medical concerns related to sleep, and you just want some old-fashioned advice on getting him off to dreamland each night, read on.

While I don't have any specific data proving that sleep difficulties are directly related to CAS, it most likely boils down to the fact that sleep and circadian rhythms are all derived from the nervous system. Since we know CAS is a motor-neurological disorder, then it can be assumed that these two systems are in tandem.

Restless sleep, difficulty falling asleep and staying asleep, being a "light sleeper," and early awakening all qualify as "sleep disturbances."

Here are some simple steps you can do to make sure your child's room is conducive to sleep:

Parents Ask...

What's sleep apnea, anyway?

Sleep apnea is best described as abnormally low periods of breathing during sleep (hypopnea) or long pauses (apnea) between breaths, which can last 5 seconds to several minutes each on an average of 5 to 30 times per hour! The disrupted breathing is usually not noticeable by the sleeper, but often by a spouse—or in this case—a parent. In which case, you may find that your child is snoring, mouth breathing, restless during sleep, a bed-wetter, or tired upon awakening.

Pediatric sleep apnea is a bit different from adult sleep apnea in that it is typically the upper airway that narrows for only short periods of time, causing frequent breaks in sleep. Kids are often quite fatigued in the daytime, which lead to crankiness, lack of concentration, restlessness, daytime inattentiveness, mood swings, and hyperactivity. If you are truly concerned that your child may have sleep apnea, it's best to have a formal sleep study done to rule it out.

➤ *Make it dark.* I know this seems self-explanatory, but some kids are bothered by the slightest amount of light creeping from under the door or peeking through blinds; you may want to consider a room-darkening shade.

➤ *Consider painting the walls tranquil and soothing colors.* There is evidence that certain colors may be more relaxing than others. For instance, blue is often used in doctors' offices and prisons because it is known to decrease one's heart rate and blood pressure. Refer to chart on page 203.

➤ *Reduce distractions.* Carefully assess your child's room and determine what items may be more distracting to him. Generally speaking, the more stuff that's in his room, the more distracting it's going to be.

➤ *Keep toys, activities, and playthings in another room.* While this may not always be possible, it's worth considering. A basement, guest room, loft, attic, or sun room makes a great place to play. You may have to be a little unconventional and repurpose your dining room for the purpose of play; you'll have to do without the formal dinner parties—at least for awhile.

➤ *Keep your child's most prized possessions in his room—just limit them.* Please don't read this as: take everything out of your child's room and paint it blue. As we talked about before, children love the idea of a place they can call their own, with their own belongings and sense of personality.

Say That Again?! Chapter Summary

I hope I have shown you that the environment really *does* shape how we feel about surroundings, and influences behavior—good or bad. Perhaps I have given you some ideas of ways you can improve your home, as well as your children's sleep, play, and work areas. When you start out overhauling—redecorating—repurposing—whatever you decide to do, keep these tips in mind:

Have fun and be sure you ask for your child's input. Even though he has apraxia, he can still share his preferences. Integrate items that are important and valuable to your child. Think of a theme, but do your best to be subtle about it, because "more" is not always "better." Take your time. Decorating is a process, not just an outcome. Shop around. Talk with other parents. Look at books and magazines and catalogs for inspiration. In fact, look at *anything* and *everything* for inspiration, even the décor of your favorite eatery. Allow your child to have some ownership of the area/room. Consider displaying his name or dedicate a spot for showcasing trophies or artwork.

Remember: clutter depletes energy. Plus, it can be downright overwhelming for kids with apraxia, whose nervous and motor systems are already overtaxed. Less is more. Consider relaxing music and tranquil wall colors, if your child needs a little extra de-stimulation. If your child has sensory issues in addition to verbal apraxia, incorporate features that let you sneak in sensory work as well. Finally, I leave you with this thought, from "apraxia mom" Holly:

"In my opinion, every place is a speech-rich environment, whether you are at the grocery store, the playground, in your own basement, or in your own bathroom. There is always something to point out, talk about, describe, sing about, look at, touch, feel, smell, etc. For us, those were richer experiences than anything I purchased with therapy on my mind."

Read On! Recommended Resources

➤ Looking for some activity-driven pieces to complete your child's playroom? Check out Weplay for items such as **balance boards, exercise balls, foam mats and blocks, trampolines, etc.:** www.weplay.com.tw.

➤ You don't have to shop in expensive therapy supply stores or catalogs to outfit your child's physical activity area. You can find many wonderful products made for kids of all abilities through HearthSong: www.hearthsong.com or 800-325-2502.

➤ *Creative Visualization with Kids: A Practical Guide* by Jennifer Day (Element Books, 2007) is a good reference guide for parents looking into trying visualization with their kids.

➤ For a book that your child can benefit from directly in terms of visualization, try **Peaceful Piggy Meditation,** by Kerry Lee MacLean (Albert Whitman, 2004). It's a sweet, simple, and straightforward approach. Adorable!

➤ For **weighted wraps,** you may want to consider these products: *North American Healthcare Hot/Cold Comfort Wrap,* which can be purchased on www.Amazon.com or the *Carex Bed Buddy,* www.carex.com/products.

➤ *Take Charge of Your Child's Sleep: The All-in-One Resource for Solving Sleep Problems in Kids and Teens* by Judith A. Owens and Jodi A. Mindell (Marlowe & Co, 2005) is a parent-friendly book on sleep problems in kids, including chapters on sleep apnea, bad dreams, and ADHD, among others.

Section Four

Off to School

Chapter Eleven

· · · · · · · · · ·

Off to School

· · · · · · · · · ·

Preparing Your Child (and Yourself!)

After being a mom for not quite three years, I wasn't expecting to be enrolling my daughter in public education. I had envisioned two more years of playgroups, parks, and Play-Doh. But after a whirlwind meeting with the SLP and special education coordinator at the school district, I was leaving the building with a stack of papers, handbooks, and registration forms. "Fill these out and get them back to us in three weeks. You will need to schedule and complete a school physical in that time, too. If the transportation department doesn't contact you within two weeks, call them. Here's their number." I painstakingly herded my two girls out of the bright and cheerful assessment room, "baby" Kelly on one hip, the papers on the other, and made my way home.

By 10:30 a.m., I was mentally and emotionally drained. My little girl, then two years and 11 months old, had just been confirmed as "severely apraxic," and because of this disability, would be attending special education preschool five days a week. She would qualify for *bus* services, too?! I tried to be optimistic for Kate's sake (and mine, too), but I desperately needed to process the events of the morning. My husband was travelling and attending an important meeting. My fingers were itching to dial someone—*anyone*—on my cell phone, but no one was available to talk at this hour. No one who *really* understood, anyway. We drove home quietly. I held back tears. My chin wobbled as I pointed out a big yellow bus, "Kate look! You'll be riding one of those soon."

I ended up calling my dad once the girls were down for their naps. Always a pillar of strength and support, he listened to me review the details of the morning and gave me his ever-reassuring words of wisdom, "Everyone wants their kids to be above average in every way, but this is the best thing for her." He told me other things too, like, "It's good you caught this when you did…you're doing the right thing…how great there's a school for this."

And he was right about all of it. But it still hurt, a lot. I did cry that day—and other days, too. But, I will tell you that it *does* get better, and you *will* get through this.

This chapter will walk you through the steps of having your child assessed through the school district, help you ease your child into the transition from being home with you full-time (or attending day care) to going to school. A special needs student and their family have, well—special needs when it comes to school. We'll explore IDEA, FAPE, and IEPs…a bit different than your 123s and ABCs.

Think of this chapter as your "Cliff Notes Guide" to sending your child with CAS to school. I will attempt to touch on your most pressing concerns, feelings, and questions, but I know you will have questions specific to your own child. Please continue to seek out all the resources you can as you navigate the school system.

The Nuts and Bolts of This Chapter

➤ General guidelines for selecting a school (but keep in mind, not all aspects may pertain to your situation)

➤ Preschool and kindergarten, as well as all of the players involved

➤ Some pros and cons of home schooling, too

➤ Ways you can teach your child's teacher about CAS, how to be an involved parent, and how to host an in-class lesson on apraxia for all students

➤ What to expect from speech therapy at school

➤ Special education jargon such as IEP and IFSP, your role in the education process, as well as how to file a complaint, and stay organized

➤ Theories as to why kids with apraxia may have a harder time academically, plus solutions and possible interventions.

➤ Learning styles, emotional IQ, and grade retention

Qualities to Look for in Schools

When we moved from the Minneapolis area to Chicago, my husband made a nice spreadsheet comparing the "new" school districts in our new suburban area with ones we were familiar with, even including some data on the public school system we attended as kids. I thought this was sweet but overly nerdy and systematic of him. At the time of our move, our two girls were just four months and barely two years old, and while I wanted the girls to attend a good school district, I was more interested in how I was going to baby proof the new digs than where we'd send them to school!

But my husband was on to something (as usual). Assuming you have a choice where you send your child to school—be it public or private, suburban or urban, "special" or mainstream, it's not a bad idea to be "nerdy and systematic" and carefully plan for the long haul. Here's a checklist for you to consider. If your child is just entering preschool, try not get overwhelmed, especially when we discuss academics. This section covers the basics for all grade levels. Hand-outs you should ask the school office for are *italicized*.

General Considerations:
➤ Find out what the school's visitation policy is like and then ...
➤ Visit the school during regular school hours. Did you feel welcome? Did the kids look happy?
➤ What were the teachers and administrators like?
➤ Is the school clean and well kept? Bright and cheerful?
➤ How are the students dressed? Do they wear uniforms? Does your child look the part?
➤ Does the school have a mission statement prominently displayed? Was the mission reflected in your first impression?
➤ Does the school accurately reflect the cultural diversity in your community?
➤ Is admission based on chronological age guidelines, and not on mastery of skills?
➤ What was your commute like to the school? Were you stopped by a train? Going against morning traffic? Now imagine the same drive in inclement weather...still do-able?
➤ What transportation options are available? Parent drop-off, bus, before and after school care?
➤ Is transportation provided if your child must attend a school that is not her "home school?"

Teachers & Administration:
➤ Do teachers take part in regular professional development? How often?
➤ Do the teachers have experience or education in child development?
➤ Are teachers ready to meet children "where they're at?"
➤ How accessible are teachers? Can they be reached through phone or email?
➤ Will teachers communicate regularly with one another and with you at home? How?
➤ Are the teachers National Board certified? Percentage of teachers that are?
➤ What percentage of teachers hold advanced degrees? Is that important to you?
➤ Are there regular school improvement days where teachers and administrators collaborate?

Social & Emotional Learning:

➤ Is there an anti-bullying curriculum in place? (More on this in Chapter 13.)
➤ Does the school support student relationships, kindness, consideration, and respect?
➤ Is there access to a school psychologist or social worker?
➤ Are social skills supported and encouraged through facilitated play, nonverbal options (PECS, Boardmaker, signing/gesturing), and social skills groups?
➤ Do kids get outside time? How often?

Student Resources:

➤ Does the library have current media and technology—computers? Books? DVDs? Does the library feel comfortable and accessible?
➤ Is the cafeteria clean? Are there healthy food choices? *Ask for a lunch menu.*
➤ Who provides speech services? What are their qualifications? How will you be appraised of developments? (Ask similar questions regarding occupational therapy, if that is a need for your child.)
➤ Where and how often do kids receive extra help (tutoring) if they need it?

Academics:

➤ What curriculum has the school adopted? It should have a formal name. Is it challenging, but appropriately so?
➤ Is there balance within the curriculum? Is it "heavy" in one content area? Does that matter to you?
➤ What special education classes are housed at the school?
➤ Is there a speech classroom, language classroom, or other special classrooms?
➤ How much homework can be expected each day?
➤ *Request a copy of a progress report and a report card.* What standards are in place?
➤ How are grades determined? What's the grading scale?
➤ Do yearly stats show a tendency for consistency? Is there improvement or not?
➤ Visit a classroom (you'll need special permission first). Are the kids actively engaged? What is the teacher doing? Is there an aide?
➤ What type of student work is on display?
➤ What is the average class size per grade? Teacher : student ratio?
➤ Is foreign language part of the curriculum?
➤ What percentage of students go on to a 4-year university?

Before and After School:

➤ *Ask for a school calendar.* What types of sporting and social events are listed?
➤ Are there before and after school clubs? What are they? Do they appeal to you and your child?

➤ Do the hours of these events fit in with your typical schedule?
➤ Is transportation available to school-sponsored events?
➤ Is there transportation to/from daycare facilities?

Parents:
➤ *Ask for a newsletter or classroom bulletin from the front office.* Read it. What other school-home communication exists? Emails? Phone calls? Website?
➤ Does the school have any partnerships with the community at large? With whom?
➤ Does the school help connect families to the community resources to promote learning outside of the classroom?
➤ Are parents encouraged to volunteer in the classroom and within the school?
➤ Is there an active PTA/PTO?
➤ Talk to other parents in the same district. Parents of older kids are a great resource. Ask, "What do you love about your kid's school? What don't you like?"

Please, listen to your instincts. If something just doesn't jive with you, there's probably a better school for you and your child (assuming you are looking at private schools or deciding what neighborhood to settle in). Obviously, if you're already settled in and looking at the neighborhood public school, you may not have a choice. You may also be interested in checking out this website: www.schooldigger.com. Here you can obtain test scores, rankings, teacher : student ratios, district boundaries, etc. for more than 120,000 K-12 schools in the United States. Of course, you'll have to hone in on the speech–language piece of it once you find a school district you are happy with.

Preschool

● ● ● ● ● ● ●

"I am so anxious about where to send my son to preschool. I know it's a drop in the bucket compared to all of the schooling he will receive in his lifetime, but I want to make sure he is in a really good program, especially because of his apraxia."

—Mom to Matthew, age 3 years.

Your child may just be three years old, but you are already thinking about her education. If you started out with early intervention services (sometimes called "Birth to Three" or "First Steps"), then your little one will be transitioning from EI to the regular school district where you reside. If that's the case for you, then consider yourself lucky. The EI program will guide you through the process of transitioning to special education services.

To qualify for preschool services through your local school district, your child will need to be evaluated just shy of her third birthday. Give yourself about three months lead to her birth date. If you are working closely with an EI therapist, she will let you know the steps involved. If you're not—then you'll likely need to call the school district where you live, and the special education coordinator will take it from there. Granted, this process is not so simple and you may need to make several phone calls or be a bit of a pest to get the answers you need. You'll also want your private SLP onboard with the plan (she may even initiate it) and for her to write a letter requesting the evaluation. If your child is seeing a private OT, consider getting a letter of recommendation from her, too.

Your child will be assessed by the school personnel—an early childhood educator, a special education consultant, and a school-based SLP are likely to be part of the assessment team. If the team concurs that your child's speech and language skills are significantly delayed, then you're in. The size of the delay required varies from district to district, but often it is 3 to 6 months (sometimes referred to as "lag time" in educational circles). Sometimes children with less significant delays in speech may qualify if they also have mild to moderate delays in others areas. According to Rhonda Banford, CCC-SLP, teams sometimes also make a professional judgment if a child is "on the cusp."

Once your child is in, you will find that what "special needs preschool" consists of varies depending on your school district, your child's needs, and sometimes your own preferences. These preschools may be separate programs housed outside of a regular school, or they may be a classroom within a public school. Then again, for some children, needed services may be provided within a private preschool or daycare that you have enrolled your child in.

Blended vs. Self-Contained: Your child's classroom may be either "blended" or "self-contained." A **blended or integrated** ("inclusive") classroom is one where students with different abilities are combined in one classroom. This is often done in public school settings. Your child with CAS may be in a classroom with typically developing peers as well as those with apraxia or other special needs. On the other hand, your IEP team may decide that your child would be best served in a **self-contained** classroom where all students have a special need of some kind (hearing impairment, Down syndrome, congenital disorders, etc.), or where the primary concern for all of the students is speech and language skills. However, note that a 2011 study in the journal *Child Development* indicated that "among children with low initial language skills, those who were placed in the lowest-ability [preschool] classes tended to lose ground during the school year, while those placed in average-ability classes tended to improve their language skills."

Be sure to discuss what kind of classroom your child will be in at the IEP meeting and make your views known about the pros and cons of different settings. (See page 243 for more information on IEPs.)

Although the term "special needs preschool" may have some negative connotations, there are instances when this is the best thing for a child—and you. Trust me, I've been there.

➤ Teachers at these schools (or in the special classroom) *know* kids and almost always have additional training in special needs, learning disabilities, and literacy.

Thoughts on Blended Classrooms

"Putting our son with apraxia in our school district's early childhood program has been the best thing we could do. It is a blended program with up to five typical kids, five kids who are considered at risk, and five kids who are considered special needs. I will not tell you this program is perfect—there is no such thing—but overall it is absolutely amazing. If you can find a blended program in your area, I highly recommend it."

—Mom to twins, one of whom has CAS.

"We live in a district that does not offer a blended ECE program and it has been a challenge to expose my son to typical peers that will reinforce all of his language and social growth. You would think that if a child has it written into his IEP that he make gains in his social pragmatic speech, the school would be responsible for creating [that] environment. Like many families we have been responsible for creating and paying for those experiences. As parents, we wear so many hats for our children. Adding the job of taking on the structural system of one's school district is just too much."

—Jessica K. Paganis, LCSW, parent of a child with mild PDD-NOS

➤ Class sizes are smaller and more manageable. Kids will receive more 1:1 assistance. Having a teacher's aide also helps reduce the teacher : student ratio.

➤ Smaller groups and individualized lessons help children adapt and make progress.

➤ Multi-aged classrooms mean kids can learn from older kids and older kids can help the younger ones feel more comfortable in a new setting.

➤ It's less likely your child will be targeted by "mean kids,"—making her feel bad for being "different." Everyone at a specialized preschool is struggling with a unique need.

If your child *doesn't* qualify for preschool through your school district (or the district doesn't provide it), you have a couple of options:

➤ *Depending on the school, your child may qualify for itinerant speech therapy services held at the school.* For example, Kate's school offered a "walk-in speech class" for children who struggled with speech, but on a more mild level. The class met at different times throughout the week for about an hour. Students received group instruction by a qualified SLP. It was offered at no cost for families who fell within district boundaries.

> ➤ *You may also consider Montessori or Waldorf preschools.* Their educational philosophies incorporate multimodal learning, which helps with speech development. Ask specifically what the school does to foster speech and language in the classroom when you visit.

Whatever form your child's special needs preschool takes, it will be geared toward getting your little one ready for kindergarten. *The goal for your child, although she has CAS, is to be on par with her classmates by the time she reaches kindergarten.* Maybe you are thinking that's a tall order, wishful thinking, or just not going to happen, but you will be wildly amazed at the progress your child will make in the two or three years she is in preschool.

Kids Cope

Preschoolers with communication disorders are more likely to choose teachers and aides (adults) as their conversation partners than fellow students. In one study, it was found that kids with delayed expressive speech also had lower socialization skills. These kids were more likely to play with toys in unusual ways and have difficulty sharing, but were less likely to play with peers.

In my personal experience, this does seem to occur. Kids with apraxia may feel comfortable with adults because they tend to be patient, give cues, and are in a position of authority/help. Peers may not "get" the language delay and give up trying to understand kids with apraxia. However, if peers are told simple things like, *"Kelly's still learning to use her words, but she's a lot fun to play with,"* it may help open the doors to friendship. Also, it may be wise to teach and encourage kids with CAS to play nonverbal games such as "tag" or "chase."

Kindergarten

Transitioning from preschool to kindergarten can be worrisome, but most often the anxiety produced leading up to the first day is unnecessary. *Remember, if you are anxious, your child will become anxious.* Parents who are positive and optimistic about a new experience will produce happy, confident kids. Communicate your excitement and hopes to your child often.

One more tip: avoid talking about kindergarten as the "real school" or the "big school" or any other term that may negate the preschool experience. Preschool was once very real and very big to your child. Kindergarten is just the next step.

So, what's kindergarten all about, *really?* Fredrich Froebel was the German educator who "invented" kindergarten, literally meaning "child's garden." And that is exactly what a *good* kindergarten is: a vital place for kids to grow, carefully tended by knowledgeable expert gardeners (educators) who water and fertilize young minds to blossom into eager and ready lifelong learners.

Five-year-olds are busy, curious little people. It takes a skilled teacher to run a kindergarten classroom with finesse. Culturally diverse and enriched programs take into account all of the strengths, interests, needs, and cultural backgrounds of students. These curriculums offer a variety of experiences that are educational, fun, and interesting.

Besides the intellectual development (basic scientific and mathematic concepts such as problem-solving and prediction, reading and writing basics such as letter recognition and handling books), kindergartners are working on social and emotional development (sharing, cooperating, collaborating, rule following), physical development (climbing, skipping, hopping, holding pencils, manipulating puzzles and other items requiring fine motor skill), and…language development.

Notice I mention language *development*? Kindergarteners are not expected to be finished developing language. *It is still in progress.* Don't despair if your kindergartener's grammar and articulation are not perfect. The good news is, the teacher will infuse the day with speech and language-rich opportunities. Teachers explain unfamiliar words and actively introduce new ones through projects and assignments. Your kid will soak it up. Plus, the teacher will engage her students in what they are doing and thinking. Your little learner will continue to develop language skills through problem solving and idea sharing.

Is Your Child Ready for Kindergarten?

As a parent, you are going to grapple with this question as your "baby" gets closer to "K-Day." You are especially concerned because your child has CAS, and with that come some other concerns: difficulties with social skills, distractibility (*sometimes* associated with CAS), and decreased verbal skills.

It's an individual—and difficult—decision to make, to say the least. Here's what I recommend:

➤ Look into your state's requirements for admission to kindergarten, as they all vary.

➤ Consider talking with your child's SLP the summer before kindergarten to get her honest and professional opinion.

➤ If there are concerns, try some summer interventions—additional private speech therapy or working on phonics, sequencing, distractibility, etc.

➤ Consider seeing an occupational therapist (OT), who can better address some of the other concerns not completely associated with CAS. Seek out social skills classes that may be offered through your private speech clinic, or ask for recommendations from your child's pediatrician.

➤ Try "beefing up" your child's social skills by role-playing potential social encounters at home: "How do you ask a question in the classroom? Let's practice!" or "Do you know how to sit at circle time? Let's try it out here at home."

Who Are the People in Your School? Seeking Out Allies

Remember that childhood jingle "Who are the people in your neighborhood...the people that you meet each day?" Well, there are a variety of faces you will soon need to become acquainted with. Who are they?

➤ **Principal:** the head administrator of the school (sometimes called the "headmaster"). Typically a principal will have advanced educational degrees (MEd or EdD) and experience as a teacher. Make sure you introduce yourself to the principal—better yet if you're on a first-name basis. Otherwise, just make sure he or she recognizes your face.

➤ **Administrative Assistant/Principal's Secretary:** This individual has a tremendous amount of knowledge of the inner workings of the school and perhaps the district as a whole. Get to know and appreciate this person—he or she is an invaluable resource.

➤ **Support Staff:** There may be additional secretaries, teacher's assistants (sometimes called "para educators"), computer/IT personnel, and custodians and cafeteria staff in the building who assist with the day-to-day functioning of the school. Always be polite. You never know when you (or your child) may need their assistance.

➤ **Special Education Coordinator:** This individual often does assessments, recommends classroom assignments for students with special needs, and generally coordinates all of the educational needs of a child with an IEP. The role may be filled by your child's teacher, a therapist, or other school staff.

➤ **Classroom Teacher:** Teaches your child according to the district's approved curriculum, makes observations, keeps records, and evaluates your child's progress.

➤ **Classroom Aide:** Often classrooms have an aide who assists the teacher. Assistance may include helping a child use scissors, complete ADLs (activities of daily living—bathroom, wash hands, zippers, eating, etc.), stay on task, or follow directions. A classroom aide is a support staff member who works within the classroom.

➤ **Speech-Language Pathologist (SLP):** Your child with apraxia will most likely have a school-based SLP who ensures she is able to communicate appropriately in the classroom. This individual may provide group therapy, individual therapy, or even run a weekly speech group for all students. She may be your child's case coordinator, if she is not receiving special services in a classroom. The SLP, your child's teacher, or the special education coordinator will lead the IEP meeting.

➤ **Occupational Therapist (OT):** Your child may or may not have an OT. If she does, it's likely to help her improve her motor planning skills and participate in classroom activities/academics that require fine motor skills in an age-appropriate manner. OTs also assess a child's sensory needs and self-help skills. In a school setting, if your child's deficit *doesn't directly affect her ability to make progress at school*, then the OT is not permitted to work with your child on it.

➤ **Physical Therapist (PT):** Unless your child with apraxia has additional concerns and diagnoses, it's unlikely she'll have an PT. If she does, then your PT is likely to help your child improve gross motor skills such as sitting or walking. In a school setting, if your child's deficit *doesn't directly affect her ability to make progress at school*, then the PT is not permitted to work with your child on it.

➤ **Social Worker (MSW):** Most schools have a social worker or a psychologist, at least on a part-time basis. Some have both. Their job is to make sure students have someone they can talk to if they need it. The social worker can help with bullies, teacher-student conflicts, emotions and concerns, and mediation skills. Some may have special groups for kids coping with parents' divorce, or for help with socialization and peer interaction.

➤ **Psychologist (PhD):** Like a social worker, a school psychologist may be the trusted individual kids can go to if they just need to talk about a problem or a concern. A school psychologist also works with academic research, testing, and evaluation of cognitive skills (e.g., IQ tests). He or she may assist students with career placement and college entrance preparation (in high school).

➤ **School Nurse:** Usually an R.N. who administers prescribed medication, mends boo-boos, completes screenings, and maintains health and medical records. She may participate in health education, especially in upper grade levels.

➤ **Bus Driver:** See text box below on riding the bus to school. You will see the driver every day. Get to know him or her. Offer a smile and a "thanks" for the important job they do each day: assuring your child's safe travels to and from school. Your school's buses may or may not be equipped with seatbelts. There are safety harnesses available for preschoolers. Make sure to specify on the IEP that your child requires a seatbelt or harness. Likewise, you'll want to specify when or if you are comfortable removing that safety parameter. In our case, Kate felt like it was "too babyish" to be in a safety harness (car seat) when she was in kindergarten. The driver told me, "Well, it's on her IEP. If you want it changed, you have to talk to the school."

➤ **Bus Aide:** See text box on riding the bus to school.

➤ **Transportation Office/Supervisor:** Make sure you have the phone number to this office in a handy location. Don't call him or her every time the bus is five minutes late, but do call if your family is going out of town during the school year, or your child is very ill and won't be riding the bus for several days. Other reasons to call: your child no longer needs to ride in a restraint system (reached a weight/height requirement), you have concerns about the bus driver, you have concerns about the kids on the bus, or your contact number is changing.

Home Schooling Your Child

Some parents choose to home school their children for various reasons. The choice is ultimately up to you. Here's a list of potential benefits to home schooling your child with apraxia:

➤ consistency,
➤ flexibility,
➤ ability to teach coping skills with academics,
➤ less academic peer pressure,
➤ no chance your child can be bullied or made fun of,
➤ ability to incorporate speech practice into lessons,
➤ ability to use a more hands-on learning approach,
➤ ability to let your child pursue individual interests,
➤ ability to spend extra time on a weakness area without the added pressure of keeping the rest of the class engaged.

Of course, home schooling is not for every parent or child. It requires a huge time commitment from parents, not to mention organizational and time management skills, as well as patience and creativity.

A few possible downsides to homeschooling your child with apraxia:

➤ Your child may not get the socialization and communication practice with other children so desperately needed.
➤ Your child benefits only from the observation and perspective of one involved school personnel (the home-schooling parent/teacher), as opposed to many at the school level.
➤ Your child may lack age-appropriate language models and you may not recognize all of your child's delays if there aren't typically developing children to compare against.

Preparing Your Child for the First Day

Where your child is concerned, start early, but not *too* early, in prepping him for school. Be sure to drive by the school ahead of time. Point it out and get excited about the place where your child will be learning and playing. Then, a week or so later, pack a picnic and head over for lunch and some time on the playground. Your child will remember that you were there with her, so when she is playing with classmates, it won't seem so unfamiliar. Teach her how to ask others to join her in play.

The building may be big and potentially confusing. Either way, go to orientation and show your child around. Remind her that she will never be walking around the school without a teacher or parent. Take photos of your child with her teacher and the classroom and some common areas of the school (ask first). Print them out and present them to her in a little photo book. Study the photos and talk about them together. Have her carry the photo book in her backpack to look at on the bus.

Speaking of which, if your child will be riding the bus, calm those fears too, but be careful not to create new ones. Kids often worry that they will get on the wrong bus or that they won't make it home. Assure her that teachers will make sure she gets on the right bus and you will meet her at the bus stop. Kids who ride the bus are often better prepared to start the school day than if Mom and Dad do the drop off. Why? It gives kids a chance to be introspective and prepare in their own way. It also lessens the separation anxiety from you.

A final tip is to get to the local library and check out some books on going to school. Read those books periodically in the days leading up to the first day.

Other ways to prepare:

➤ *Describe the school-day routines* (get a copy of the schedule from the teacher). Discuss what happens first, where her cubby is located, the bathroom, snack, and lunch routines, and going-home procedures. Answer any questions your child may have. This helps prevent any surprises.

➤ *Make sure you attend the "sneak peek day" with your child before classes start.* Get to know people who may be able to help your child and point them out to your child. "If you ever need help being understood, look for this nice lady at the front desk. She will help you."

➤ *Practice saying these feel-good confidence boosters:*
   ● "I know you can do this!"
   ● "I trust you will do well at school."
   ● "You are very important to me."
   ● "I will always love and care for you."
   ● "If you want to talk, I will listen."
   ● My youngest daughter liked this one: "Parents always come back [for pick-up]."

➤ *Make your own Social Story about a child going to school for the first time.* It's simple. Draw pictures (or have your child draw them) and then write a brief sentence on each page about what's happening in the picture. Page one might go like this: "This is Kate. Today is her first day of school." Page two: "She is going to kindergarten. Hooray!" Go through general steps and feelings. The book should be no more than 10 pages.

➤ *Kids with CAS have special concerns, of course.* Practice saying the teacher's name several weeks before school starts (or as soon as you know it). Depending on your child's verbal skills, you can teach her how to ask others to join them in play, "I'm Kylee. Want to play?" Or offer a variation. The more you model statements like these, the more equipped your child will be to try them on her own.

➤ *Kids with CAS need to be reminded about safety identification.* By the time children reach kindergarten, it is important they know—and are able to recite—their parents' names (first and last), their address, and telephone number. In fact, many kids are unable to do this, simply because they haven't been taught. However, your child with CAS is different in that she *can't* do it. For your child's safety, consider writing her name on the inside of her clothing, or sew on labels, attach a label to her shoelaces, create a necklace she wears, or some other identification system. Folks will need to know who your child is and how to get hold of parents in an emergency. Teach your child how and where this special identification is if a "safe" adult inquires. See "Read On! Recommended Resources" at the end of this chapter.

➤ *Talk to your child about "strangers."* On the other hand, you don't want your child's personal identification broadcast to the world. Keep it as discreet as you can. Remind your child to only ask adults with a school nametag for help, or other individuals you specifically list and describe. Know, too, that schools these days are carefully monitored, but there is always the potential someone with less-than-noble intentions is lurking around.

➤ *Together, determine a special "'Twas the night before school" tradition you create for your family.* How about a family night at the ice cream stand or a back-to-school bonfire with marshmallows?

➤ *Plan a special way to say good-bye the morning of the big day.* Will you walk her to the bus stop? Drive her? Decorate the car with balloons? For other mornings, your good-bye ritual should be simple, yet meaningful for her. A quick hug and kiss and a reminder that you will be there when she gets home from school may be all she needs.

Once your little sweetie is established in her school and has found activities—and friends—she likes, *have a play date with some of her new peers.* Invite her parents and siblings, too!

Your Child on the Bus

The idea of your child riding a bus may frighten you or make you jump for joy. Likely, you're somewhere in the middle. On the one hand, it's nice *not* to have to do the drop-up and pick-up every day, especially if you have younger kids at home to care for. On the other, you could quickly morph into a high-maintenance worrywart following behind the bus to ensure its safe arrival at your child's educational institution.

Bus drivers are required by law to follow a standardized set of safety rules and guidelines. Get a copy of your school district's school bus safety policy and consider adding a few transportation and safety goals to your child's IEP.

Bus drivers hold a commercial driver's license (CDL), and must have demonstrated their skills to drive a school bus and have passed a knowledge test. They must be able to read and speak English well enough to prepare daily or weekly reports. Generally, bus drivers are at least 21 years of age, but many employers prefer them to be 24 years old or older.

Your school transportation department will likely request your child's height and weight measurements to ensure she is placed in the proper safety restraint. They will tell you about the route, the bus number, who your child's driver will be, and if there is an aide (there often is—this person greets the children at the door and helps with their belongings and gets them buckled in properly). Our aide even sang songs with the kids!

Since your child has limited verbal communication, you worry. Of course you do. Teach her to say a few things like, ***"Wait!" "I'm Here!"*** or something of that nature. **Make sure she has proper identification on or in her backpack, as described above.**

There are a lot of friendly and familiar school faces ready to greet your child when she gets off the bus. Teachers, classroom aides, SLPs, and even the principal are involved in ushering kids to their classrooms.

Riding the bus helps your child prepare for her school day (giving her a buffer between the transition of home and school), provides some down-time on the way home, and even encourages the socialization that's so important to incorporate into her day.

Preparing Yourself

And now for us parents…. Ease your fears by taking control of the things you can control. Did you read that right? *Worry about what you can control, not what you can't.* Sure, make some calls to the school if you have to, but chances are the school knows what they are doing. Make a list of all the things your child has learned to do in the past—independently. Kids are pretty amazing and resilient creatures and going to school is just another event. If you make a big deal out of it, your child will fear that school is scarier than it really is. So, have fun with the idea that your little one is going off to school and let that fun shine. Do you adore the fall clothes and shoes or maybe the smell of fresh vinyl school supplies? Make a date to take your child shopping for the essentials. She'll pick up on your excitement and feel good about the process.

On the other hand, it's perfectly normal to feel sad that your "baby" is growing up. Saying good-bye will get easier every time. It's also perfectly OK to be excited or relieved.

One more tip, parents: slow down. The days leading up to the first day of school can get hectic. There are last-minute forms to fill out, meetings to attend, school supplies to gather, and fall schedules to arrange. Kids feel this pressure too. They are fueled by your anxiety level, which may mean they rev up their own activity, resulting in problematic behaviors. Talk less, stretch out and play, sip lemonade, and hit the pool one last time.

Teaching Your Child's Teachers about Apraxia

Do you wonder what you should tell your child's teacher about apraxia? Not all teachers will have specific knowledge on *all* special needs. Kate's preschool teacher admitted that she didn't know much about apraxia, but she was very willing to learn. She knew it had something to do with verbal skills, but that was about it.

It helped a little to give Kate's teacher the scientific explanation: "It's a motor-neurological communication disorder in which she knows what she wants to say, but just can't quite get it out." What really helped was when I said, "It's like being totally exhausted and not able to carry on a conversation." She got it then. I further explained that Kate had to work really hard to have even a *simple* conversation.

Rhonda Banford, CCC-SLP, gives this explanation to parents, and you may be able to relate to it as well: "Can you wiggle your ears without touching them? Most folks will say, 'no.' I then tell them that my mother can. When I ask her how, she shrugs and just says, 'the same way I wiggle my fingers. I don't have to think about it.' I go on to tell these parents that there is no way I would know what muscles to access or even how activate them. I know what I want to do, but I just can't figure out how. That's how apraxia is—these kids know what they want to say, but they can't figure out how to make their muscles move."

Other explanations from parents you may consider adapting:
➤ "You know that feeling of being tongue-tied, or having a thought on the tip of your tongue? Well, that's how Adam feels most of the time."
➤ "Ask someone how their day was, and then tell them they can't use their words to tell you. That is what my little man faces every day," says the mother of Drew in Frankfort, IL.
➤ "Aidan has a speech disorder called Childhood Apraxia of Speech. He knows what he wants to say, but has trouble coordinating his mouth to say the words," says one Naperville, IL mom.

What's a Parent to Do?

Meet with the teacher as early in the year as possible and share with her specific information about CAS and how it affects your child. There is a fabulous **"Dear Teacher"** letter on the Apraxia-Kids website written by Sharon Gretz, M.Ed., the founder of CASANA (Childhood Apraxia of Speech Association North America). I urge parents to print it and give it to your child's teacher. You can find the letter at www.apraxia-KIDS. org. Once on the page, head to the search field, type "teacher letter." You'll get several hits, but the one you want is a letter that is downloadable in PDF format. The neat thing about this letter is it gives suggestions on how teachers can help your child at school.

While you're on the Apraxia-Kids site, look at the brochures about apraxia written with a layperson in mind. Like the "teacher letters," these brochures are downloadable and printable. Consider including one with the letter you give your child's teacher. Make it into a little "welcome to my child packet." Including a brief write-up on things about your child is very helpful, too. It doesn't have to be long or fancy, just a few bullet points like this:

- ➤ Fun, outgoing child
- ➤ Likes art and being creative
- ➤ Excels at gross motor activities
- ➤ Slow to warm up, may need to be drawn into social situations with specific questions or play
- ➤ Loves books

Of course, your descriptions may be different than mine! Now, if every parent would do something like this for their child's teachers (whether or not they have CAS), it would take a lot of guesswork out of teacher's lives.

Here are some *more tips on putting together an information packet for the teacher:*

- ➤ *Give her a book (like this one) or DVD* on Childhood Apraxia of Speech ("Hope Speaks" is available on the Apraxia-Kids website: www.apraxia-kids.org).
- ➤ *Provide a list of easy ideas* that may help with speech in the classroom (refer to Chapter 9).
- ➤ *Remind the teacher that* while your child sometimes has a hard time communicating, or takes longer than usual to respond to a question, *apraxia does not affect her intelligence.* She does not have to simplify things for your child if she only has CAS. (Of course, if she has Down syndrome, fragile X syndrome, or another disability in addition to CAS, you will want to advise her about any learning difficulties related to the other condition.)
- ➤ *Offer to create a communication notebook or worksheet that can be shared between parent and teacher.* We made worksheets on the computer. I printed out five of them Sunday night and placed them in Kate's backpack for Monday morning. Each day her teacher filled them out and sent them home with Kate. This daily report gave me some talking points for Kate about her day.

➤ *Be open and available.* In *The Complete Guide to Special Education,* authors Dr. Linda Wilmshurst and Dr. Alan Brue recommend that you keep your ears and mind open to new ideas from your child's teacher or other school professional. They typically have lots of experience and ideas in working with kids that just might help yours. If you disagree with a suggestion, ask more about it. It's part of their job to explain it.

➤ *Consider communicating some tidbits from the home front.* For example, "Papa and Nana visited this past weekend," or "Kate really enjoys the unit on frogs—ask her what we saw last night when we visited the neighborhood pond." This gives your child's teacher something to ask her about and encourages verbalization on things that are meaningful to your child's home life.

Parents Ask...

What was on your parent/teacher communication sheet?

I wanted to know who the helper was for the day, what the snack was (did she eat it? How much?), where she played, who she played with, what songs were sung, what book was read, what the speech therapist did, how verbal Kate was (I used a 10-point scale), and finally—I wanted to know what she struggled with that day (couldn't sit still during circle time, got frustrated when she practiced writing her name).

It sounds like a lot of writing for a busy teacher, but you can streamline your worksheet by providing "circle me" options. For example, the "who did she play with?" question can be a copy of the class list. The teacher can just circle the names of the students your child played with. Do the same for snacks—that is, if they have the same snacks available day after day. Or, you could say something like, "Snack today was ____. Kate ate: all   some   none ." You get the idea.

Tips for Teachers

If you are a teacher reading this, then hooray! I applaud your efforts to learn more about the kiddos in your classroom. I'd like to give you a few pointers for teaching a student with apraxia.

➤ Read the child's IEP.

➤ *If parents challenge your knowledge, make special requests, or argue for a special IEP meeting, remind them that you are on their side and please don't take it personally.* As parents, we just want the very best for our children and we might get a little passionate about it.

➤ *Communicate privately with parents and never in front of other classmates,* unless it is to give really good praise that will make your student feel proud. These kids often *know* they can't communicate as effectively as their peers and they may feel a bit defensive about it. Help build their self-esteem in every opportunity you can find.

➤ **Give parents advice and insight you learned from teaching their child.** For example, "Kate did a great job teaching another student about how we sit at Circle Time. She loves to be in the helper role." Parents love to hear praise and stories about their child doing well.

➤ **You may need to do a bit more "pre-teaching" when working with a child with CAS.** Let her hear and practice vocabulary words ahead of time (send them home in backpack with a letter to parents indicating the upcoming unit).

➤ **You might need to work a bit harder to engage a student with apraxia in group activities.** Don't take it personally if she doesn't respond right away (or at all); just keep trying.

➤ **Each day is a new beginning.** What this student struggled with yesterday could be a nonissue today. Please don't hold grudges.

➤ **Be sure you give your students with CAS lots of praise.** It helps their confidence level and self-esteem. While you're at it, praise her parents, too. They're working really hard all day, every day, to help their child.

➤ **Relate something special about your student to the parents.** I can't tell you how happy it made me to receive an out-of-the-blue email from our teacher saying something like, "Kate was really cute today in class when she started dancing and singing, 'Mama Mia!'" Small accomplishments mean a lot to us parents.

➤ **Respond to parents in one way or another (phone, email, "I'll get back to you later"), even if you don't have an answer.** Parents do not like feeling like they have been forgotten.

➤ **Realize that we all get burned out.** Parents need encouragement and motivation, just like teachers. If we can encourage one another, then all the better!

Parent Involvement at School

There's one more aspect of sending your child to school we should cover before jumping into the nitty-gritty school stuff like speech, IEPs, and all of those other intimidating acronyms. It's called parent involvement.

Studies show that parents who are *actively* involved in their child's education promote kids who enjoy school more, get better grades, and don't have as many behavior problems. Tons and tons of research point to parent involvement as the #1 predictor of a child who does well in school. (It's actually *not* natural intelligence, parent education, or income, although those things do *influence* a child's education).

What's a Parent to Do?

It may be as simple as helping your child with her science fair project, brainstorming with her on her essay about "what I did this summer," or reading aloud from a book each night before bed. You don't have to be the fundraiser chairperson or run the school carnival to make a difference. Little things add up. Volunteer in the library once every couple of weeks, go to literacy night, attend parent-teacher conferences, or work the book fair for a two-hour window. We're all busy, and yes, you have your plate especially full with speech therapy and CAS-related issues, but if you are serious about your child's education, I urge you to get out there.

Here are a couple of points to remember:

➤ *Your involvement boosts teacher morale.* When they see you take an active role at school, they feel more valued.

➤ *Kids develop better social skills*—and isn't that the whole idea, especially with our children with CAS?

➤ *Kids feel supported and valued when Mom and Dad walk into their place of learning.* This develops kids' sense of self, thus increasing self-esteem and confidence.

➤ *You will benefit, too.* It's empowering to be a part of your child's school day. You'll feel more confident in the lay-out of the building, plus gain confidence in parenting and educating your children.

➤ For more information and helpful tips, see www.SchoolFamily.com.

Should You Volunteer in the Classroom?

Volunteering in the classroom offers a fantastic opportunity to see what happens there each day—a plus for parents of kids who aren't able to communicate well. But Dr. Linda Wilmshurst and Dr. Alan Brue point out a few caveats in *The Complete Guide to Special Education*. First, keep in mind that young kids who have a tendency to be clingy may find your classroom volunteering difficult. Your child may expect to see you in the classroom every day, even if it's only Wednesdays that you volunteer. Also, she may not perform as well because she just wants to play with you. Know your child and anticipate how she may react if you choose to volunteer.

Talking about CAS with Your Child's Classmates

Here's another way to increase your involvement at school, help your child, her classmates, and her teacher at the same time: go into your child's classroom and give a little lesson or presentation about CAS. This works well for kids in pre-K through 3rd grade. It's easy and you don't have to be a professional speaker to do it.

First, check with the teacher and establish a good day and time. Plan to be in the classroom for twenty minutes or so. With your teacher's permission (run it by your child, too), get started with your lesson plan.

You might consider reading *My Brother is Very Special* by Amy Glorosio-May, or *I Want to be Your Friend* by Angela Baublitz. Both authors share intimate feelings and experiences their own children with CAS experienced as a way to teach other kids about the disorder. Bring along copies of the *What You Should Know about CAS* (as mentioned earlier in the chapter) and type up a brief letter for kids to take home to parents indicating why you were in the classroom and what you told their children.

The lesson might focus on strengths and weaknesses: "What are you good at? What are you not so good at?" Make a list on the whiteboard. Depending on their age, most kids will think of things they are personally good at. Turn the table and ask students about their classmates: "What is _____ (say a child's name) good at?" They may or may not know.

Introduce yourself as your child's parent. Explain that you are in school because you want to tell them what your child is good at and not so good at. Start with the good. Make a list. See if others can identify what she does well. Your goal is to let others see your sweetie as any other "regular" kid. Then tell them about apraxia. Start with a simple explanation: "She knows what she wants to say; it just takes her longer. She has a hard time getting the words out."

Let them ask questions. Do your best to answer. You might even ask if the kids have noticed your child leaving the classroom at times (to attend speech therapy). Do they know why? Ask if the kids have any ideas on how they can make your child's day easier. I'll bet they do. The apraxia lesson you present to the classroom will hit on things like diversity, sensitivity, and self-esteem.

Give yourself a pat on the back! It takes guts to go into the school and talk with a bunch of kids—your child's peers—about something so close and personal to you.

Having Your Child Explain Apraxia to Her Classmates

Now that Kate is in first grade, I haven't found it necessary to go to her school to talk about apraxia. But, one day her class was discussing similarities and differences, in response to a reading comprehension activity. Kate announced that she had apraxia and proceeded to ask if anyone else had apraxia. According to Kate, everyone shook their head. She related that they asked what apraxia was, but she was unable to tell them. When I probed further, she said, "Mom, I couldn't get the words out. I didn't know what to tell them about apraxia." Well, if you are chuckling right now as I am—then you understand the irony of this example. Later we came up with a plan: "You can just tell them it's hard to talk sometimes," and we also agreed that apraxia is sort of a private thing that we don't have to share with the entire classroom.

Speech at School

Make friends with your child's school SLP. Get her contact information and use it. Consider giving her hand-outs and a letter (see "Teaching Your Teacher about Apraxia").

Let her know you are available to answer any other questions about your child. Even though her expertise is in speech and language problems, she may not be an expert in CAS. Like your child's classroom teacher, she may need a little tutorial in "Apraxia 101."

Your child's IEP (see next section) will indicate how many minutes a week your child is to receive speech services. It may be 60 minutes or 90 minutes—maybe as many as 120. If you get more than 60, consider yourself lucky. I know it sounds kind of puny, compared to the hour or more you might receive two to three times a week in a private setting, but school is a different beast.

The school is required only to provide a free appropriate public education (FAPE) to children who qualify for special education. What that really means is "adequate" and not "superior" or even "really good." Schools really have no standard they are to meet (you'll see this in variations from district to district), so that puts the responsibility back into parents' hands. We have to be proactive and advocate for services that are in our child's best interests.

Although your child may not receive as many minutes of therapy as you would like, bear in mind that CAS is best remediated in numerous short sessions, rather than one long session. Short, intensive sessions five days a week are preferable to one long session once a week. The key is "intensive," meaning lots of intervention and plenty of practice.

What you probably want is for the SLP to come into the classroom, smile and wink at your little precious, and motion for her to come to speech room for a full hour of uninterrupted therapy. Unfortunately, that's probably not going to happen. Your child will miss way too much of general classroom instruction (days in preschool and kindergarten are short—an hour away is too long), not to mention the SLP has a busy caseload.

A more likely scenario is this: your child and one to three peers (also with speech or language delays or disorders) are pulled out to work with each other and the school SLP for 20 minutes or so. That counts toward your child's 60 minutes a week. The SLP may also come into the classroom a couple of times a week to work with the class as a whole. She might do some verbal exercises and games, read a book, or something of that nature. This counts, too. In addition, your child *may* receive a private session with the SLP if she has goals that can't be worked on in a group.

With that in mind, it's not a bad idea to give the school SLP a few tips that will help his or her time with your child be as productive as possible. Type out a list of things that you and your private SLP have done that have been particularly successful. Sign any releases between the school and your child's speech clinic so the two therapists can communicate. Please ask, if they don't offer. Our private therapist even made a school visit. Ask if yours will, too. The goal is to get both therapists working on the same skills, or at least working together so that skills your child is learning from one therapist are easily transferred to the other setting.

Our school SLP did a fabulous job of keeping parents in the loop. She sent home a weekly speech newsletter describing what she did with the kids (even if it was whole group work) and suggestions to try at home. Since Kate received some pull-out therapy, too, she'd often email me with progress Kate made, or she'd tell me directly when she saw me pass through the school. Ask your school SLP what communication style would work best for her. Perhaps you can develop a special speech notebook that you can pass back and forth? Or perhaps you can designate a weekly or daily email schedule.

As you get more comfortable (and confident) with your child's school day and SLP, the communication may dwindle. Don't take it personally. At the same time, your child's speech is improving and she just might be able to share some of these things with you on her own!

Kids Cope

"Now that Aidan is in kindergarten [and no longer the speech-intensive preschool], he wonders why he is sometimes singled out to go to speech therapy. I think it kind of bothers him."

What can you tell your child who asks why she needs speech and the other kids don't? Remember, no two individuals are alike. Telling your child this is often a good place to start. Keep the conversation positive and as light-hearted as you can: "We all have things we need extra help with. It's no big deal." If you know the other children in the class, you may be able to use them as an example: "Erica gets reading help and Chris needs extra help with math."

You may be interested in reading Ronda Wojcicki's book, **Speech Class Rules**, with your child (best suited for ages 4-8). It's a great picture book designed by a school-based SLP in which speech therapy is introduced in a kid-friendly, "cool" manner (The Speech Place Publishing, 2007).

Individualized Educational Programs (IEPs)

We've been alluding to IEPs throughout the book, but what exactly *is* one? In short, it is a written document that all children who qualify for special services under the Individuals with Disabilities Education Act receive. The IEP document is developed by parents, therapists, teachers, and other school staff during an IEP meeting.

An IEP is a legally binding contract between the school and your family. It lays out:

1. What your child's qualifying disability is (in this case, a speech-language disorder called Childhood Apraxia of Speech, though there may be other diagnoses you child is also struggling with).
2. Your child's present level of functioning (this is where assessment results are reported—are her receptive language skills at the level of a six-year-old, while her expressive language skills are at the level of a four-year-old?)
3. What goals the IEP team thinks she should work on, over and above what is covered in the regular school curriculum (does she need specific

244 ■ Off to School

goals related to expanding the length of her sentences? related to being able to respond to another child's greetings? Does she need goals related to bringing her reading skills up to grade level?).

4. What special services ("related services") your child needs to help her reach those goals and make progress in the general education curriculum (speech therapy, occupational therapy, social skills group, special education instruction).

5. What accommodations and modifications your child needs to access the general education curriculum. (See below for definitions.)

6. Where your child should receive the instruction and therapy she needs (should she receive all her instruction and therapy in the classroom? leave the classroom for 30 minutes a week for speech therapy?).

7. How the school will monitor your child's progress and report that progress to you.

8. Who will provide your child's speech therapy. You may assume it's the school speech-language pathologist (SLP), but that may not always be the case. Look at your IEP very closely. If it reads that speech services should be provided by the SLP, then that is a "good thing" (legally correct and legitimate). But, *if* your child's IEP says speech language services will be provided by "SLP/Staff," "SPED staff," "special education staff," or a "speech language assistant," then your child *may* receive speech therapy from an untrained, unlicensed individual, including substitutes, aides and paraprofessionals, or any staff member willing to do speech therapy. They are not licensed by your state Department of Education, nor are they accredited by the American Speech-Language-Hearing Association (ASHA). *Make sure your child's IEP states that speech therapy will be provided by an SLP.*

Note that the school is not required to develop an IEP that will "cure" your child's apraxia as quickly as possible, or provide everything you think would help her reach her potential. *The school is only required to provide services to allow your child to "access the curriculum" and not to perfect his or her speech.*

Whoa…what does this mean, exactly? It means that schools want our kids with CAS to be able to participate in classroom activities and to be intelligible. And if your child has another disability in addition to apraxia, the IEP will address how your child can "access the curriculum" and participate in classroom activities despite that disability—but not necessarily to "fix" every single difficulty your child has.

You will be able to propose the goals that will help your child "access the curriculum" and participate in classroom activities. A possible preschool goal may be:

➤ Connor will use a variety of means to request items and actions within the classroom (e.g., signs, single words, two-word phrases, pictures, and gestures) 80% of the time, which will be evidenced in quarterly data charting by teacher observation.

Another might be:

> ➤ Angela will verbally approximate the words for common objects within the classroom setting in the following categories: food, classroom items, toys, and actions *without* a model with 80% accuracy. This will be measured by teacher observation and charted quarterly.

You will also get to discuss and agree upon the **least restrictive environment (LRE)** for your child. This means the classroom setting where she will have the maximum contact with typically developing children while still being able to meet her individual goals. For most children with CAS in kindergarten and above, the LRE will be the regular education classroom in the neighborhood school. For children with additional disabilities such as learning disabilities, Down syndrome, or autism, the LRE may be a combination of the regular classroom plus time spent in a resource room to receive extra help in some academic areas.

Every year, you will be expected to attend a new IEP meeting to discuss your child's progress and re-discuss all the issues above, setting new goals, rehashing the LRE, determining what related services and accommodations and modifications are needed. You can also request an IEP meeting at any time you think one is needed.

Parents Ask...

What's the Difference between an Accommodation and a Modification?

> ➤ An *accommodation* is a change to the way information is presented to your child, the way your child responds to that information, or the setting where your child learns. Accommodations do not affect the content of what she is learning. For example, if your child can't respond orally to the teacher's questions about days of the week, she might be given written words or pictures to use to respond instead. If your child is having trouble paying attention, she might be seated near the teacher's desk.

> ➤ A *modification* is a change in the content of what a child is learning. For example, if a child struggles with spelling, she might be given a list of easier words to learn each week than the rest of the class.

Prior Written Notice

Before we get into the heart of IEPs, I'd like to introduce you to a term you will likely encounter on your special education journey: **Prior Written Notice (PWN).** Perhaps one of the most overlooked, yet powerful tools for parents to keep in their special needs tool box, PWN requires the school district to provide written notice and explanation of any changes—even proposed changes—to your child's IEP. The school is also required to send you prior written notice before your child's very first IEP meeting—which will probably happen either when she is transitioning out of early intervention, or when you ask for her to be evaluated before kindergarten.

These changes can include your child's identification as a student who requires special services, notice of evaluation techniques to be used, or changes in educational placement within the school, among others that may affect the school's ability to provide FAPE (free-appropriate public education).

PWN forces educators to stop, think, and write things down. It's assurance that their decision is not just an off-the-cuff remark or decision. It's formal and meaningful. PWN provides a written history of exchanges between the school and family, resulting in a paper trail that cannot be denied.

PWN works both ways. Parents can and should write down (typing is best) their questions, complaints, compliments, and requests for clarification regarding their child's education. If you want a written response, start with a written request. This is exactly why you should know about and use PWN. Of course, you'll want to keep copies of all of the written communication between you and the school, no matter how big or small the comment (more on organizing later in this chapter).

Parents Share...

What happened with our family

It was the beginning of the school year for Kate (early October). She had completed one full year of special education with an IEP plus Extended School Year (more on that at the end of the chapter). She had just started in a new classroom with a new teacher. Her new SLP stopped me in the hall one day and told me that she thought Kate was doing great and needed a reassessment.

I was dumbfounded. We had just started private OT and Kate was continuing with private speech therapy as well. I didn't like what the school SLP was implying—that Kate no longer qualified for services. The SLP continued: "I'll be sending home a letter with Kate indicating what we are seeing and have you sign it." Ah ha—that's the PWN! I could have *not* signed it. But after reading the large packet of information, I agreed that Kate probably did need a reassessment. After all, she *had* made a lot of progress. After Kate was reevaluated and the treatment team met with us, Kate's IEP was discontinued, as were her speech services at school. I was told that Kate's apraxia was not affecting her progress in the classroom, though her speech was certainly *not* perfect. We celebrated the accomplishment with dinner out and a scooter Kate had been eyeing for some time. Yes, the event was filled with uncertainty and emotion, but in the long run, I'm glad things worked out as they did.

Advice about IEP Meetings

Be Prepared! Do not just show up for your child's IEP meeting expecting the school staff to handle the whole process without any input from you. Here are some guidelines in prepare for the meeting:

1. Ask if you can see any assessment results the school has done *before* the meeting and then review the report so you have a good picture of your child's strengths and needs.
2. Ask your child's teacher(s) and therapist(s) to tell you what goals they are considering for your child. (In some school systems it is common for staff to go into the meeting with preliminary goals already written down. If so, ask to see these preliminary goals before the meeting.)
3. If the teachers and therapists haven't written goals about something you think is important, try your hand at writing your own. Share them with the staff before the meeting if you want their input; if not, bring them to the meeting to discuss.
4. If you think your child needs a service she isn't presently receiving, or needs more of a service she is receiving, try to articulate *why* so you can advocate for the service at the meeting. Has she fallen further behind? Failed to achieve goals set for her in the last IEP? Been bullied or become depressed due to her speech difficulties?
   - If this isn't your child's first IEP, read and review IEP progress reports, which should be sent home throughout the school year. Keep them and compare them. Bring them to the meeting, along with other supporting documents (more later on organizing the boatload of paper you have for your child).
5. Educate yourself about the IEP process. Research IEPs from trusted sources. You may want to spend some time reading *From Emotions to Advocacy* by Pam and Pete Wright, both of whom are adjunct law professors at William and Mary Law School. Together they have written several books, built websites, and have a blog. Their website is professional and helpful. Check it out at www.wrightslaw.com. Another good resource that has stood the test of time is *Negotiating the Special Education Maze* by Winifred Anderson, Stephen Chitwood, Deirdre Hayden, and Cheri Takemoto.

Do Some Classroom Reconnaissance

One parent I was in contact with while writing this book suggested that one of the best things a parent of a child with an IEP can do is to spend an entire school day observing their child at school. Look at academics, socialization, scheduling, distractions, and how your child fits into the microcosm of school—or doesn't. Then make sure all your concerns about your child's functioning in any of these areas are addressed during the IEP meeting. That said, it's still a big time commitment for a busy parent to make—but doing so just may help your child's school experience.

Pointers on Writing and Evaluating Goals

An IEP is a blueprint for your child's education. It should address your child's needs related to academics and social and physical functioning. Deficits (such as in speech) are identified and annual goals are made by breaking things down into manageable steps.

Please note: *Only goals that the SLP or teacher feels the child can achieve in a year are written.* If the child achieves the goals sooner, new ones can be written. It is better to write achievable goals than goals your child has little chance of meeting, no matter how much you may want your child to accomplish them.

As a parent, your job is to **make sure goals are meaningful to your child, specific, measurable, and attainable.** Merely writing "Kate will learn to talk" as a goal is laughable. What will you do to get her to talk? How much talking is enough? How will we know if she's making progress? What incentives are in place to push her along? Granted, you probably won't see this written as a formal goal in an IEP, but you get the gist. A better goal is something along these lines:

> ➤ "Kevin will imitate 1- to 2-word phrases to comment within the classroom." (If Kevin needs a certain type of prompt or model to imitate phrases, that should be noted in the goal as well.)

Teachers are well trained at "catching students being good," and often praise or otherwise acknowledge their attempts. It may work for some children to receive a sticker or token as an incentive and as a way to measure their own progress. Be sure you mention to your child's teacher what may help with your little one's progress.

Remember to separate the forest from the trees. The IEP is the trees; your child's overall education is the forest. If you are trying to figure out goals to propose for your child, ask yourself, Where do you want your child to be educationally? Work backwards from that ending point. What baby steps does your child need to get a "Ph.D. in Linguistics?" Get those skills in the IEP as early as possible.

Make sure goals are addressing meaningful progress. OK, your little one is talking more. But is she speaking *well*? How are her pragmatics and social skills? Can she effectively ask others to join her in play? Does she know how to stand up for herself?

Pointers on Participating in the IEP Meeting

It's overwhelming and intimidating to go into the meeting with a bunch of folks from the school staring at you. *Bring support*—your spouse, a friend, and/or your private SLP. Consider asking a third-party special needs advocate to go with you (they usually charge for their services). Don't go alone.

Be familiar with the terminology they may use. If the teachers and staff use words you don't know like "benchmark," "goal-directed," "outcome oriented results," ask what these things mean to you in plain English.

Don't just sit there. You are an active member of the IEP team. Did someone say something you don't agree with? Speak up—diplomatically, of course. You don't want to wait until after the meeting to express concerns.

Bring up everything that concerns you about your child's education and progress with communication skills. That includes such topics as making friends and preventing meltdowns.

When I was practicing nursing, it was drilled into us, "if it wasn't charted, it wasn't done." Even if I knew I did something for a patient, but I didn't chart it in the medical record, there was no proof I had done it. *Get it in writing,* no matter how small the request, idea, or action seems.

Make sure you have read all of the forms and double-checked all of the boxes. If the boxes are pre-checked that you agree with something that you don't (sometimes they are), then DON'T SIGN it. Add to the existing paperwork that you don't agree with something you see. Sign or initial it. Then ask for a clean copy and set a date for another meeting in the near future.

Afterwards, give yourself a special treat. Stop for ice cream on the way home or pick up a magazine. While you're at it, consider giving your child an extra-special treat, too. After all, she's the one who really deserves a job well-done.

Tech-y Tools to Help

Just when you thought technology couldn't get more individualized, there's a new iPhone app[lication] offered from the Parent Education Advocacy Training Center (PEATC) called the "IEP checklist." It comes in English or Spanish and helps tech-y parents become better informed and gain easier access to school-related goals. For more information, to see it in action via YouTube, or for a free download, go to www.peatc.org/peatc.cgim?template=IEPChecklistiPhone.

Transitioning from Elementary School to Middle School or Junior High

If your child still needs an IEP when she is getting ready to transition out of elementary school, you will want to make sure everything in the document is up-to-date and ready to go from day one.

Valle Dwight, a parent and disability writer, lists these pointers in her article "Getting Off to the Right Start: Ten Tips to Make Sure Your Child's IEP is Ready":

➤ *Meet early.* Meet with your preteen's team before school even starts so you can hash out the details of the IEP. Keep it casual, and remember, this meeting sets the tone for future conversations.

➤ *Talk to your child.* Ask, "What worked for you last year? What didn't? What changes would you like to see?"

➤ *Go to the pros.* Get to know other parents who have walked this road before. Parents of older kids can be a great resource, if you know where to find them. Start with your neighbors.

➤ *Make it stand out.* Make copies of the IEP on brightly colored paper for all of the teachers, even the P.E. teacher—emphasize how important it is to read it (you'd be surprised).

➤ *Check in.* Schedule a meeting a few weeks after school has started to chat with your child's homeroom teacher or school counselor. See if he or she has any questions about your child's IEP now that he or she has gotten to know her a bit. Tell your child's teacher how she learns best, offer to answer questions about CAS, and suggest ways to help.

➤ *Make a plan.* Set up a communication system with the teacher(s) or counselor to stay in touch with daily concerns, homework, behavioral issues, or social skills. Many folks do this over email. You can make a habit of checking in the first of the month, or if a problem or change should occur. Whatever you decide, stick to it. Be persistent but polite!

Filing a Complaint about Your Child's IEP

Remember, most teachers and SLPs just want the best for your child, but they have to work within parameters you may not know about. Be sure to ask why they are proposing something if you do not agree with it.

With that in mind, you do have the right to file a complaint if you still don't agree with something the IEP team has done. If services were decreased or changed in any way without your knowledge or you don't agree with the change in services or if you disagree with where your child is receiving her services, then you absolutely have the right to address it. (However, in some states, IEP teams are allowed to make changes without the parent's permission—as long as it is not the first IEP.)

Here are the steps in filing a complaint:

➤ *Send a letter by certified mail or with a receipt.* Better yet, hand-deliver. To whom should you address your letter? That depends on what kind of complaint you are filing. If you are just not happy with a decision the school has made, then make sure it gets into the hands of the Director of Special Education at the school district. If the school has broken a law, file a complaint with the state for noncompliance. To cover your bases, go ahead and send a copy to both the school and the state.

➤ *Each state differs in this process.* Visit your state's Department of Education website, look for a contact number, call them up, and ask about your state's mediation process or how to initiate a due process proceeding. The Wright's Law website has some good information and articles on due process hearings: www.wrightslaw.com/info/dp.index.htm.

➤ *Some states will want you to start with a mediation process.* You and the school staff will meet with a mediator (without lawyers) to present your sides of the issue and the mediator will try to get you and the school to reach a compromise. Generally, it's the "nice" way to go, and hopefully you and the school can settle on a compromise.

➤ Otherwise, *you might have to go ahead with due process.* A due process hearing takes place in a courtroom with both sides using lawyers to present evidence, calling upon witnesses, etc. It can be extremely expensive and emotionally draining for parents. Each state has an advocate to guide you (the parent) through the process. They will help you understand the law and your rights.

➤ *The state will take procedural violations (violations of the right to FAPE and LRE) very seriously.*

➤ *You'll need to include evidence*—so review and include bits and pieces of your child's educational records, as well as speech therapy progress notes.

➤ **Check in periodically**—but don't be a pest—to make sure things are being monitored and implemented. You may have to do this as the due process case is underway; but continue to check in with your child's school after the case is over.

Parents Ask...

How can the iPad and iPhone help my child with CAS?

Technology can be a blessing and a curse. But the parents I've heard from *love* the benefits an iPhone and iPad bring. One mom I know was so pleased the first time her son took his iPad to [speech] therapy and "read" an interactive story with his speech-language pathologist. Another mother notes that the iPad was less frustrating for her son because the large size makes fewer demands on fine motor skills. Still another parent says that her son *loves* his, and was thrilled that an AAC specialist came to school to help find more apps for her son to use during peer play within the classroom.

   If you are brave enough to venture into the ever-growing world of technology, then I urge you to look into a program called *TouchChat*, adapted for iPhone/iPad by Nancy Inman (creator of *WordPower* and *Picture WordPower*). Go to www.silver-kite.com/touchChat for more information.

   One Place for Special Needs founder Dawn Villarreal has put together this comprehensive list of apps that may help your child with communication, among other concerns. It just may give you more information than you bargained for! Find it at: www.oneplaceforspecialneeds.com/main/library_special_needs_apps.html (link shared with permission from One Place for Special Needs).

Organizing All of That School-related Paperwork

There are mounds of papers and emails and all kinds of stuff you'll need to keep straight when your child is enrolled in school. Don't rely on your own brain to make sense of it all. What you need is a *system*. If you don't have one in place yet, it's time.

Don't put this off too long, like I did, or you'll really feel overwhelmed when you do get around to it. Pick a system that you will use. You don't need anything cute or fancy.

Here are some ideas to consider, keeping in mind that you will need both an electronic and "real" file:

➤ A large 3-ring binder, 2- to 3-inch size (my personal favorite)
➤ Filing cabinet with carefully labeled hanging file folders
➤ An expanding file
➤ A word-processing program on your computer with a special folder for all letters and correspondence specific to your child's apraxia-related issues
➤ A folder in your email account for your child's speech therapy emails (cc yourself so you always have a copy of what you send), and another folder for your child's school communications
➤ Ask for your child's IEP to be emailed to you, and also ask for a paper copy. You can easily send the digital copy to private SLPs or access it if you misplace your hard copy.
➤ Put your system in an area where you will see it and use it. (What good is a really great filing system if you can't find it or have to climb into the crawl space to get to it?)

You'll soon be receiving lots of school-related documents—newsletters, progress reports, sample pieces of art work or assignments. Some items don't require keeping. If you have decided to use the binder method, lightly mark each "save-able" piece of paper that comes out of your child's backpack with the full date written in pencil. Pop the papers in the binder in chronological order. What's on the top page of the binder will be the oldest document and the bottom page will be the most recent, that way your binder reads like a book. You can look back on the binder as a way to measure progress.

Avoid using staples or page protectors; they just cause confusion and delay. Even dividers can slow things down. What you can do is use those nifty little page tabs that stick to paper (but can be removed easily) for pieces of paper you want ready access to (like the most recent IEP).

Avoid writing directly on the papers in your binder. Use a sticky note if you must. You never know when you'll need to make a photocopy or scan that document. You wouldn't want the name and number of the pizza place you ordered from last weekend to appear on a letter you are sending to your child's speech clinic, would you? Questions, comments, and thoughts you have about particular document also go on the sticky note. Once you get answers to your questions, remove the sticky and move on.

Wrightslaw has some great suggestions for making your binder work for you. Head to their website, www.wrightslaw.com, or look for a copy of their book, *From Emotions to Advocacy*.

Parents Ask...

Do you combine school and private speech into one binder?

That's up to you. I combined ours into one mega-binder (that's where I used dividers) and dubbed it, "Kate's School and Speech Binder." I kept everything in there, even the receipts from private therapy and EOBs from our insurance company. It cost little to nothing to create and maintain.

You may appreciate *"An IEP Toolkit,"* a binder system that can help you get all of those school papers organized, which can be purchased at www.organized4kids.com.

How Does Special Education Work in Private Schools?

Private schools vary in their ability and willingness to accommodate children with developmental or learning differences because they aren't given funds or guidelines from the state. They are also not required to provide a free and appropriate education in the least restrictive environment for children with disabilities, as public schools are required by IDEA to do.

Things worth asking your prospective private school about:

➤ Are there other students with learning/developmental differences?

➤ What special accommodations do they currently have? What other changes is the school willing and able to make to ensure the best learning environment for students with special needs?

➤ Is there a care team, tutoring team, or group of therapists and specialists available? If so, are their services included in tuition?

Keep in mind that *every* child is entitled to receive any therapies/support services they are found eligible for. However, *where* those therapies are given can vary from district to district and state to state. Some school districts may be willing to send therapists to a private school, day care, or other educational facility to give therapies. In this case, you will need to consider and discuss with teachers and administrators the impact of removing your child from her daily schedule at the private school to receive the services from the public school specialists. In many other instances, you need to take your child to a public school district facility to receive "itinerant" or "walk-in" services. (These services may be during normal school hours, or possibly after school. Often public school employees are restricted from entering any "faith-based" educational setting, and often they are not allowed to travel outside district boundaries.)

Even if your child does not attend the public school for her main educational needs she will need an IEP if you opt for her to receive *any* services through the public school.

Receiving Supports for CAS in Private School

"Since my daughter's Pre-K program is both faith-based and outside our district boundaries, she receives itinerant services at one of the district's early childhood centers. If she were to continue needing speech therapy into kindergarten or beyond, her services would likely be given at an elementary school."

—a St. Louis mom of a daughter with CAS

"We went from a public school to a private Lutheran school. I was extremely worried about support in the classroom. The private school is working hard to accommodate children with special needs. We attended orientations, open houses, anything that would help familiarize [my son] with the school. The director of Special Services had us do a walk thru of Zach's day the day before classes began. That helped immensely."

—a mother of a son with CAS

School Is Hard

I wish I had better news, but studies have documented that there are relationships between early speech-language problems such as CAS and reading/writing difficulties. Researchers have proposed a few theories for this connection:

➤ **Theory #1:** Kids who aren't making many sounds (or saying the ones they do have correctly) don't have a very good mental/visual representation of the sounds. Without this, they have a harder time developing the sound-letter correspondence that helps them sound out the words they are reading and writing.

If you believe this is to be the case for your child, I highly recommend the *Jolly Phonics* program for teaching sound-letter correspondence. It's systematic, sequential, research-based, and multisensory. The program incorporates a body movement piece to learning the sounds as well, which we know by now is huge for these little people with apraxia. If your school doesn't use Jolly Phonics, consider buying their products for home use at www.jollylearning.com.

➤ **Theory #2:** Kids who have speech-language disorders have difficulty reading and understanding symbols (think about it: letters are a pretty abstract way of representing sounds). This could translate into having a difficulty with manipulating numbers and symbols in math as well.

➤ **Theory #3:** Kids with apraxia have "differently-wired" brains. Speech is one area of the brain that is affected, but other areas that contribute to learning might also be affected. This theory might explain why not all kids with CAS have the same strengths and needs: their wires are all connected uniquely.

Reading, (W)riting, and 'Rithmetic—The Three R's

Reading might be hard for your little one with apraxia. In fact, it's hard for *many* kids. The next chapter gives some specific suggestions for helping your child at home and school. But since this chapter is on school, and reading is a big part of school, I want to give you a brief overview.

In the U.S., kids are typically taught to read in kindergarten or first grade. You can start preparing your preschooler by reading to her every day, teaching her the alphabet and the sounds the letters make, and playing word and rhyming games. The idea is to get her comfortable with written language. Your child with apraxia may also have difficulty reading aloud because she skips the smaller, supportive words in a sentence—it's as though the brain doesn't register them. (*If your child has fallen significantly behind in literacy skills, it's time to look for a reading specialist. Chapter 12 covers specific reading programs.*)

One resource to consider is the Riggs Institute of Reading (www.riggsinst.org), along with Jolly Phonics, mentioned in the section above.

Handwriting is hard for kids with apraxia, too. No surprise there. Letter recognition, plus the motor planning piece of getting from brain to hand to paper, can be difficult due to the underlying neuro-motor issues of apraxia. What can you do? Ask if the program *Handwriting without Tears* is an option for your child at school. It may need to be done with a school-based OT (if there is one and your child qualifies). Otherwise, you can work with her on handwriting at home with some of the *Handwriting Without Tears* products you can find on-line at www.hwtears.com. The earlier you correct those handwriting mistakes, the better off your child will be as academics get more and more challenging. Note: Some children with CAS also have limb apraxia, which makes the motor aspects of writing very challenging.

Math: Kids with apraxia *may* have difficulty with mathematics because symbols (numbers) represent even more abstract concepts. Plus, it takes a whole new set of vocabulary words such as addition, subtraction, and factor. In addition, it's hard to draw from real-life experiences when the language of math is so obtuse (another math word)!

Kids with apraxia may also have difficulty sequencing (even following two-step directions from parents and teachers can be tricky) and that makes it especially hard to assess and apply problem-solving skills to mathematical problems.

Note that not everyone believes that CAS can be intertwined with math difficulties. According to Rhonda Banford, CCC-SLP, "In my experience, most kids with CAS do not have trouble with math; in fact it may be a strength!" Remember kids with CAS are all unique.

Please don't get the wrong idea about CAS. There is no reason to expect that apraxia will *most definitely* cause difficulty with math! I present this to you so you can keep a watchful eye on your child's mathematical skills.

What's a Parent to Do?

There are lots of programs and curricula for teaching math. Find out what your school uses. In the mean time, you may consider looking at *Everyday Math* for some inspiration and tips: www.everydaymathonline.com. Its educational philosophy is to teach students to play with numbers, suggesting a variety of methods of correctly solving the problem, hoping your child will pick the option that "fits" her best. You might prefer another program called *Math U See* (www.mathusee.com), which was developed by a former math teacher for homeschooling and special ed students. It's clear, systematic, and multisensory.

Another simple thing you can do at home to help your child with sequencing is to practice digit spans (remembering increasingly long series of numbers) for "fun." What you do is this: go on a little walk and say, "I am thinking of three numbers: 3...6...4. Do you "see" those numbers in your mind?" Then quiz your child on what those numbers were. Did she remember? Did she get them in the correct order (sequence)? You may need to start with just two numbers. Once your child can repeat the sequence correctly, add in another digit. Mix it up. Have your child quiz you.

Why bother? It's a fun game to do while you pass the time on a family walk, in a waiting room, or in the car. Plus, if you are practicing while you and your child are doing something active (jumping on the trampoline, walking, swinging), you are activating that vestibular system that is so important in speech development *and* sneaking in a little exercise. Your child will be none the wiser. Well, actually she *will* be: she'll be able to sequence better!

If your child is struggling with mathematical concepts, you may be interested in checking out these research-based programs (which is just a sampling, in alphabetical order):

- ➤ *Addition the Fun Way* (www.citycreek.com): The creators want kids to know that "math is a story to be told," so there are books, music, and even coloring pages in which addition facts are worked into stories intended to make those facts easier to learn.
- ➤ *Everyday Math* (www.everydaymathonline.com): Their educational philosophy is to teach students to play with numbers, suggesting a variety of methods of correctly solving the problem, hoping your child will pick the option that "fits" her best.
- ➤ *Memorize in Minutes* (www.multiplication.com): This program combines stories, activities, and pictures to make math meaningful and memorable.
- ➤ *Right Start Math* (www.alabacus.com): Joan Cotter developed the double-sided ALabacus and then, with her husband, developed this curriculum combining visual, auditory, and kinesthetic systems to "help children understand, apply and enjoy mathematics."

➤ *Sequencing in a Flash* (www.licketysplitlearning.com) has a variety of products (computer games/software, flashcards, and workbooks) that may help kids struggling in math, as well as reading. Their programs work best for auditory and visual learners.

➤ *Touch Math Method* (www.touchmath.com) is the leading multisensory mathematical program. It involves teaching kids to recognize "touch points" on each number, adding up to the value of the number (e.g., 5 touch points on the number 5). Then children are taught to touch each touch point on the numbers that they are adding, subtracting, etc.

➤ *Math Graphic Organizers:* There are numerous graphic organizers that help school-aged students learn to visualize mathematical concepts and word problems. One that may be helpful to your child can be found through The Creative Teaching Press (www.creativeteaching.com) by Davilla Harding. You may also be interested in looking at programs on www.luminosity.com and Nintendo DS's Big Brain Academy.

Parents Ask...

What about standardized testing at school?

Your child will undoubtedly complete some testing in school—at the state level—which measures kids at their school as compared to other schools in the state and across the nation. Tests that may be included are the *Stanford Achievement Test*, *Iowa Test of Basic Skills*, and tests developed by your state to comply with the No Child Left Behind Act (NCLB). You can ask for accommodations to assist your little one on these tests. For example, some students qualify for extra time, or a smaller, less distracting test-taking setting, or someone to read the tests aloud to them. Talk with the IEP team and see what might be appropriate for your child.

Helping Your Child Focus at School

You may think you've got it all figured out as far as the school system goes. Sure, you've had some bumps along the road, but you've worked them out. Then a curve ball is thrown at you: you're told your child can't focus at school. She can't keep herself organized, either. Her backpack is a junky mess, and homework somehow never makes it in on time. The fancy word for all of this is "executive functioning" difficulties.

Again, ***apraxia does not cause a child to have executive functioning problems.*** A child can have both CAS and executive functioning concerns, but they are not the same thing!

If your child's teacher is concerned about executive functioning, then:

➤ *Consider requesting an extra set of textbooks for home reference.* You will be glad you have them, especially if your child gets into the middle elementary grades (3-6) and continues to struggle with CAS and executive functioning skills.

➤ *Consider asking for some accommodations at school.* Perhaps worksheets that have clutter and unnecessary visuals removed would be helpful?

➤ *You may want to get an occupational therapist (OT) on board,* either through the school district or privately. They often have a wealth of ideas for helping kids regain focus. Perhaps your child just needs some oral stimulation (like chewing gum) to stay in the game at school. Weighted vests, background music, even a reminder note or image taped to the desktop might help.

➤ If you are truly concerned about your child's executive functioning skills, please refer to Appendix A. We'll cover executive functioning disorders (like ADHD) in more detail. *Again, just because your child has CAS, it does not necessarily mean she also has ADHD!*

Learning Styles

No two people learn in the exact same way. Often, kids with CAS do best when using their hands and bodies to learn, but not always. For example, kids with apraxia *do* benefit from visual cues because auditory cues in speech are not enough; and sometimes just a visual cue is all that's needed without adding a tactile one.

What's a parent to do?

The chart on pages 259-60 lists some ways to incorporate early academic skills into a fun-filled at-home activity. You can use these ideas for any child, not just a child with apraxia. All of these suggestions work well with a more physical learner.

What about IQ Tests?

I don't really believe in formal IQ testing. The tests can be frustrating and can unfairly affect how children are perceived and what expectations others have for them. Plus, they tell parents of kids with special needs little about their child's long-term learning potential. Why? These tests are scored according to the mean performance of children without disabilities (*Science Daily*, Dec 2008).

Some school districts insist on administering standardized IQ tests when children are being evaluated for special education eligibility under IDEA. If your school insists on an IQ test such as the WISC-IV (Wechsler Intelligence Scale for Children, 4th edition) or the Stanford-Binet, then you may be stuck with it. Just keep in mind that the results may not be an accurate assessment of your child's abilities now, or in the

Early Academics the Fun Way

Pre-reading	Writing	Math	Listening & Focus
Create a reading fort and use it for a cozy reading spot (e.g., drape a blanket over some kitchen chairs, or find another suitable area at home).	Work on writing something together, especially something "real" like a grocery list or your daily to-do list. Ask her to practice saying sounds/words/ phrases that go to-gether with food.	Search the house for common, everyday shapes like circles, squares, triangles. Throw in some tough ones like ovals and cylinders. Ask her to tell you about them or say them in unison with you.	Play "Simon Says" or "Follow the Lead-er." See if she can imitate your words or gestures.
Host a book-related party or play date. Ask her to help select the book or theme.	Use sand, glitter, glue, or Play-Doh to spell out words and names like your own and your child's.	Play with puzzles, blocks, and other building type materials.	When you are cook-ing, read the recipe out loud and have your child gather the ingredients. Practice saying the word, sounds, and phrases that go with that ingredient.
Make an ABC post-er or collage with your child. Ask her to practice saying the sounds, words, and phrases on your collage.	Keep a travel log of your outings and errands—stash it in the car and talk about it on longer trips, or allow your child to look at it while you drive. Ask her to talk about it with you.	Allow your child to experiment with vol-ume—think: kitchen sink with plastic measuring devices.	Suggest your child go on a household mission for you. Tell her 2-3 items you need help gathering. Have her repeat the item's name as she looks, if she is able.
Attend story time at the library or book-store and then talk about it.	Buy a composition book for your child and encourage her to keep a journal. Even better if the book has blank spaces for drawing pictures and lines for practicing handwriting, just like at school. Talk with her about what she draws.	Look for patterns at home, or develop your own. Have your child say the pattern back to you, "plate, bowl, plate, bowl."	At the grocery store, ask her to get very specific items to put in the cart: for example, 3 yellow apples; the big blue bottle of detergent on the middle shelf; the tub of butter with the red lid.

Pre-reading	Writing	Math	Listening & Focus
Act out a scene from a book.	Get a whiteboard and assorted colored markers for a family message board. Encourage your child to "write" her own messages, even if they are picture messages.	Stage a math game at snack time. "You have five grapes. If I take away two, how many do you have?"	Ask your child to help you remember a list of objects for a shopping errand; e.g., "paint, sandpaper, and string."
Use or make finger puppets to go along with a story.	Encourage your child to talk about and make a list of her daily activities.	Categorize and talk about small objects such as rocks or hair clips.	Ask your child to repeat a series of numbers you make up. Start with the numbers in your address.
Serve a meal from a book, like *Green Eggs and Ham*. It is fun to connect books with everyday experiences. Target words like "ham," "green," "Sam," as well as work on rhyming activities, which can be challenging for kids with CAS.	Have your child practice writing and saying her name *at the same time*.	On the road, add up all the school buses (or other type/color of vehicle) you see on an outing. "I saw One bus on _____ road plus (+) two buses on ____ road, which equals (=) three buses total." See if your child can say a target word/phrase from this activity (bus, yellow, two, etc.)	Say a variety of words you know your child knows. Tell her to remember them; you'll ask again what they were (e.g., hi, park, sun). Quiz her on those words in a few minutes.

future. The standardized IQ tests that schools routinely use are *language-based*, and require children to respond verbally to the test questions. That's a tall order for any child and obviously "penalizes" kids with CAS from the start.

One option is to pursue IQ testing through an independent evaluation, not from your school district. An independent evaluator—child psychologist or neurodevelopmental psychologist—is unbiased and won't make specific recommendations that could affect your child's education. He or she will give you a long list of ideas you can take to the school. A thorough psychological evaluation will cost several thousand dollars, though, so make sure the results are worth the financial investment to you.

Any IQ test given to a child with apraxia should not require a verbal response. Consider the TONI-4 (Test of Nonverbal Intelligence, for kids 6+ years old), the Leiter-R (Leiter International Performance Scale-Revised, best for kids 2-20 years old), or the UNIT (Universal Non-verbal Intelligence Test, ages 5-17, or K-12).

Extended School Year (ESY)

Just because you made it through the school year successfully doesn't mean you and your child are home-free when it comes to summer vacation. IDEA mandates an Extended School Year (ESY) for students at risk of losing their skills during the summer break. It is *not* a program to increase skills or develop new ones. Participation in ESY is determined by IEP team recommendations. It must be documented in the IEP. Generally, these programs are held for a portion of the summer—maybe six weeks of half-day reinforcement.

The Wright's Law website (www.wrightslaw.com) discusses a federal court case (Ruesch v. Fountain) in which eligibility standards for ESY were determined. These factors are what the educational team should consider when determining whether or not students are eligible for ESY:

1. **Regression and Recoupment:** Is the child likely to lose critical skills or fail to recover them in a reasonable time should there be a break from school (regression in life skills)? If you want your child to be included in the ESY program for the upcoming summer, start making a list of any and all regression noted over breaks from school, especially the longer ones like Winter and Spring Break. Give specific examples if you can, like "Forgot how to say /st/ blends."

2. **Degree of Progress toward IEP Goals and Objectives:** The team needs to look at how the child has progressed on established goals; if the child is having difficulty keeping up, then ESY may be necessary.

3. **Emerging Skills with Possible Breakthrough:** If formal instruction is halted or interrupted, will there be a problem, regression, or future difficulty, especially with significant skills like reading?

4. **Interfering Behavior:** Does the child have ritualistic or self-injurious behavior (SIB) that may prevent her from benefitting from her IEP? If so, ESY may be best.

5. **Nature and Severity of Disability:** Does the child's educational team believe that the nature and severity of the disability warrants summer services?

6. **Special Circumstances:** Are there situations beyond your control that interfere with your child's ability to participate and benefit from special educational services?

Your child may *not* qualify for services, and that may be a good thing. It means she is progressing and doesn't need reinforcement over the summer—at least, according to your IEP team. To learn more about the requirements for ESY, go to your favorite search engine and type in:

your state name + extended school year regulations + students with disabilities

The results will help you understand how your state generally handles ESY. Keep in mind that CAS falls in a continuum of severity and kids with moderate to severe CAS will be most likely to qualify. If you feel that your child really would benefit from ESY, be prepared to state your case and come with supporting documents to any meeting that may be held to discuss the issue. Please refer to "Standards for Extended School Year" on the Wright's Law website (www.wrightslaw.com/info/esy-standards.barlev.htm) for more information.

Our Experience with ESY

When Kate didn't qualify for ESY one summer, I was a bit perplexed. She had in the past, and it had been good for her. Her teacher and the rest of the team pointed out that she *could* receive ESY if I *really* wanted her to, but I needed to be aware that she would probably be the highest functioning kid in the program. At the time, I thought that might not be such a bad idea. Perhaps it would boost her confidence, as she might be able to help other kids. After more thought, we ultimately decided against it. If Kate was to continue to progress in speech and social communication, she needed to be surrounded by typically developing peers to serve as motivation. See Appendix C for some guidance on selecting a summer program for your child.

Grade Retention (Being "Held Back")

A big concern for parents who have a child with CAS is when and whether a child should be retained in a particular grade level. Hopefully, you will receive guidance from school staff if things get to this point. You will also have some IEP meetings where you can discuss the pros and cons. Questions to consider include:

➤ What do you (and school staff) believe will change in the school environment that will address your child's needs, if she is retained?

➤ What changes in your child do you think will improve her progress (social maturity, academic maturity, better communication)?

➤ What, if anything, are you and the teachers willing to do to assure that things move along at the "right" pace if she spends another year in the same grade?

➤ How would it affect your child socially and emotionally to stay behind while her classmates are promoted?

Many school systems actively discourage grade retention, even if children have very significant disabilities. So, even if *you* believe your child would benefit from being held back, you may not be able to convince the school to do so.

I should mention here that not all kids with apraxia continue to struggle with speech and language issues for their entire school years. Childhood Apraxia of Speech is a *dynamic* (ever-changing) disorder specific to the *childhood* years (up to about age 10). Sure, remnants of speech/language issues may resurface at times, but for the most part, if you are aggressive in getting your child the appropriate speech therapy, and she doesn't have another disability that affects communication, your child will be a typically speaking tween, teen, and adult.

Say That Again?! Chapter Summary

We've certainly covered *a lot* in this chapter! From what to look for in a school to navigating an IEP, this chapter was loaded with tips, ideas, and resources I hope you have found helpful. Of course, I can't possibly include everything you may want or need to know about your child's education. I urge you to do more research on your own so that you can develop an individualized educational guidebook for your child. Remember, each individual is unique and we all learn in our own unique ways. I'll leave you with this favorite quote:

"All students can learn and succeed, but not all on the same day in the same way."
–William G. Spade

Read On! Recommended Resources

➤ Here are some websites that may offer ideas for easing your child into the first day of school:
  - ➤ *Helping Your Child Adjust to Preschool:* http://kidshealth.org/parent/positive/learning/adjust_to_ preschool.html
  - ➤ *A Successful First Day of Preschool:*
  - ➤ www.teachingstrategies.com/pages/page.cfm?pageid=131
  - ➤ *My First Day at School:*
  - ➤ www.timberland.lib.wa.us/kids-booklists-school.pdf
  - ➤ *Preparing your Child for the First Day of School and Separation Anxieties:*
  - ➤ http://ali.apple.com/edres/parents/firstday.shtml
  - ➤ **Ready for School? Books to Share with Your Child:**
  - ➤ www.santacruzpl.org/kids/bibs/preschool/school.pdf

➤ Your child may like this book: *First Day Jitters* by Julie Danneberg (Charlesbridge Publishing, Whispering Coyote Press, 2000).

➤ Other children's titles that may help ease the separation and anxiety are: *It's O.K.—Tom's First Day of School* by Beth Robbins (DK Publishers, 2001) and *What to Expect at Preschool* by Heidi Murkoff and Laura Rader (Harper Festival, 2001).

➤ If you are interested in having your little "teacher" participate in some role play to prepare for school look in the HearthSong for the "Let's Pretend School": www.hearthsong.com or call 800-325-2502.

➤ If your child is a fan of the Maisy storybook character, then look for **Maisy Goes to Preschool** by Lucy Cousins. The simple illustrations and text are a sure way to comfort and pave the road to a successful first preschool experience.

➤ Read **Choosing a School for a Child with Special Needs** by Ruth Birnbaum (Jessica Kingsley Publishers, 2009).

➤ You may find the **Homeschooling Catalog Site** helpful for additional resources, even if you choose *not* to homeschool: www.rainbowresource.com.

➤ Here are some online resources you may be interested in when seeking **personal identification/safety awareness** for your child:
  ➤ Kid's Vital IDs: www.kidsvitalids.com
  ➤ Kidsafe ID: www.kidsafeid.com
  ➤ Petite Baubles Boutique: www.petitebaublesboutique.com

➤ Rich Weinfeld and Michelle Davis present an excellent and information-packed resource on what you can do to help influence your child's education in **Special Needs Advocacy and Resource Book: What You Can Do Now to Help Advocate for Your Exceptional Child's Education** (Prufrock Press, 2008).

➤ **The Complete Guide to Special Education: Expert Advice on Evaluations, IEPs, and Helping Kids Succeed** (Jossey-Bass, 2010) by Linda Wilmshurst, Ph.D. and Alan W. Brue, Ph.D. Includes tools, checklists, forms, and advice, plus expanded coverage on autism spectrum disorders as well as RTI (response-to-intervention), a "new" way of identifying students with learning disabilities.

➤ **The Complete IEP Guide, 7th edition** by Lawrence Siegal (Nolo, 2011) explains the intricacies of IEPs in a clear, concise way; includes sample documents and pull-out forms.

➤ The All About Adolescent Literacy website has some tips for **summer programs**. It indicates it's for grades 4-12, but I am sure you can glean something for younger kids, too: www.adlit.org. Also, Reading Rockets has a great article on the same topic you'll want to check out: www.readingrockets.org/article/2342.

➤ If you are interested in **retaining your child in a particular grade**, then read: www.greatschools.net/cgi-bin/ showarticle/1213?cpn=3D20090512my2.

➤ *The Discovery Center in the UK* offers a website by Professor Amanda Kirby that may provide you with valuable advice and ideas for home and school: www.boxofideas.org.

➤ *Kiz Club* has some great resources for parents and educators alike. You may especially like the flannel board pictures for familiar books. Check them out at www.kizclub.com.

➤ Looking for *parenting articles and fun ideas for home and school?* Check out www.PreschoolRock.com.

➤ Check out *Dr. Jean Feldman's website:* www.drjean.org. She has been in education for over 35 years and is the author of many books on topics ranging from transitions and games to self-esteem.

➤ Older kids with more homework and projects to keep track of may benefit from a *graphic organizer* such as those available at: www.eduplace.com.

➤ *More on Graphic Planners*—Kidspiration and Inspiration software has a 30-day trial you may want to consider. www.inspiration.com/themes/inspiration/video-player.php?nid=953.

➤ *Lost at School: Why Our Kids with Behavioral Challenges are Falling Through the Cracks and How We Can Help Them* by Ross W. Greene (Scribner, 2008) is a nice resource for kids with social, emotional, and behavioral challenges who lack important thinking skills.

➤ *All Kinds of Minds: A Young Student's Book about Learning Abilities and Disorders* by Dr. Mel Levine (Educators Publishing Service, 1993) includes narrative short stories about kids with learning disabilities *written for kids*. It reviews feelings and thoughts about the first day of school, ADD, reading disorders, memory problems, language disorders, and poor social/motor skills.

➤ *Taming the Recess Jungle: Socially Simplifying Recess for Students with Autism and Related Disorders* by Carol Gray (Future Horizons Press, 1993). Although this book focuses on kids with autism, it can be applied to just about any child. It discusses transitions at school, how to ask the "right" questions, and how to help a child who may be socially impaired.

➤ *The Anti-Bullying and Teasing Book for Preschool Classrooms* by Barbara Sprung and Merle Froschl with Dr. Blythe Hinitz (Gryphon House, 2005) is a nice resource for teachers, but may also give parents a peek inside teasing within the classroom.

➤ *The Mislabeled Child: How Understanding Your Child's Unique Learning Style Can Open the Doors to Success* by Brock Eide and Fernette Eide (Hyperion, 2006) may be useful if your child has additional concerns with vision, attention, sensory processing, or autism.

➤ *Different Learners: Identifying, Preventing, and Treating Your Child's Learning Problems* by Jane Healy (Simon and Schuster, 2010) discusses current changes in education, the case of difference vs. disability, and genetics vs. environment, all with a research-based background. She writes in a straightforward, no-nonsense way busy parents can appreciate.

➤ Laura E. Berk's *Awakening Children's Minds: How Parents and Teachers Can Make a Difference* (Oxford University Press, 2001) includes lots of good information on why and how children talk to themselves, learning in classrooms, as well as a chapter devoted to helping children with deficits and disabilities.

Chapter Twelve

· ·

Phonological Awareness

· ·

Learning to Read and
Reading to Learn

You know the scene well: your child is sitting comfortably on his bed or the floor and "reading" a favorite book. I remember walking into Kate's room one day when she was about four and seeing her in a similar situation. I proudly remarked, "Oh look—you're reading!" In her broken language, she replied, "No read, mom. Look pictures." I was doubly proud. My little girl with apraxia was able to string a few words together to tell me she wasn't really reading, but instead just looking at the pictures.

This wasn't the *first* time she was able to say more than a few words together, but she was doing several things I was especially pleased about: looking at books and studying their pictures (a pre-reading skill), giving herself (and me) some down-time, exhibiting insight (she knew she wasn't really reading), *and* communicating that insight to me. Of course, I had to give her a hug, lie down on the floor, and join her for a little mother-daughter book reading.

In fact, what we were doing is what researchers and educators refer to as strengthening "children's memory for words and literacy." Think back to your own childhood for a moment. I am sure you have some favorite books and literary characters that really stand out in your mind. Who and what were they? What did you love about them? Do you remember where you read those books? Who read with—and to—you? Do you look back on those memories with fondness and delight?

Those memories shaped your childhood and they continue to shape your adult reading life as well. Other memories may not have been as positive when it came to

> ### The Nuts and Bolts of This Chapter

> ➤ An overview of why kids with CAS tend to have more difficulty learning to read—and how you can help

> ➤ Research-based interventions to give you specific ideas for enhancing literacy at home

> ➤ Suggested books to read with your child and activities to promote excellence in reading

> ➤ Handwriting and story writing tips and ideas for your eager young reader to write on her own, without frustration

> ➤ Potential reading concerns for children with CAS, and when to bring in a specialist

> ➤ Types of home-based reading programs available

reading: the material selected may have been too challenging, you may have been bored, or perhaps the story lacked imagination.

Essential Terminology

Before we get started, let's get a couple of definitions out of the way.

Phonological Awareness: This term was first used in research in the late 1970s and early 1980s. It replaced "phonetic analysis of spoken words" and "linguistic awareness," which referred to: "Children's knowledge of words as comprised of smaller, discernable units" (Gillon, 2004). Simply put, phonological awareness is an individual's awareness of the sound structure of spoken words. It includes the ability to recognize rhyming words, or to identify how many syllables there are in a given word. Without the awareness of sounds in words, it's much harder to learn to read and spell correctly. That's why phonological awareness is an important and reliable predictor of later reading ability.

Phonemic Awareness: A phoneme is the smallest unit of sound that influences the meaning of a word, regardless of how that unit of sound is spelled. For example, the phoneme that we perceive as a /k/ sound can be written as a "k" in kitten or a "c" in cat. Phonemic awareness refers to the ability to hear and manipulate the individual sounds in a word (for instance, to recognize that "soup" and "sand" begin with the same letter, or to understand that if you take the /n/ sound and put it in the front of the /o/ sound, you get "no." When we speak, listeners aren't saying to themselves, "I hear the /r/ and the /i/ sound. Instead, they blend those sounds into syllables; they have learned to *perceive* the phonemes in spoken language. In the English language, there are 41 phonemes (25 consonants and 16 vowels).

Phonemic awareness is a component of phonological awareness. They are not the same thing, but are often used interchangeably.

Children with CAS and Reading

Let's not beat around the bush. You should know that many kids with CAS *probably* will have *some* difficulty with phonological and phonemic awareness—the precursor skills that are needed to understand how speech sounds translate into written words on the page. In addition, kids who have persistent speech difficulties such as CAS, with no other medical cause, are at-risk for related literary problems such as trouble with reading comprehension (Puranik et al., 2008; Stackhouse, 1997). Some more proof:

➤ The following researchers concluded that a "large percentage" of kids with a speech pathology diagnosis in the preschool and kindergarten years encounter difficulty learning to read and spell: Lewis, Freebairin & Taylor (2002), Catts, Fey, Zhang & Tomblin (2001), Larrivee & Catts (1999), Johnson et al. (1999), and Boudreau & Hedberg (1999).

➤ Kids with speech-language impairment are 4 to 5 times more likely to have reading difficulties than children from the general population (Catts et al., 2001).

➤ Of course, not all kids with spoken language impairment have reading problems. But those with a *specific speech-language impairment* just may.

➤ In addition, 50 to 70 percent of kids with spoken language impairment will have some academic difficulty in their school years, according to Felsenfeld, Broen, & McGrue, 1994 and Shriberg, Tomblin, & McSweeny, 1999.

I don't mean to be all gloom and doom, but I do want you to have the facts. There is a light at the end of the tunnel. Follow along in this chapter and I think you'll start to see it.

Why Is Reading Difficult for Children with CAS?

We touched on this a little bit in the last chapter. To review, kids with apraxia may have these problem areas related to reading:

1. Kids who aren't making sounds accurately (or at all) may have a decreased visual representation of what letters look and sound like.
2. Kids with speech-language disorders may have a distorted sense of what the symbols (letters) represent (letters are symbols which represent words).

3. Kids with apraxia may have "differently-wired" brains, affecting the way they read, learn, and interpret information.
4. Children affected with CAS may have a decreased ability to coordinate the vocal track in producing a word.

When it comes to *reading comprehension*, researchers say that some kids with apraxia and other learning difficulties lack the appropriate strategies to allow them to understand what they just read. It's complicated. Reading requires a lot: decoding words, visualization, understanding context, activating prior knowledge, a large vocabulary, and the ability to comprehend what you just read. For example, if a kid has to work really hard to understand (decode) the words on the page, then he may not have much energy left over for defining an unfamiliar word.

In a 2009 study published in the *International Journal of Communication Disorders,* the researchers set out to compare the phonological awareness and reading development in twelve children with CAS and twelve kids with inconsistent speech disorder (ISD), and twelve other "typically-developing" kids. They found that kids with CAS did indeed have less-than ideal ("inferior") phonological awareness (letter-sound knowledge and decoding) compared to the ISD and typically-developing kids.

Parents Ask...

What's an Inconsistent Speech Disorder (ICD)?

Kids with ICD have a high degree of variability (40 percent or more of the time) in the way they say a word. For example, a child with ICD may say "rabbit" like "wab-bit" one time, "babbit" another, and even "tabbit" another. See the similarity it shares with CAS?

This research supports that **kids with CAS need early intervention in learning to read**—because they are more likely to develop a reading delay. It also suggests that parents, caregivers, and educators really ought to help these kids develop underlying skills to improve their written and spoken language, as well as the words they read on a page. Of course, we can't base a claim on just one research study with 12 kids with CAS. Just know that there is a correlation and this study helps support that correlation. We definitely need more research, though! See Appendix E for additional research on reading difficulties in children with speech and language delays.

What Can We Do?

Research can give us great insights, but we need some clear guidelines as to *what to do right now* with our struggling kiddos. If your child is at reading age (5-8 years old) then I *know* you are curious as to what to do. I bet you have some of your own ideas and hopes (goals). What are they? What do you consider to be realistic for a "typical" child at this age? How might you need to adjust your expectations for *your* child?

Here are a few suggestions to stoke the fire:

➤ To have your child with CAS reading at a level that is appropriate for him, even if he is considered "behind" when compared to his peers.

➤ To improve his sequencing skills in activities of daily living (ADLs) such as getting dressed, bathing, and eating. After all, being able to follow steps in a sequence has a lot to do with reading.

➤ To work with your child to make sure he is "up to speed" on pre-reading such as rhyming words, alliteration, sound segmentation, and isolating sounds.

➤ To incorporate some of this pre-literacy work into speech therapy, school, and home environments.

Spend a few moments jotting down your goals on your child's reading and writing life. Go ahead, dream a little. Now, brainstorm about how you can help your child with the resources you already have (consider time, effort, and your own special skills and talents; not just money, books, and tutor centers as resources).

Want to know what educators say the real goal is? The "real" goal is getting the child to break the code from sounds to letters (writing the correct letters that represent the correct sounds) and from hearing what is said to reading what is written (auditory to visual). I know, it sounds daunting. This next section will focus strictly on working with your child with CAS on reading.

Breaking the ABC Code—Reading with CAS

As discussed above, some researchers say that kids with CAS have difficulty understanding the abstract idea that letters represent words. Sometimes these kids don't even have a good visual of what that letter looks like. You can say, "That's the letter h," and your child still won't get it. Finally, kids with apraxia may have "differently wired" brains altogether and process information in a totally different way. That doesn't mean it's impossible; it just means you need to take a different approach.

The approach that is most beneficial to all kids is simply this: read to them and read to them often. That's not all, of course—if you want to raise a reader, then you need to read yourself. And your kids need to *see* you reading for this monkey-see, monkey-do approach to work. I know you likely don't have the luxury of time to plop down with a great novel while your children quietly play at your feet. Here are some ideas:

Pick up something quick and easy that you can do within the eyeshot of little ones. Glance at the headlines in a newspaper, flip through a magazine, bring a book along to a waiting room, and establish a fifteen-minute reading time at home for everyone.

Beyond reading to your kids and setting a good example, there are two other winning strategies, according to Joy Stackhouse's text *Persisting Speech Difficulties in Children: Children's Speech and Literacy Difficulties.* Teach phonological awareness skills and add strong literacy skills (reading strategies) and then you've got a kid ready to learn to read.

Phonological Awareness + Reading Strategies = Ready to Read

How do you do that? Well, there are five specific learning abilities necessary for reading:

1. **Phonemic Awareness:** rhyme, syllable knowledge, sound manipulation, onsets, and rhymes
2. **Phonics:** sound-syllable correspondence, invented spellings
3. **Text Comprehension:** ability to decode symbols and sounds, understand syntax, vocabulary, and semantics
4. **Vocabulary:** expressive, reading, and writing vocabulary.
5. **Fluency:** the ability to read a text smoothly and accurately, to be able to understand what one reads without having to stop and decode words.

Check out the chart on pages 273-75 to understand what this really means. The top of the chart depicts skills that are typically more advanced, while the bottom of the chart shows earlier literacy skills.

Lisa Circelli, M.Ed., early childhood educator at The Brokaw Early Learning Center, advises parents, "Focus on letter sounds rather than letter names. This helps children correlate and discriminate letter-sound recognition."

Encouraging Phonological and Phonemic Awareness at Home

Now that we've covered some of the nitty-gritty of how kids learn to read, here are some activities you can do together in the comfort of your own home.

➤ *Read, read, read, and read some more.* Books are multisensory learning media. Think of your senses when you read a book—you can hear the dialog, see the scenery, feel the emotions, and almost taste the salty sea air. Frequent practice of hearing and saying, even seeing words print in familiar books, can help kids with CAS.

➤ *Start out with repetitive books.* According to speech-language pathologists Michelle Soloman and Lavinia Pereira, repetitive books are an effective therapeu-

Building a Foundation for Reading

Learning Ability	What It Is	Example	What You Can Do	Check Progress
Phonemic Awareness	Knowing linguistic sounds. Having the ability to hear different sounds by the way letters are grouped together.	Knowing the difference between the /p/ and /b/ sounds in *pat* and *bat*; being able to distinguish between the /sh/ and /s/ in *show* and *sow*	Say, "Is show and sow the same word?" Ask your child to listen carefully as you emphasize the unique sounds. Can he tell you the difference?	Look at words in print that are similar in spelling—*mat, pat, cat, sat*— and ask if your child knows what's different and the same about them.
Phonics (*Not to be confused with phonetics, which is the range of possible sounds in languages, and not used in teaching and education-land*)	The *instruction* piece of building on kids' phonemic awareness. Knowing that letter symbols have sounds.	Knowing that when the sounds of /b/, /a/, /t/ are put together, they make *bat*.	Word-Slam! Sit with your child and with one hand say, "I have a /ba/ sound." With your other hand say, "I have an /at/ sound…put them together and you get, "bat!" Clap your hands together (with the different sounds "in" them) for a slamming sound.	Ask your child to do some word-slam activities with you. He may be able to make up some of his own. Accept it even if it is a made-up word.
Segmentation and Blending	Pulling apart and putting together different combinations of sounds and letters.	Think phonics in reverse. Knowing that the word bat can be broken down into /b/, /a/, /t/.	Cover part of a printed word and ask your child to sound out what he sees. In the word *Jump*, you can cover up the /ump/ and have your child sound out the /j/ sound, add in /ump/ and make a word.	"Hey, look! Here's a "b." Tell me what sound a "b" makes." Then ask, "If we add the "at" sound to the "b" what word do we make? That's right—"bat!"

Learning Ability	What It Is	Example	What You Can Do	Check Progress
Letter Identification	Knowing that the letter "names" of the letters in the alphabet correspond to a symbol. There are also blends of two letters, called "digraphs" such as ch, sh, br, bl, fl. Dipthongs are the vowel combinations, such as "ow," "aw," "oy."	You know that A and S have different names and sound different.	Talk about the letters whenever you see them. Environmental print (out and about in the community) is great for this.	Quiz your child when you see a letter on a coffee cup, at the newsstand, while driving. Ask, "What letter(s) do you see? I see an "m"—do you?"
Letter Sound Identification	Knowing what sound each of the letters in the alphabet makes.	Awareness that the letter /i/ can sound like /i/ in pit, but sound different in ice.	Sing a little jingle with all of the different sounds one letter makes. "E makes the 'ee' sound, it also goes like 'eh.' Now you say it!"	Practice and listen carefully to your child!
Visual Discrimination	The ability to discriminate between letter shapes and words.	Being aware that b and d and p are different, even though they kind of look the same. Also, knowing that h and z are unique because they appear so unalike in structure and sound.	Have some alphabet flashcards (make your own!) and present two at a time; ask "Are these two letters the same?" You're just looking for "yes" or "no" at this point. Do the same with other print material.	Kids love to see parents make mistakes! So have your child play teacher and see if he can trip you up. Let him win sometimes!

Learning Ability	What It Is	Example	What You Can Do	Check Progress
Print Awareness	Knowing that printed text has meaning.	When your child brings you something and says, "What does this say?"	Read whatever your child brings you. "Oh that's an invitation to Sara's party. It says …."	Show your child a book or scratch paper with words on it. Ask, "What does this say?" Let him elaborate or talk nonsense. He will make a connection to print, regardless.
Book Knowledge	Knowing how a book "works" (cover, spine, how to hold, left-to right orientation, page-turning).	Hold a book by first looking at the cover. Talk about what you see. Turn the book page by page and follow from left to right.	Show your child the parts of a book. "Here is the spine. It tells us the title and author's name." Point to the words as you read them. Let your child use a finger to follow along with the words. Ask him to turn the pages for you.	Get goofy. Hold the book upside down and see if your child can correct you. Start reading from the back of the book. Read a few pages out of sequence and see if he notices.

Adapted from *The Young Child's Memory for Words,* Daniel R. Meier (Teachers College Press, 2004).

tic tool for kids diagnosed with CAS. That's because repetitive books are usually highly predictive. This helps kids grasp the sense of the story early on and there is less to think about and more opportunity to verbally express their thoughts and the actual words from the book. So, if you are reading a book that has the same phrase page after page, pause every once in a while and see if your child can "fill in the blank." Also do this with words or character's names. This lets your child participate more in story time and allows for more turn-taking opportunities and possibly decreased frustration. More ideas for repetitive books:

- Give your child time to respond. Remember kids with CAS may need a longer time to retrieve those speech-motor sequences.
- Read a favorite repetitive book repeatedly. Redundant? I know. It helps, I promise.

Some Repetitive Books to Try

➤ Boynton, S. **Red Hat, Yellow Hat** and **Snuggle Puppy.** If you like this author, you're in luck—she has many to choose from!

➤ Brown, M. **Goodnight Moon.** This classic is sure to hook your child, as is **Home for a Bunny.**

➤ Campbell, R. **Dear Zoo: A Lift-the-flap Book.**

➤ Carle, E. **Have You Seen My Cat?** along with **123 to the Zoo.**

➤ Carlstrom, N.W. **Jesse Bear, What Will You Wear?**

➤ Christelow, E. **Five Little Monkeys Jumping on the Bed.**

➤ Eastman, P.D. **Are You My Mother?**

➤ Guarino, D. **Is Your Mama a Llama?**

➤ Kalen, R. **Jump, Frog, Jump!**

➤ Katz, K. **Where Is Baby's Mommy?** among others. Great lift-the-flap fun, illustrations, and repetition.

➤ Rosen, M. and Oxenbury, H. **We're Going on a Bear Hunt** and variation, **We're Going on a Nature Hunt**.

➤ Williams, L. **The Little Old Lady Who Was Not Afraid of Anything.**

➤ Of course we can't forget about good ol' Dr. Seuss books as well! Lots of his stories not only repeat, but rhyme. Both are skills needed to help kids learn to read. Check out classics such as **Green Eggs and Ham** or **Hop on Pop.**

➤ *Read wordless books.* Wordless books are important in getting kids to be the storyteller. Each time a child "reads" a wordless book, the story changes slightly. Of course, this may be harder to do if your child isn't saying much. But the more you present the book, the more he will attempt. For kids who are more verbal, you will almost "see" their creativity, vocabulary, and knowledge grow as they add to and elaborate the story. Some wordless titles you may want to look for: *Pancakes for Breakfast* by Tomi dePaulo, *The Surprise Picnic* by J.S. Goodall, and *Good Dog, Carl* by Alexandra Day, as well as books by these authors—Emily Arnold McCully, Mercer Mayer (the author of the Little Critter series), Peter Spier, and Nancy Tafuri.

➤ *Engage in dialogic reading.* What this means is you stop and ask your child questions about the book you are reading. "Oh, look. I see a little girl who is ready to go to school. She has a backpack. Can you say 'backpack?' What else do you see?" You don't have to do this type of reading on every page, but once in awhile as you read. Plan for extra reading time so you can point out things in the illustrations and allow for your child to engage with you.

➤ *Read riddles.* Riddle books are great for long car rides or an after-dinner family activity. Riddles provide good exposure to, and practice with, the nuances of language. Kids have to really listen to the story and hear that some words have multiple meanings. Riddles also help develop a rich vocabulary and improve reading comprehension.
- Talk about the structure of a riddle. It's a question/answer "story" in which words "play" with one another.
- The answer makes silly sense if you understand the multiple meanings of words.
- Share your thoughts on how the words work together so your child can understand the riddle more clearly.

Keep in mind that riddles are tricky. It may be best to wait on these until your child is developmentally more mature. Generally, kids who are in the kindergarten to 2nd grade levels find them hilarious.

➤ *Explore letters and sounds.* Develop a "Letter Center" at home if you have the space. Supply it with magnetic letters, alphabet puzzles, sponge letters, foam letters, sticker letters, rubber letter stamps, clay/Play-Doh and cookie cutters shaped like letters, and perhaps even computer software that focuses on the alphabet. In the same area, it may be a nice extension to offer different types of literacy materials: catalogs, labels, newspapers, empty cereal boxes, recipe cards, junk mail, and greeting cards. If it has print on it, it counts!

➤ *Clap it out.* You may want to start with a simple adaptation of clapping out syllables. Say, "I am going to clap my hands in a pattern. Repeat after me." Then clap out a simple little sequence. Your child is listening to the rate and pattern of your claps. He should repeat it back to you. Make them more complex as he grasps the idea. Then, add in clapping out syllables to words. Remember, a syllable will always include one vowel. "Momma" becomes "Mom"-clap-"ma"-clap. Do this often with words you and your child say. Have your child try it. You can vary this activity by stomping or jumping.

➤ *Try body cues.* Rhonda Banford, CCC-SLP, shares this idea for teaching about syllables: "I like to have kids put their hands on their heads for the first syllable, shoulders for the second, waist for the third, knees for the fourth, and toes for the fifth. I find this helps more than clapping when I ask them how many syllables there are. It is easier for some kids to remember which of these different movements they made when they count the syllables than remembering how many times they clapped."

➤ *Play the "Letter a Day" game.* Pick a letter and have it be the focus of your day. "Today we are going to focus on the letter B. Let's see how many letter Bs we can find. Let's try to say words that begin with the letter B. But first, let me show you what the letter B looks like." Everywhere you go, point the letter out in its uppercase and lowercase form. Practice making the /ba/ sound. Make a collage with the letter B. Play ball and say B words as you bounce or roll it to each other. Practice writing the letter B. You can adapt this idea, too. Rhonda Banford, CCC-SLP, suggests, "Make the activity multisensory in other ways, too. Write it in pudding, construct it out of Play-Doh, trace it with the finger on a piece of sandpaper you've cut into the letter shape, paint the soles of the feet and have the child 'walk' the shape of the B on a large piece of butcher paper (available at craft supply stores)."

➤ *Shop at home.* Give your child a shopping bag. On the bag, write or attach a letter. Tell him to go around the house and collect things in his bag that begin with that letter sound. Talk about what he shopped for together.

➤ *Make a name collage.* Start by writing your child's name on a large sheet of construction paper. Then look in old magazines and catalogs for items that start with the sound of his first name. Steven=stove, stop, stick, stone, stay, story. Let your child do some of the work.

➤ *Match letters to toys.* Grab a few of your child's favorite toys. Spread them out on the floor and make your own alphabet cards, making sure that you include some "correct" as well as "incorrect" cards. For example, say your grouping of toys consists of ball, doll, car, puzzle, and jump rope. Your alphabet cards would include the letters Bb, Dd, Cc, Pp, Jj. Throw in a couple of random letters as well, Mm, Zz, Hh. Have your child match the correct card to the correct toy. Practice saying the name of the object, as well as the sound the letter makes with your child.

➤ *Does this rhyme?* Play this simple game in the car, in a waiting room, or even in the grocery story. Say, "I am thinking of three words. They are cat, bat, and ball. Which words rhyme?" This works on short-term memory as well as rhyming skills. You may first have to describe what a rhyme is. Your child will get good at this and begin developing his own list of three rhyming words. Praise your child for attempts at creating a rhyme, even if it isn't 100 percent correct. A simple and fun book to read to your child that uses rhyme is *There's a Wocket in My Pocket,* by Dr. Seuss. But don't forget about your classic nursery rhymes, too!

➤ *Play with your food.* At snack time, consider playing with your child's food. Pretzel sticks, carrot sticks, or any other "stick-like" foods work well with this type of activity. You can create many letters this way—M, N, E, K, to name a few. If you need the circular part of a letter, try using bendable foods like licorice or string cheese. Consider making pancakes in the shape of different letters. This may be the perfect breakfast for your letter day fun!

➤ *Find letters in nature.* Go on a hike and look for natural formations that look a bit like letters. Need a little inspiration? Check out ***ABCs Naturally: A Child's Guide to the Alphabet through Nature,*** by Lynne Smith Diebel and Jann Faust Kalschuer. You can start with the letter A and work your way through the alphabet by having the first person find something that starts with A (acorn, anthill), the next person does the same thing that begins with B (bug, bluebird), and so on. The second person needs to remember what the first person found/said and add that to his list of B words…anthill, bug…This helps with observational skills, recall, and phonological awareness. Of course, modify if this recall portion is too tricky.

Making Reading Fun

While some kids love to read, others may grow to dread it. Here are a few ideas that you might consider adopting as you impress upon your child(ren) that reading is fun:

➤ *Pick books that are easy for your child to read.* Give him some success early on and he will find that reading really isn't as difficult as it seems.

➤ *Sit with your child as he reads a book for the first time.* I know, we're all busy—who possibly has the time? Your child needs to know that you value reading, and may need help with some of the more difficult words.

➤ *Find—and help your child find—different kinds of books.* That means wandering into the children's nonfiction section at the library. Let him peruse the shelves for something that piques his interest. Consider poetry, mysteries, biographies, among others.

➤ *Read harder books to your child than he could read himself.* Researchers and educators have found that kids can understand stories about three to four grade levels above their reading level. It introduces them to the story structure of more complicated tales, along with vocabulary, plus it's motivation to continue reading on one's own.

➤ *Make connections to books and real-life experiences.* Reading the *Little House on the Prairie* series? Visit one of the historical centers that honors Laura Ingalls Wilder's life or a pioneer village in your area. Other examples could be as simple as visiting the bakery in your grocery store after reading a book about cookies, or touring the pizza parlor. Call ahead, of course.

➤ *Suggest having your child read books aloud to practice expression and inflection.* Hard skills for anyone to master, but even more so for kids with CAS.

➤ *When your child comes across a word he doesn't know, have him pre-dict what it could be: "What makes sense in the story?"* This not only teaches prediction skills, but also the concept of context.

➤ *Extend reading activities* by suggesting your child create a play around the story with neighborhood friends, draw a picture of what you just read (especially helpful if mom and dad are reading to a child from a chapter book), or make your own "book."

➤ *Consider hosting a book play date.* Decide on a theme based on a book, book series, or character your child is particularly drawn to. Make it meaningful—and set the stage—by sending out an appropri-ately themed invitation to the guests. You can decorate accordingly, and prepare food that the storybook character might also like (green eggs and ham, anyone?). Have a reading of the book, followed by a short dis-cussion (depending on the age of the kids), throw in a few book-related games and crafts, then call it a day.

➤ *Look into creating a parent-child book group in your neighborhood or school.* Depending on your child's grade level, you can read all kinds of things—start with picture books, pick a favorite author, or go with a theme (animals as the main character, children's books that focus on feelings and self-esteem, for example), then set a schedule—say once a month. Everyone reads the same thing—or pick a few titles—then come together and share what you learned.

What Is Guided Reading?

Guided reading helps kids develop important concepts as they read and helps lay down the foundation for writing stories of their own. What is it, exactly? Guided read-ing is the process of supporting reading in a small-group setting by first introducing the book and story in a pre-reading exercise. Our teacher called this a "book walk." It could simply mean talking with your child about the author and title, and identifying the spine, table of contents, etc. Next, you might introduce characters, new vocab-ulary, and prediction-making skills. Supporting your emerging reader with context clues, letter-sound recognition/relationships, and word structure would be the final step. It's not as easy as it appears, but this is a very important part of learning to read.

You'll also want your child to be able to retell a story (narrative skills) and follow the general structure of a story. You can practice and build these skills by asking the right ques-tions after a reading session. Or, try the Guided Reading Beach Balls by Carson-Dellosa (www.carsondellosa.com), which just might be the perfect formula for kids with CAS:

vestibular stimulation + verbalization = possibly a more chatty kid

You can make your own, too! Purchase a beach ball and write questions about books in general on each of the colored wedges with a marker. Examples may include:

Who is the author? Is there an illustrator? Who is the main character? My favorite part was ____. The story was about ____

Mention the beach ball activity at the beginning of the book: "We're going to read a book and then play this game with the ball. The ball will "ask" some questions about the book we just read. Some questions will be ____ (read them). Pay attention as we read so you are prepared to answer the questions." Read the story, then sit in a circle (with multiple kids) or across from your child. Toss or roll the ball back and forth. Answer the question on the part of the ball your hand touches first.

Working on Reading When Your Child's Speech Is Lagging

I was concerned about Kate's ability (or inability) to read when she was about five. I asked members of a listserv, "Is this a bad time for my daughter to learn to read? Her speech still isn't that great. Does her speech have to improve before she can read?" Another parent advised me that Kate's speech might actually begin to improve once she began to read. Whether this is supported by actual research, I'm not entirely sure, but it worked in this mom's experience and it just may work in yours. Could it be that reading and hearing and articulation are all somehow connected?

What Should Schools Be Doing?

Is your child's teacher doing the right thing when it comes to teaching his or her students the basics of reading? Here are a few pointers to keep in mind. You can find answers to these questions by asking directly during a conference, sending an email to your child's teacher, visiting the classroom, or asking to review the school's reading curriculum.

➤ Does the teacher read aloud frequently?
➤ Are favorite stories read again and again?
➤ Is "pretend" reading encouraged? Do kids have the opportunity to do so?
➤ Does your child have access to a variety of books in the classroom?
➤ Do kids practice writing? Is there a writing center in the classroom?
➤ Does the teacher teach phonics? Does he teach that there is a relationship between letters and sounds?

Teachers will likely keep a portfolio of your child's literacy growth over the school year and talk with you about this at conferences or whenever you inquire. Generally, teachers are looking to see if your child:

➤ can handle books properly (e.g., knows when a book is right-side-up, "reads" from left to right, etc.);
➤ is aware of story sequences;

- ➤ recalls details from familiar stories;
- ➤ expresses a preference for a specific story;
- ➤ uses pictures to "read" a storybook;
- ➤ is aware of print-meaning associations/permanency/orientation;
- ➤ recognizes his own name in print;
- ➤ records ideas (by using drawing as writing, then pictures and scribbles for writing);
- ➤ makes letter-like forms for writing;
- ➤ uses random letter forms for writing;
- ➤ practices with invented spellings;
- ➤ finally uses conventional spellings.

Teachers also have a form on literacy awareness they complete as children are transitioning from preschool to kindergarten. This gives your child's kindergarten teacher a sense of "where he's at" in terms of literacy growth. Modifications, special assistance, and instruction, if needed, can be made from there.

Reading Problems? There's a Program for That!

If you think that your child has a reading disorder, or a difficulty with reading, by all means, bring it to the teacher's attention! The good news is, most schools have a reading specialist who can home in on those skills. Plus, you can have many reading issues addressed by your child's SLP, especially in the case of moderate-severe CAS. If you are interested in specific reading programs for your child, here are some well-known and researched programs:

➤ *Visual Phonics.* Originally developed for kids who are deaf or hard of hearing, this program can be used in a range of settings from the classroom to a speech clinic. Visual Phonics is a method in which kids can *see* the phonemes in action. It's quick and easy to learn, can be used with any reading curriculum, multisensory, and interactive. Visit www.sensorysound.org for more information.

➤ *Lindamood-Bell.* Do you ask yourself or your child, "What do the words help your mind see as you read?" If so, then this program may be right up your alley. Patricia Lindamood and Nanci Bell have been helping kids and adults read, spell, comprehend, think critically, and express language since 1986. Their model encompasses three "rights": "the right evaluation, the right instruction, and the right environment." It is often used for children with significant dyslexia (diagnosed reading disabilities). For more information: www.lindamoodbell.com.

➤ *LiPS Program.* Part of the Lindamood-Bell program for reading, the LiPS program targets phoneme sequencing for reading, spelling, and speech. It can be especially helpful for kids to *feel* the mouth movements involved in the decoding process of speech sounds. See Lindamood-Bell above. Look for the LiPS manual and DVD at www.ganderpublishing.com/LiPS.

➤ *Immediate Intensive Intervention.* Designed and customized reading instruction in small groups or 1:1. It's systematic and explicit, requiring 90-minute reading blocks and calling its approach, "balanced literacy."

➤ *Florida Center for Reading Research (FCRR).* The FCRR presents a multimodal series for beefing up reading skills. The three modes consist of: 1) Core (all kids, comprehensive, small group, re-teaching methods); 2) Supplemental (like the core program, only these kids need a bit more instruction in vocabulary, phonics, and strengthening of existing skills); and 3) Intervention instruction (kids who are lagging behind their peers in critical reading areas). For more information, visit www.fcrr.com.

➤ *Phonics Faces.* Phonics Faces is a nice program for kids who are still working on basic sound and alphabet skills. This collection of flashcards focuses on phonemic awareness, rhyme, letter-sound association, phonics, and articulation. There is a clip on YouTube which shows a child with CAS working on this program. Look for it at www.tinyurl.com/drmoo. For more information: www.elementory.com.

➤ *Directed Reading Thinking Activity (DRTA).* A strategy that guides kids in asking questions about a text, making predictions, and then continuing to read to see if their prediction is correct. DRTA helps produce active, thoughtful readers. For more information, see: www.readingrockets.org.

➤ *The DuBard Association Method.* This is a phonetic, multisensory teaching-learning strategy for children with language deficiencies that was originally designed by the late Mildred McGinnis, a teacher at Central Institute for the Deaf in St. Louis. It has been successful for children with severe CAS. See www.usm.edu/dubard/associat.html for more information. Ask your child's SLP if she is familiar with this program.

➤ *FastForWord.* FastForWord is an expensive software program for home computer use that has a series of fun, engaging games. These games are meant to "retrain" the brains of struggling readers to improve attention, memory, and the ability to process the sounds in words. However, to be effective, this program must be used consistently for a long period of time (90 minutes a day for weeks). The website (www.scilearn.com) has many studies about its effectiveness in helping children with disorders of language and reading. Other studies suggest it may be an effective treatment for kids with Auditory Processing Disorder. However, according to research, it is not a cure-all, and other programs were just as good, as was direct therapy. For more information see www.gemmlearning.com, where you just might be lucky enough to find some online coupons.

➤ *Earobics, Step 1.* Earobics is a fun-to-play interactive computer software program designed to teach the fundamental listening and sound awareness skills that research has proven is the best prediction of reading success: www.earobics.com.

➤ *Wilson Reading Program.* Like the Lindamood-Bell program, the Wilson program is frequently used by schools to help children who have a diagnosed learning disability in reading. It is a very rule-intensive, multisensory program for kids of all ages who are not progressing in reading skills. Teachers ideally should be formally trained in the method. Check them out at www.wilsonlanguage.com.

➤ *ABeCeDarian Reading Program.* This is a multisensory decoding program that focuses on phonemic awareness, phonics, and fluency. This program has an easy instruction model for parents and teachers to use with their children, but it can also be used for adults who have reading difficulties. It's less expensive than many other programs. For more information: www.abcdrp.com.

Keep in mind that these programs may or may not be able to be implemented by a parent at home. They may require training and certification to implement. You can start with asking your SLP about them, research them online, and then determine if your child will benefit.

In addition, these programs aren't cheap! If you have a network, group, club, or listserv you frequent, consider posting a message looking to purchase an older program someone is no longer using. If you're lucky, someone may allow you to borrow their copy or just give it to you! We borrowed *Earobics* from Kate's preschool teacher. It never hurts to ask.

Determining If Your Child Needs a Specialized Reading Program

Hopefully, your child won't. But if you have concerns, you'll want your child to have a comprehensive and accurate evaluation to begin with. Your child's school may do one for free if they suspect your child has a learning disability in reading. However, they will likely put off evaluating your child while they try various types of "response to intervention." RtI is a procedure detailed in IDEA that requires schools to gradually provide more individualized, intensive help to students who *may* have learning disabilities before actually labeling them as having a learning disability.

If you don't want to wait while the school is trying RtI and you have the money, get an evaluation done outside of school by an educational psychologist, if possible. SLPs don't typically evaluate children formally for reading problems, although they may do an informal assessment with phonological awareness skills. Independent evaluators typically have no other motivation for doing the assessment and evaluation. Schools, on the other hand, might. Funding, teacher and evaluator availability, and other resources may all come into play.

Here's a sampling of tests that evaluate reading behavior:
➤ Gray Oral Reading Test/Gray Silent Reading Test, 4th Ed (GORT-4)
➤ Test of Phonological Awareness
➤ Test of Early Reading Ability
➤ Test of Word Reading Efficiency
➤ Woodcock Reading Mastery Test (WRMT-R)
➤ Kaufman Test of Educational Achievement, 2nd Ed (KTEA-2)

Your own thoughts on your child's reading progress should also be an important part of any evaluation.

There is not one test that measures reading skills comprehensively. Different reading tests measure different types of skills. It is up to the evaluators and educators to synthesize the results into an individualized package. They assess your child's passage comprehension, word comprehension, ability to read nonsense words, letter identification, decoding fluency, and word recognition. Even if your child is not communicating well verbally, you can still have an evaluation of his reading skills. There are many nonverbal components to these tests. Keep in mind, however, that not every diagnostic test is given equally (code for "well or appropriately").

One more thing about any evaluation: don't interpret it as a "label." Use the results of an evaluation as a baseline. You need to know where your child started before you can begin to assess any progress.

Visual Tracking

Another thing to keep in mind with your young reader with CAS: he may have difficulties learning how to track visually. That is, he may have a hard time following the words on the page because he is unable to track where he was reading, even in a short paragraph. OR he may have difficulty switching from looking at the chalkboard or Smartboard to looking at the paper on his desk (reading print from far and near). It all has to do with convergence of the eyes, the inward movement of both eyes toward each other at the same time. Not all children with CAS have difficulty with visual tracking. There is no known connection between the two, although it *can* occur in children with CAS.

What's a Parent to Do?

A Pediatric OT can help with some simple visual exercises. Tracking, for example, can be practiced by having your child follow a finger tip back and forth. Convergence can be practiced by having your child follow a light source (such as a pen light) from two or three feet away from his face to his nose. Do it several times in a row several times throughout the day. Another idea is to have your child follow an object around the room with his eyes only. It doesn't "count" if he has to move his head or body to track the item. Move the item up, down, right, left. Keep him guessing. Let him "test" you, too. It's fun for kids when they can play therapist.

Tell Me Something That Makes Me Feel Good

All right—I will:

The key to working with your child with CAS on reading is to remember that he will get it!

It might be challenging at times, but you'll both get there. Treat him as though he is any other kid in terms of how you go about teaching it, and try not to get too hung up on the apraxia piece.

Here's another "warm fuzzy" to keep in mind as you travel down the road less-read: in many other countries, kids don't learn to read until the third grade. For some reason, the U.S. seems to think we need to be ahead in this area, often attempting to teach kids to read at an earlier-than-ready age.

I leave you with this analogy: You are in an intense exercise class but your knee is killing you. You can't do lunges and squats as your instructor would like, so you modify. You do something similar that stills gives you the benefit, but with less strain. As a parent, and as an educator, *you may just have to modify how you teach your child with CAS to read.*

Write On!

Learning to write is a complicated process. First you need a basic understanding of the alphabet and the fact that letters represent sounds and sounds make words, and then you need to know how to order those letters so that they spell recognizable words. Here are some more steps that need to happen for the "write" stuff:

➤ Lots of reflexes need to come together to control the rate and rhythm of writing. Your child's body needs to be anchored in time and place.

➤ Your child will need to be able to cross the midline of his body with his dominant hand—the one that holds the writing utensil.

➤ He should understand that his fingers are controlling the writing utensil…sort of an abstract concept, but important nonetheless.

➤ Eyes must focus and move along the paper he is writing on.

➤ He must be able to control the fine muscles in his fingers.

➤ He will need to have the motor planning to draw the letters correctly.

➤ Most of all—he needs to have the ability to sit still!

I present this information to you because some kids with CAS also have limb apraxia and fine motor delays. Not all children with CAS will exhibit the above concerns.

Where to Begin

It may be helpful to start by teaching large arm movements. Swing those arms around in big arm circles, flap them like a bird, get creative and have fun (this is because large motor movements come before small motor movements in typical development). You don't even have to tell your little one what you're up to. He'll be none the wiser.

Some folks suggest it may be best to start writing on a vertical surface (up and down), rather than on a traditional horizontal writing surface such as a table. Again, this is strengthening those large arm movements of the body, trunk, arms, and shoulders.

Try taping paper to a wall, having your child write on an easel or the fridge—just make sure you are using washable markers or dry-erase materials.

Another fun activity is to use "window markers." Just as they sound, these markers are safe to use on windows and patio doors. Look for them at craft stores or the kids' art aisle at your favorite discount store. Have your Magic Eraser handy for those inevitable accidents.

Kids can "paint" the house with a bucket of water and a paint brush when the weather's nice. Sidewalk chalk presents similar opportunities and works the whole body.

Try "writing" in various outdoor settings such as on a gravel driveway or mud using a stick, a shoe, or your finger. Your kids will think you are very cool if you do this with them. They love when we get down and dirty while at the same time being instructional. "Sneaky" parenting, but it works!

Another aspect of writing is fine motor control. So, find toys and manipulatives that your child can squeeze and twist (fidget toys), as well as toys common in your household, like Polly Pockets and Transformers. Get some Wikki Stix or Bendaroos at craft stores and toy stores.

What You Can Do at Home

Assuming that all is "good to go" after a period of warm-up writing activities as outlined above, then it's time to jump in. Most kids learn to print their names first. Start by encouraging your child to write his name with a capital letter followed by lower-case letters. Upper-case letters are easier to master, but don't get in this bad habit of allowing your child to write in all caps. It's a hard one to break. When he's in kindergarten and first grade, lower case letters will be encouraged, if not required. He may think, "If I know and can write in all caps, what's the point in complicating matters with these pesky lower-case letters?"

Once your child learns to write his name in upper and lowercase letters, it's time to move on to the alphabet in all capitals. But here's a trick you may not know: it's not best to go in order. Start with straight letters and then work into curvy ones. That's the order of progression from easy to difficult. You'll want to give your child some success early on, right?

Here's a chart to refer to as you move through the ABCs, in order of difficulty (adapted from our experience with the *Handwriting without Tears* program):

Sequence of Difficulty in Forming Letters

FIRST	SECOND	THIRD
E, F, H, I, L, T	B, C, D, G, J, O, P, Q, S, U	A, K, M, N, R, V, W, X, Y, Z

You will also want to encourage your child with some tracing exercises. It doesn't necessarily matter if he's tracing letters—although that could be part of your approach. Sneak it in by starting first with those coloring books with tracing paper. Move on to tracing dotted line pictures and letters, which you can make yourself. Other prewriting skills include mazes and dot-to-dots.

Handwriting and Apraxia

A lot of components come into play as our kids learn to write—visual-motor coordination, motor planning, strength, sensory processing (proprioception), and cognitive processing, to name a few. You know your child best, so observe and see if you can determine where in that process things are breaking down. For my daughter, I would bet that it is visual-motor coordination and motor planning. Your child may also have something amiss in this sequence (but not always). Not all kids with CAS have motor planning problems beyond verbal or oral apraxia, but they *could*.

Think back to how you deal with the motor aspect of speech. You'll need to apply similar principles to helping your child lay down the motor pathways to handwriting. *Verbal cueing* and *verbal feedback* may be just the ticket, "Big line down, big line up, little line across the middle…that's it—you got it!"

Of course, just as with speech, **you'll need to provide many repetitions of the writing movements so that they become automatic.** Also, be sure to provide lots of positive feedback in the form of results: "I like the way this letter looks," and knowledge: "To make an /o/ you need to connect the top of the circle."

Need Some Handwriting Intervention?

Your child may require some 1:1 writing intervention that you alone—at home—can't accomplish. Teaching handwriting is complicated and time-consuming and it will test your patience. Don't lose heart and try not to feel like a failure if you can't help your child be successful. You may need an occupational therapist to step in and do an evaluation of your kiddo's writing abilities. Some writing evaluation tests are:

➤ The *Print Tool* by Jan Olsen, which is part of the *Handwriting Without Tears* program
➤ *Diagnosis of Remediation of Handwriting Problems*
➤ *The Minnesota Handwriting Test*
➤ *Children's Handwriting Evaluation Scale-Manuscript*
➤ *Evaluation Tool of Children's Handwriting-Manuscript (ETCH)*
➤ *Test of Legible Handwriting*
➤ *School Function Assessment* (looks at *all* school-related skills and functions)
➤ *The Miller Assessment of Preschoolers* (can be administered to kids up to age 5.8 years)

Most of these evaluation tools look at the eight basic handwriting skills:
1. Memory—remembering and writing letters that are dictated by another person
2. Orientation—Making sure all letters face the same direction
3. Placement—putting letters in the right direction
4. Size—how big or small a child writes
5. Start—where each letter begins
6. Sequence—the order and stroke direction of the letter parts
7. Control—the neatness and proportion of letter parts
8. Spacing—the amount of space between letters and words

As you go about seeking an evaluation and interpreting the results, keep in mind some very important pieces—how the test was administered, the scoring, reliability, and validity of the tool. Ask questions, seek answers.

If your child needs the help of an OT, get to it as soon as you can. Our therapist used *Handwriting without Tears (HWT)* for Kate and it was quite helpful. The basics behind this program is that most letters can be "drawn" with straight lines, with a few exceptions (P, O, C, and D, for example). Initially kids work with a group of wooden sticks that look a bit like 12-inch rulers to "make" letters. Next, they draw them on a small chalkboard. It's whole-body and multisensory—something our kids with apraxia can appreciate and excel at. See www.hwtears.com for more information.

Loops and Other Groups: A Kinesthetic Writing System helps kids visualize and feel the movements in writing. It's good for those who require more attention to detail, and kids learning cursive handwriting.

Scribblenauts may be more up your child's alley. It was designed for Nintendo DS to get kids to work on bringing their writing to life. It's a game in which one can, "Write anything. Solve everything." It may just be what your child needs to motivate and improve his writing. Plus, it sort of disguises "work" as "fun."

You may want to try *Mead Writing Fundamentals: Learn to Write with Raised Ruling,* a notebook containing paper with raised lines. It may provide enough of a tactile cue for your child as he learns to navigate the intricacies of print. Look for it where school supplies are sold.

Finally, Kid-O makes a product called the *A to Z Magnatab Magnetic Writing Tablet*. This fun, multisensory tool may help your child focus on forming letters correctly and consistently. The magnetic stylus works to pull metal balls to the surface, snapping into place to form the letter. To reinforce the "feel" for each letter, kids can lightly trace over the letters with the tip of their finger, pressing the metal balls back into the base. Look for it at www.kidoproducts.com or where educational toys are sold.

Writing to Communicate: Stories

At some point, your child will move into more independent storytelling and story writing. I know, it may seem eons away from the here and now, but before you know it, his imagination will be taking him to "far, far away land." Look for ways to promote writing for fun.

Provide him with notebooks and pens. Have a time of day that you let your kid experiment with "writing" books, cards, newspapers, diaries, journals, letters, checks (old, out-of-date), grocery lists, to-do lists, whatever you can think of. It's an important step in teaching kids to learn to love writing for a purpose.

Kids with apraxia may have a harder than usual time getting their thoughts from their brain to their hands and out of their writing instrument. It's just like the underlying neuro-motor issue with verbal communication. Only now it's with written communication. There are some software programs that can help your child get his internal narratives out of his head and onto the paper or screen and organize them. These include *Draft Builder, Co-Writer,* and *Write Out Loud* (www.donjohnston.com). There are also software programs such as *MacSpeech Dictate* (www.MacSpeech.com) and *Dragon Naturally Speaking* (www.Nuance.com) that convert speech to text.

Remember, if your child's expressive language is still rough in terms of correct syntax and morphology, it will show in his story-writing abilities. "Encourage him to read what he has written aloud. This will help him catch missing and extraneous words," says Rhonda Banford, CCC-SLP. Again, your child's classroom teacher, reading/writing specialist, or SLP can also assist with these skills.

What about Spelling?

So, you finally got your little one to progress from scribbles to more meaningful letter development; maybe a few words or two have emerged. But there seems to be one little problem: your child isn't spelling correctly! No worries. What your child is doing is referred to as "invented spelling." It's a term that was originally coined by linguist Carol Chomsky, and used by many others, even the prominent child development psychologist Jean Piaget. It's the young child's unpressured efforts to write words of his own communication before learning the correct spelling. Invented spelling is a way of self-expression and it's not something to stress about.

Invented spelling reveals how your child *thinks* words are spelled. It's actually a step in the right direction. It's like putting phonics on paper. Your child is using the symbols he knows or makes up to "write" words. Invented spelling gives children a window to their own awareness. Your child will spell correctly when he is cognitively ready. Look at this period in his writing life as inquiry, experimentation, and growth.

Say That Again?! Chapter Summary

I hope you found this a jam-packed source of information and encouragement when it comes to helping your child succeed in reading and writing. These are two skills he will undoubtedly need in his academic career and beyond. Please don't give up. These skills are extremely difficult and time consuming to teach for the parents of any kid, with or without CAS. They will test your patience. But you don't have to go it alone. Remember, you can always call on the assistance of your child's school, his SLP, his OT, or an educational psychologist. And remember, your child will be successful in his own way.

Read On: Recommended Resources

➤ While it's a huge book, *The Mislabeled Child: How Understanding Your Child's Unique Learning Style Can Open the Doors to Success* by Brock and Fernette Eide (Hyperion, 2006) covers a lot of good information on learning and memory, autism and giftedness, handwriting and dysgraphia.

➤ A book you may find helpful in your journey is *Different Learners: Identifying, Preventing, and Treating Your Child's Learning Problems* by Jane Healy, Ph.D. (Simon and Schuster, 2010). It does a great job of discussing current changes in education, the case of difference vs. disability, and genetics vs. environment, all with a research-based background.

➤ If you'd like more nitty-gritty reading research, look for *Phonological Awareness: From Research to Practice* by Gail T. Gillon (Guilford Press, 2004).

➤ *The Young Child's Memory for Words: Developing 1st and 2nd Language Literacy* by educator Daniel R. Meier (Teachers College Press, 2004) is a good resource for getting a grasp on literacy development, teaching, and learning.

➤ *Early Speech Language Issues and Late Literacy: Will Slow to Talk Mean Slow to Read?* is a CASANA-sponsored DVD with Dr. Ruth Stoeckel of the Mayo

Clinic. It details the reasons kids with apraxia and other types of speech-sound disorders are at risk for later reading, writing, and spelling difficulties. It gives evidence-based intervention for those emerging literacy skills. Find it at the Apraxia-KIDS store, www.Apraxi-KIDS.org.

➤ *Ready Bodies, Learning Minds* by pediatric physical therapist Athena Oden (David Oden, 2006) is a small, spiral-bound resource you may find helpful in understanding how to help your child learn to read and write from a motor-planning perspective: www.readybodies.com.

➤ *Miss Brooks Loves Books (and I Don't)* by Barbara Bottner (Random House Children's Books, 2010) is a fun and adorable book that even the most resistant reader will appreciate.

➤ *The Living Classroom: Writing, Reading and Beyond* by David Armington (NAEYC, 1997) presents lots of examples of invented spelling and drawings done by pre-literate children. It's a great resource for parents and teachers alike when it comes to teaching the basics of writing and spelling.

➤ *Mosaic of Thought* by educators Ellin Oliver Keene and Susan Zimmerman (Heinemann, 1997) offers a step-by-step approach to developing thoughtful, independent readers.

➤ *Learning to Read and Write: Developmentally Appropriate Practices for Young Children* by Susan B. Neuman, Carol Copple, and Sue Bredekamp (NAEYC, 2000) gives concrete examples of how to teach reading and writing to kids before the 3rd grade. It's mostly geared toward early childhood educators, but parents can glean something from it as well.

➤ *First Sound Series* is an interactive series of children's books developed by SLPs Michelle Soloman and Lavinia Pereira that encourage the development and growth of speech and language skills: www.firstsoundseries.com.

➤ *Over 1000 Games, Activities, Tongue Twisters, Fingerplays, Songs, and Stories to Get Children Excited about Reading* by Pam Schiller and *The Complete Book and CD Set of Rhymes, Songs, Poems, Fingerplays, & Chants* by Jackie Silberg and Pam Schiller (Gryphon House, 2006) suggest some great ideas for things to do at home to build phonological awareness.

➤ The Zaner-Bloser website is dedicated to *early literacy*. The site includes information on reading, leveled books, vocabulary, spelling, and handwriting: www.zaner-bloser.com.

➤ *365 Phonics Activities* (HTS Books, 1998) by Sandra Fisher, Carole Palmer, Susan Bloom, and Joyce Stirniman with consultant Elizabeth C. Stull will give you *at least* 365 ideas.

➤ Lakeshore Learning has some great products for teaching **phonemic and phonological awareness** skills. My favorites are: *Rhyming Big Book, Phonemic Awareness Activity Card Library and Chart, Match a Sound,* and *Rhyming Sounds Basket.* Visit their website at www.lakeshorelearning.com.

➤ Here are **some great books** you may want to read with your children. They have been recommended by parents of kids with CAS:
  - *If You Give a Mouse a Cookie* and any other *If You Give* books by Laura Numeroff
  - *Cornelius P. Mud* series by Barney Saltzberg
  - *Dinosaur Roar* by Paul and Henrietta Strickland
  - *Polar Bear, Polar Bear* and *Brown Bear, Brown Bear* by Bill Martin, Jr.
  - *Pout-Pout Fish* by Debra Diesen
  - *Something from Nothin* by Phoebe Gilman
  - *Mr. Brown Can Moo, Can You?* by Dr. Seuss
  - *It Isn't Easy Being a Bunny* by Marilyn Sadler
  - *Curious George* books by H.A. and Margaret Rey
  - *Go Dog Go* by P.D. Eastman
  - *Runny Babbit* by Shel Silverstein (best suited for older kids with CAS)

➤ Pam Allyn's **What to Read When** (Avery Trade, 2009) may be helpful in your search for the perfect books to entertain and motivate young readers.

➤ *Reading Magic: Why Reading to Our Children Will Change Their Lives Forever* by Mem Fox (Mariner Books, 2008) is a fantastic book written by an educator and reading specialist. It provides lists of books to consider reading to and with your children, and does a great job of surveying the literature.

➤ *Reading Together: Everything You Need to Raise a Child Who Loves to Read* by Diane W. Frankenstein (Perigee Trade, 2009) has great tips, tools, and suggestions for raising a reader.

➤ For more **suggestions on books to read with your children**, visit the Time Out to Read website: www.TimeOutToRead.com.

➤ *The Read Aloud Handbook* by Jim Trelease recommends books that are fun for parents to read and engaging for kids.

Section Five

Coping & Hoping

· · · · · · · · · · · · ·

Chapter Thirteen

CAS Affects Us All

· · · · · · · · · · · · ·

Coping as a Family

It was a stressful time when we learned about Kate's childhood apraxia of speech diagnosis. We had recently relocated to the Chicago area from Minnesota. My husband was starting a new job that took up lots of time and involved considerable travel. I was in charge of getting the new house in order and unpacked while raising two young girls. Kate was only two and a half years old and baby Kelly was nine months.

I was also adjusting to the demands of being a full-time at-home mother, a change we'd made out of necessity. I'd considered going back to work as a psychiatric nurse, even interviewing for a job or two. But who would watch the girls in a strange new city while I worked? Plus, Jim's travel schedule made it nearly impossible for him to keep regular hours. I couldn't rely on him to be home on evenings and weekends due to "extra work" and the learning curve of starting a new job. Meanwhile, the housing market was going south and our Minnesota home was still on the market. We were making two house payments on one income. And Kate wasn't talking.

Growing up, my dad had always said, "Worry about the things you can control, not what you can't." His fatherly advice resonated at this point in my life. The move, the house not selling, my husband's travel schedule—they were all out of my control. What I could do, though, was get Kate evaluated at a speech clinic. My spirits started to lift.

While it was hard to hear the diagnosis, it was also a relief. I could at least check one thing off my list—"help Kate learn to talk"—by getting her to and from speech therapy. And the ironic thing was, hearing the therapist tell me Kate had apraxia wasn't nearly as stressful as hearing, "I'm sorry but the buyer of your home backed out at the last minute and now you have two house payments." Everything is relative.

Of course, my example is extreme. I don't want to imply that it's "no big deal" that you suddenly have been thrust into this world of apraxia. It is very real and very challenging. But you *will* get through it. This chapter will help.

> ### The Nuts and Bolts of This Chapter
>
> ➤ A discussion of how it is still possible to develop a healthy, happy family life when your child has CAS
>
> ➤ More on the grief process (it was covered briefly in Chapter 4) and ways you and your family can work through your feelings
>
> ➤ Differences in reactions and coping styles
>
> ➤ The unique stressors of raising a family in which one member (or more) has special needs, plus tips on remaining strong and developing positive coping strategies
>
> ➤ How to look after your own physical and emotional needs

Happy Families Struggle at Times, Too

The previous chapter talked about how we just want our kids to be happy. Well yes, that is true. But even the happiest of families can hit some bumps along the road. Everyone will be affected in some manner by the apraxia diagnosis.

This chapter will break it down by family member, but generally you will all feel a sense of loss. Why do you feel this way? Well, it's as though you are grieving the loss of the child you thought you would be raising, a normally chatty kid who doesn't have to struggle to put her words together. It's akin to moving away to a new city or state, the loss of a job, the loss of a marriage through divorce, or the loss of a loved one through death. The stages that parents go through in coping with a child's diagnosis have been compared to the stages of grief identified by psychiatrist Elizabeth Kubler-Ross. Not everyone who experiences a loss goes through these stages in order, but you can expect to go through *some* of these stages at *some* point along your apraxia journey, even if the amount of time you spend in one stage or another is variable.

Denial: You may be experiencing denial if you are "waiting and seeing" in regards to your child's lack of communication. Deep down inside, you *know* something's amiss, but you aren't ready to hear it. After you hear the diagnosis, you may question the competence of the evaluator, or seek a second opinion because "they don't know what they're talking about."

Anger: You've heard the news—your child has apraxia. And now you're just plain ol' angry. Next you know, you're picking a fight with the receptionist at the front desk of the speech clinic, your husband (because it's his "bad" genes, after all), and your mom because she doesn't know what apraxia is and therefore thinks it must not be "real."

Bargaining: You pray, you put your faith in God, you promise you'll do everything you can if the apraxia will just go away.

Depression: You're overwhelmed, you feel powerless, you feel vulnerable and drained. You may even feel guilty ("It was my speech problems she inherited. It was because I had that glass of wine when I was pregnant"). You may begin to feel uncertain about your child's future or your ability to pay for speech therapy, and that can be downright depressing.

Acceptance: You have allowed yourself to feel your emotions and process all of the new information, and now you can accept the new diagnosis. The good news is, you are in the very best position to help your child when you enter this stage. Hooray! And since we all want to help our kids be their best, you can finally feel empowered. It's time now to hop on the Internet and join online support groups so you can offer advice and ideas to other parents. It's time to join local groups on apraxia. It's time to do something big like write a blog, a book, or attend a conference. You've got the power!

Don't get discouraged if you periodically go through feelings of anger, depression, sadness, or bargaining even though you've reached the "acceptance" stage. It's perfectly normal to regress at times. When Kate had to go back to therapy after a six-month break, I felt cheated in some ways. When her little sister, Kelly, started talking a mile-a-minute, I felt a sense of loss—I'd never heard Kate's sweet little voice at that age because she wasn't talking. Although Kate is older and has had more experiences than her little sister, I often felt protective of her when she couldn't keep up verbally. I felt it especially necessary to build up her self-esteem by acknowledging her other strengths when she faltered in communication: "You are a really smart girl, Kate. Let's try saying that again."

What's a Family to Do?

➤ *Realize that you are in this together.* How much, what, and when you share with your other children about their sibling's apraxia is a personal decision based on lots of variables—how old they are, their maturity level, how much involvement they are expected to have in the day-to-day aspects of apraxia. We'll get into more specifics later in this chapter. The bottom line is to let your other children know you love them and you'll always be their parent, too.

➤ *Use coping strategies that worked for your family in the past.* What did you all do when Dad lost his job several years ago? You made it work somehow. What can you draw on from the past to help you in the present?

➤ *Teach your family about CAS.* Hold a family meeting or two. Get out a whiteboard or have a Power Point presentation. If your kids are old enough, assign them some Internet searches on CAS that they can present to the rest of the family. Younger kids may appreciate reading Amy Glorosio-May's book, *My*

Brother Is Very Special or Angela Baublitz's *I Want to be Your Friend,* or watching movies on accepting differences (see Resources at the end of this chapter). Allow family members to ask questions. Give them the best answers you know or promise to follow-up when you have the information.

➤ *Appreciate the little things.* Instead of focusing on the "big news" that your child has apraxia, look for the little things in life that make your family fun. The bike ride you all enjoyed, the family hike, the trip to the county fair. I will never forget the first time I heard Kate say, "I love you." That was a small moment in the grand scheme of things that we all celebrated as a family.

➤ *Remember that all members in your immediate family (and perhaps your extended family) will go through the stages of grief.* It's common to feel like you are the only one. Be alert to the stages of grief and help your children and spouse work through them.

The Care and Keeping of Mom

"When Momma's happy, we're all happy." I know you've heard this saying before. Is there any truth to it? Yes!

It was no surprise that I was particularly stressed in the time surrounding Kate's diagnosis. I wanted to crawl under a rock and stay there. I wanted to scream. I wanted to pull all of my hair *and* eyeballs out. Interestingly, I wasn't the only mom who felt that way.

Researchers in Germany thought that the emotional state of mothers of kids with speech impaired children would make an interesting research study. So, they designed and ran a study, "Anxiety and Depression in Mothers of Speech Impaired Children" (see References). Fully 11 percent of mothers of speech impaired children (unknown whether these kids had CAS or not) met criteria for depression and anxiety, whereas only 2.5 percent of moms in the control group (children who were not speech impaired) met those criteria. The researchers also found that:

➤ Mothers often take on the largest part of the extra care a child with speech or language problems requires (arranging therapy, transporting to therapy, communicating with therapists).

➤ In order to take care of those special needs, mothers often have to give up their personal interests and their job.

➤ Mothers often feel additional pressure and strain because they now have the responsibility of supporting speech therapy at home.

➤ Moms worry that their children with speech impairments won't be socially accepted.

➤ Mothers fear that their children with speech impairments will develop other disorders such as ODD, ADHD, depression, and anxiety.

➤ Finally, moms worry about their child's future and whether he or she will ever be able to talk "normally."

That's not to say that dads don't feel this way, too. When I asked my own husband how he felt about all of this, he said something like, "Sure, I think about those things, too. But I am not overly worried about it. I don't lose sleep over it. I know Kate will get the help she needs. She's going to speech [therapy]." And he's right. She will get better. It's the way of a woman, and particularly a mother, to process these events differently than a man. Men are typically solution-focused ("she's going to speech therapy"), whereas women are more concerned with immediate feelings and understanding the "whys" of the event ("Why did this happen to Kate? Aren't you worried, too?").

I should point out that while 11 percent of moms in the study meet the criteria for anxiety and depression, the majority (89 percent) did not. Don't feel you are bound to be diagnosed with anxiety or depression just because this study says you *might*. It's a good idea, though, to keep your antennae up should you start to feel a little "off," especially if you have a family history or a personal tendency to suffer from depression or anxiety.

It's downright hard work to be a mother. Some will say, "It's the hardest job I ever loved." If you're a mom reading this, congratulate yourself. It's a great step towards understanding and educating yourself on apraxia so you can be even better at the important job you already do: being mom.

Are You Depressed? Anxious?

Curious as to what some symptoms of depression/anxiety are?
➤ Lack of interest or enjoyment in things you previously enjoyed
➤ Eating too little or too much (appetite changes)
➤ Weight gain or loss
➤ Jittery feeling; heart feels like it's beating "too fast"
➤ Feeling as though you are always holding your breath
➤ Sleeping too much or too little (restless sleep)
➤ Headaches or other bodily aches and pains that are "new" for you
➤ Excess worry or guilt
➤ Poor concentration
➤ Loss of energy

If you find yourself saying "yes" to more of these points than not, it may be time to see your physician. You are not alone. It is estimated that 14 million folks in the U.S. suffer from depression and anxiety. Many physicians are comfortable treating your symptoms. (Family practitioners and internists are becoming more comfortable discussing mental health.) It never hurts to share your concerns with your doctor. He or she is there to help.

The road of parenting is spotted with bumps and potholes. There will be others in your parenting journey, too. Understanding and helping your child with apraxia is just one of those bumps. Go ahead and whine and cry about apraxia if you need to. I know you weren't expecting it. But know, too, that there are ways to cope.

What's a Mom to Do?

Amy Baskin and Heather Fawcett, authors of *More Than a Mom: Living a Full and Balanced Life When Your Child Has Special Needs* (Woodbine House, 2006), offer a multitude of helpful suggestions:

➤ *Get the most out of life.* Even though moms often bear the brunt of the work involved in raising special needs kids, they need to have a happy and fulfilling life for themselves. Ask yourself: what's important to me? Make a list. Keep a journal. Write down what it is you want out of life. Most folks will divide their lives into these categories: friends, marriage/intimate relationship, physical/exercise, sleep, work, volunteer work, church/spirituality, housework/maintenance, education/knowledge, and health (not listed in any significance).

➤ *Draw a pie chart of the things in your daily life, add a percentage to how much time you think you spend on them.* Are some pieces of the pie too small? Too big? How about making a chart with two columns—"Before we knew about apraxia" and "Now we have apraxia" and compare and contrast what has changed. Determine your new priorities (getting your child to and from speech therapy, home practice) and find places where you can make compromises (I'll take her to therapy, if you [husband] can pick her up). *Looking to find more hours in the day?* Then you may like this book, *168 Hours: You Have More Time Than You Think,* by Laura Vanderkam (Portfolio, 2010).

➤ *Determine how you keep your pitcher filled.* We all need to fill our personal well from time to time. How do you do it? What do you need to feel energized and ready to go? It's different for everyone. For you, it may be a morning jog, an afternoon nap, time on Facebook, a crafty enterprise, a phone call to a good friend, or daily prayer. You need to find and make the time to keep your pitcher filled.

➤ *Know that you need breaks, too.* You will feel better if you schedule a break for yourself. Did you know that employers are supposed to give employees a fifteen-minute break for every four hours of work? Even if you are an at-home mom, you are still working and you deserve a break.

➤ *Reclaim past hobbies or explore new ones.* Perhaps before you had kids, you loved to make handmade cards. Then kids came and you no longer had time or a place to store your craft supplies. Find them. Dust them off and start working on a card for your friend who just had a baby. Always wanted to learn about spelunking or knitting? Why not absorb yourself in learning about something new? You may find that you become less focused on the problems (of apraxia) and more interested in something that revs you up.

➤ *Schedule time away.* It doesn't have to be a trip to the Virgin Islands, but go somewhere, even if it is just to the hotel down the road for a night (or your parent's or friend's home). Put it on the calendar. You are that important.

➤ *Connect with your friends.* No doubt you will meet others who have a child with apraxia or other speech-language needs. That's great. Share stories and feelings about your unique experience, but remember that you have other friends, too. It's like when you first had a baby and all you wanted to do was hang out with other new moms; your childless friends felt jilted. Connect with friends who aren't all about apraxia, too.

➤ *Join a Support Group.* You may want to look into a support group for parents and caregivers of children with apraxia. You'll learn a lot, connect, commiserate, and have a unique bond with others. You can start by joining listservs at Apraxia-Kids (www.apraxia-kids.org) and Speechville (www.speechville.com). There may be one in your local area like Windy City Apraxia (www.windycityapraxia.com) in the Chicago area. For help finding a support group, ask your SLP or early intervention team or even consider starting your own (see Chapter 16).

➤ *Remember that you are not alone.* You have friends and family. Rely on them. Ask specifically for their support. Try this, "Honey, I know you and I don't always respond to stress/change in the same way. But right now I really need you just to listen to me as I work through Kate's diagnosis." Periodically, check-in with your sweetie; ask what he needs/wants right now in the apraxia journey (don't be surprised if he says, "nothing."), then share your needs/wants. We'll cover more relationship/marriage concerns later in this chapter.

➤ *Learn about CAS and brush up on terminology that goes along with the diagnosis.* You may want to seek out more information than this book provides. Go for it. If you don't understand something your therapist is sharing with you, ask. You weren't born knowing everything about speech and language issues, were you? You will uncover lots of terminology and abbreviations. Don't ever think your question is "stupid"; it's stupid *not* to ask for clarification.

➤ *Use coping strategies that have worked for you in the past.* Whatever it is—getting a massage, heading to "Fatblaster" at the gym, eating a bucket of popcorn at the movies, or reading a juicy new book—it's important that you take care of yourself.

What Stage Are You In?

We're often so concerned about what "stage" our kids are at, but moms have stages, too. According to Ann Pleshette Murphy in her book, *The Seven Stages of Motherhood: Making the Most of Your Life As Mom* (Knopf, 2004), they are:
- ➤ Stage 1: Altered States—Pregnancy, Birth, and the 4th trimester
- ➤ Stage 2: Finding Your Footing—Finding Yourself (months 4 - 12)
- ➤ Stage 3: Letting Go—The Toddler Years, One and Two
- ➤ Stage 4: Trying to Do It All—The Preschool Years (ages 3 - 6 years)
- ➤ Stage 5: Reading the Compass to God-Knows-Where (years 6 - 10)
- ➤ Stage 6: Living in the Gray Zone: The Preteen Years (10 - 13 years)
- ➤ Stage 7: It Gets Easier…and Then They Leave: The Teen Years (13 - 18 years)

Can you see how there are some parallels between these stages and Elisabeth Kubler-Ross' stages of grief? Can you see how sometimes you vacillate between several stages at once?

Dads Cope, Too!

Since I'm not a dad, I can't give you a blow-by-blow account of how it feels to be a dad who's just heard that his child has CAS. I can recall, though, how blasé my husband seemed to be at hearing Kate's diagnosis, "Oh, hmmm…well, now we know." I cocked an eyebrow and looked at him like, "What?! That's all you're going to say?" And then he proceeded to flip through the mail looking for the big check from Ed Mc-Mahon. Just as the German study on mental health mentioned at the beginning of the chapter found, mothers often take on the lion's share of the work in taking care of a child with speech and language difficulties.

But that's not to say dads never do. There are househusbands and dads who decide to quit their full-time jobs-for-money to tend to the daily needs of such a child. There are families who make a conscious decision to co-parent—literally in a 50/50 fashion, job-share, and other arrangements.

Dads worry, too. Their list of concerns may differ from a mom's, though. Dads often worry about the financial costs of speech therapy. They may be concerned about insurance issues and logistical problems such as who will take your little one to and from therapy. They may fear for their child's future—but they haven't gotten as far as visualizing her socializing in college. Their fears may be more immediate—like whether she'll be reading at an age-appropriate level or attending kindergarten with her peers.

I don't want to stereotype here; there are all kinds of people out there. Generally, though, men don't share their emotions as freely as women. Men typically aren't as chatty as women. Men often like to *solve* problems. Women often enjoy *talking about* problems. Men may gather their information differently than women. Not all men will go to their friends first for information about apraxia. They will likely go to the Internet. Men may shut themselves off from the family (playing golf, working longer hours) while processing information about CAS. Men care just as deeply as women, but need time to absorb it all.

If you are a father reading this, take your time to process the information in your own way, but please discuss it at a later time with your wife/partner. If you are the mother, give your husband or partner some breathing room. You might try scheduling a time to talk—e.g., "After your golf game, I'd really like to talk about Carson's apraxia."

Your Marriage—Seeing Things Eye to Eye

You knew it was coming. We can't talk about Mom and Dad in separate sections and call it done. Not if you are married—or in a partnered, live-in arrangement. As a joint force behind your child's success and rearing, it's important that we not ignore the marriage relationship.

By now, you know just how hard it is to be a parent *and* be a couple. Having kids puts a strain on your relationship (constant care, finding private couple time, finances, and equitable division of "work"). Add in a kid with CAS, and it's *really* no walk in the park. You can do it; you just may have to try a bit harder and use creative tactics.

In *Married with Special Needs Children: A Couple's Guide to Staying Connected,* authors Laura E. Marshak and Fran Pollack Preznant identify these common stresses on relationships:

- ➤ *Lack of diagnosis:* In the early stages, you just knew your child wasn't communicating like she should be. I bet you argued about this in some form or fashion. Now that you have a diagnosis, do you argue about that? "She does. She does not!"
- ➤ *Information overload:* You may be hearing conflicting information from specialists, other parents, or your relatives. This ultimately leads couples to confusion and delay, and sometimes anger.
- ➤ *Financial issues:* One parent may feel the apraxia burden more than the other and may have had to quit work. The family is now unable to draw on that income. Plus, products, books, resources, testing, and therapy all cost money. With less income, it's no surprise that financial stress can come between couples.
- ➤ *Time constraints:* You need time to do the basics in running a household like paying bills and cooking. If your children are school-age, factor in time for assisting with homework and communicating with teachers, as well as IEP meetings. Now that you have a child with CAS, there are therapy appointments to keep and speech practice at home. You may have to rearrange your work schedule or negotiate with daycare providers for a flexible schedule that will accommodate therapy.

➤ *Mental and physical fatigue:* Exhaustion can bring out the worst in marital partners. You're cranky and your needs aren't getting met. Who *wouldn't* snap?! Take turns being "on," look for respite care (Grandma and Grandpa—see later section in this chapter), teach independence skills for your child so you don't have to do *everything* for her.

➤ *Dealing with reactions from others:* Others may tend to identify the apraxia and not your child. You may deal with pity, curiosity, rude comments. It's completely natural to feel stressed by hearing these comments, and figuring out how to deal with them. Come up with a joint plan with your spouse/significant other so you're on the same page. Refer to the section, "Do You Feel the Need to Justify Your Child's Apraxia?" in Chapter 14 for additional guidance.

Parents Share...

"I felt the need to justify speech therapy so much. I had to decline play dates often. "No, we can't because we're at speech therapy [at that time]." I wondered if apraxia was in his school record and how that would affect how teachers looked at him. My anxiety level just kept going up."

—Small Talk: All About Apraxia parent participant

A study in the *Journal of Health and Behavioral Science* (March 2009) reported that parents of children with disabilities face more daily stress. Through a parent survey and a clinical measure of stress (measuring the amount of cortisol—the stress hormone—in parent's saliva), it was found that 50 percent of their days are considered "stressful" as compared to 40 percent of the days for parents who did not have a child with a disability. Stress was referred to as time, daily hassles, positive events, and physical symptoms of fatigue. The disabilities in this study did not include apraxia specifically, but did include ADHD, Down syndrome, and bipolar disorder, among others.

Parents Cope: What's a Couple to Do?

➤ *Know that you and your partner may deal with emotions differently.* How do your coping styles differ? Do you even know *your own* coping style? Be honest. How does your partner cope? If you don't know, ask.

➤ *Let your spouse hear the information about CAS from someone other than you.* Try not to be "Brainy Smurf" when it comes to apraxia. Whether your spouse hears something about CAS from your SLP directly, or through the Internet or a listserv, it gives him or her some control in your child's progress. You might try printing out an article or forwarding it to your sweetie's email. Make a date to discuss it. Consider learning about your child's apraxia together as a way of bonding.

➤ *Speaking of dates, have one!* Put it on the calendar and secure a sitter, and go on an old-fashioned date. It doesn't have to be fancy or involved; just alone time with your spouse. Go on a walk, see a movie, chat at a coffee shop, have a picnic. Make it something you two enjoy doing together. Try not to talk about the kids, if you can help it.

➤ *Have a "date" at home.* You can schedule a weekly date night right at home after the kiddos have gone to bed. My husband and I have a standing agreement that every Saturday night we don't do anything but hang out with each other. That means no laundry folding or Internet surfing. Instead, we may get takeout and play a game of Scrabble. Have a fire, watch a movie, try a new wine. No chores and no kids. Plan it now.

➤ *Dream build.* One mother whose daughter has apraxia mentioned she and her hubby like to "dream build"—talk about future ambitions and family goals. Your version of dream building may be walking the aisles of The Home Depot and dreaming of the home improvement ideas you'd like to tackle. Or you may enjoy thinking about retirement plans or how you're going to create that tree farm you've always wanted.

➤ *Know when to say "enough."* We all need time alone. Find time to pursue your own interests apart from your spouse. Believe it or not, parents who connect well when they are together have other emotional and social outlets besides one another.

➤ *Laugh!* Humor is the balm to a stressful or worrisome situation. Laughter increases endorphins (feel-good hormones) and opens the nasal passage so your brain gets more oxygen. Even smiling has a similar effect. Look for situations in your life—be it an "apraxic moment" or not, and laugh at them. I'll never forget the day a couple years ago when Jim took Kate to the mall for a cookie. They were sitting in the café area of a bakery that opened to the mall. It was spring, so the Easter Bunny had replaced Santa. Kate's eyes got as big as saucers as she pointed to the bunny hut and exclaimed, "No Ho Ho...Big Hop Hop!" We still laugh about it to this day.

Leaving Your Child with a Sitter

You desperately need a date night, but Grandma and Grandpa aren't available. You need a sitter you can trust and feel at ease with. Make sure you tell your babysitter about your child's difficulty in communicating. You don't even have to call it "apraxia." Simply say something like, "Olivia has a hard time using her words. She can understand everything you say to her; she just might not be able to respond—right away, or at all. Just have fun with her and if you get stuck, ask her to show you [lead you to] what she means—that usually works for us." Of course, tell the sitter what works for *your* child.

If you are "shopping" for a babysitter, consider asking at your speech clinic for a student who may be interning, or a local college's nursing, education, speech pathology, or child psychology department. Most college students appreciate the extra money, and if you start with these departments you're almost sure to find a sitter who likes kids.

> ### Could You Benefit from Couples' Counseling?
>
> That's a tough decision involving lots of emotions. Generally, couple's counseling can provide you with:
> - ➤ New perspectives, an unbiased approach, a third person's point-of-view;
> - ➤ Help in questioning your assumptions, goals, and intrapersonal dynamics;
> - ➤ Ways to break dysfunctional patterns in your relationship.
>
> (From *Married with Special-Needs Children* by Laura Marshak and Fran Prezant)

Practical Matters—The Logistics of Parenting a Child with CAS

Let's go ahead and hammer out some boring, household maintenance things that need to happen before we jump into how the rest of the family (other children, grandparents, etc.) are dealing with your child's apraxia. First of all, you will need to take stock of your family goals, schedule, and routine at some point in this journey. You may formally sit down and hash this out with your spouse. Or you may need to deal with it on the spur of the moment. For example, your kid needs to get to speech therapy at 3 p.m. on Mondays. Getting her there may be relatively easy if you are a stay-at-home parent, but what if you're not?

➤ *Consider changes to your job.* It's an important part of who you are and helps keep the family living the lifestyle you've chosen. You may find that the only way you can give your child the time and attention she needs, however, is to cut back on your work. In my case, I wasn't working because I was on maternity leave, and then we relocated to a new city. When we learned of Kate's diagnosis, I saw it as a "sign" that I needed to be home with the girls. I didn't go back. But I missed interacting with adults, plus I had a hard time understanding just how important my being home was for Kate. Look for options for making it work: cut back to part-time, work a condensed week so you can have a three-day weekend, job-share, work evenings or weekends if you can, telecommute, or start your own business.

➤ *Map out your household chores.* What goes into running your home? Make a chart. Who usually does what? Add in your new duties: schedule therapy appointment, drive to therapy, observe therapy sessions, read and learn about apraxia and therapy techniques, research and purchase products to help your child with communication, follow up with therapists (in-person, over the phone, via email), connect with teachers and special education specialists at the school. Now, determine how these things will be divvied up.

➤ *Maximize your peak energy time.* Learn to manage your time better by finding your peak energy times. It may not be a specific time of day like 2 – 5 p.m.—instead, it may be more like two hours after you wake up, or after you've exercised. Tackle the things you hate to do first and then reward yourself with something more pleasurable. Don't deliberate on the task. Just do it!

➤ *Document everything!* You will be making more phone calls and seeing more paper come through your door. Keep notes on calls and other pieces of paper in a file or binder. Keep a journal or blog on your child's progress and day-to-day changes, because it gets difficult to recall specifics later. Even just marking sample things on the kitchen calendar can trigger a memory: "Said a 3-word sentence today!"

➤ *Keep your eyes peeled for fine and gross motor development.* Children with CAS may also have global apraxia (AKA dyspraxia, developmental coordination disorder, limb apraxia, or motor incoordination). You may get so focused on the lack of communication that you fail to recognize that she is having difficulties in other areas of development. If so, occupational and physical therapies may be just what your child needs.

You and the Family Medical Leave Act (FMLA)

What It Is: A federal law that protects parents' jobs if they need to take time off to tend to a child with a health concern, including a speech-language disorder.

How It Works: Parents can take an unpaid leave of absence (LOA) for as little as a few hours to as much as three months and be guaranteed a job to return to. If you need to take regular time off to get your child to speech therapy a couple of times a week, your employer has the right to make reasonable job reassignments. However, they must maintain your current salary and benefits.

How to Qualify: You must have been working in your current position for at least 12 months, and also must meet these additional conditions: you have worked at least 1,250 hours in the last 12 months and your employer has at least 50 employees within a 75 mile radius, and you intend to return to work at the end of your LOA. Talk to your manager or HR representative about securing the proper paperwork.

Your Other Kids

● ● ● ● ● ● ● ● ● ● ●

It's hard enough to parent your children equally anyway. It's even more challenging when one of them has CAS. It's hard not to think about apraxia when you are interacting with your child with apraxia. You wonder what it is (again). What caused it (will we ever know)? What can we do? How can I help? And the granddaddy of all questions, will she ever be okay? So, we cater to our child with apraxia. We try to make life easier for her. And in doing so, our other kids may get—or feel like—they get the short end of the stick. It's not intentional; it just is. The bottom line is this: sibs worry too. They need support and a peer group and they need time with you—their parents. Specifically, though, siblings are struggling with lots of questions, concerns, and feelings.

Debbie Feit, author of *The Parent's Guide to Speech and Language Problems,* advises parents to look out for feelings of confusion and worry, anger and jealousy, embarrassment and guilt, and protectiveness and pride.

Confusion and Worry: When we learn of our child's apraxia diagnosis, we're confused and worried, but have skills in place for coping. Our other children may not. Try to keep discussions about apraxia between you and your spouse. Little ears hear a lot. If you feel comfortable—and your other children are at an appropriate age—share with them a bit about what's going on: "Kristen has a hard time using her words. We go to speech so she can get better." Consider taking your other children to the clinic so they can see what's happening. You may or may not want to label the disorder by referring to it as "apraxia," depending on your other child(ren)'s age(s) and maturity level.

Anger and Jealousy: Even though you've explained your child's apraxia to her siblings and told them why it's important for you to spend extra time with her, they still may not think it's fair. That's completely normal. Talk to them about their feelings: "I know it's hard for you to see me working with Grant on his speech issues all the time. I wish things were different, too. I love you very much, too." Make a date to spend with your other child(ren) on something important to them—studying for a science test, shopping for new school shoes.

Embarrassment and Guilt: Your other children may not know who to turn to when they want to talk about their sibling's apraxia. Sometimes siblings are embarrassed when their friends make fun of their sister who "doesn't talk." Other times, they may feel guilty when they lose their patience with their sibling because they just can't understand what she's trying to say. Let your other children know that this is normal, and give them the opportunity to talk to you about it.

Protectiveness and Pride: Some siblings, especially older ones, may become protective of your child with CAS. They may become good "speech therapists" to your child with apraxia, quizzing her on words or reaching her in a way you or your child's therapist may not be able to. For example, a mother in Illinois named Courtney shares this:

"My daughter is 3 ½ and a little 'advanced' in terms of speech development. She will help her 5-year-old brother when he says something incorrect.

*For example, 'No, Ryan. The 'p' comes from your lips. Say 'up' with your lips.'
Or, 'go comes from your throat,' and she points to her throat. It's cute and helps
some of the time; but sometimes Ryan won't have anything to do with it."*

(Examples and descriptions of common sibling feelings were gleaned from *The Parent's Guide to
Speech & Language Problems* by Debbie Feit).

Coping Corner for Sibs

➤ Let your other children know you love and value them.

➤ Talk about how everyone in the family has strengths and weaknesses. List them for each family member.

➤ Be open and honest about your child's disability and how it affects the family. Give concrete examples: "We'll have to spend an hour or so each week at Ms. Jen's office. You can bring your homework and we can work on it together while we are there."

➤ Teach your children about apraxia. As mentioned in the beginning of this chapter, you may want to hold a family "in-service" on CAS. Enlist older kids to do a little research on it and present it to the family. You may be surprised how eager they are to participate.

➤ Give them an explanation to share with others, should they ask. Practice saying something like, "My brother has apraxia. It's a speech disorder. He can't say what he wants to say because his brain and mouth have a hard time working together."

➤ Role play what they may say if someone says something hurtful. For example, your other children are taunted on the playground: "Oh your sister is dumb. She can't even talk right." Yikes! How can your children respond in a diplomatic way?

➤ Suggest they connect with other kids who have a sibling with special needs. It doesn't have to be apraxia, but they can validate and share feelings anyway.

➤ Here are some resources for additional guidance:
  ● "Brothers and Sisters of Children with Disabilities: Family Relationships with a Complicated Diagnosis" (www.bellaonline.com/articles).
  ● *Views from Our Shoes: Growing Up with a Brother or Sister with Special Needs,* edited by Donald J. Meyer (Woodbine House, 1997), is a collection of 45 short essays written by kids ages 4 to 18, who share what it's like to be a sibling of someone with a disability.
  ● *The Sibling Slam Book: What It's Really Like to Have a Brother or Sister with Special Needs* (Woodbine House, 2005) edited by Donald J. Meyer. This book includes 80 teenagers' views of what it's like to have a brother or sister with special needs in the vein of a "slam book" passed around school. It tackles tough questions such as "Do you like hanging out with your sib?"

- Younger siblings will find comfort in these titles:
  - *My Brother Is Very Special* by Amy Gloroiso May (Tafford Publishing, 2004) doesn't mention apraxia by name, but is a great introduction to speech and language disorders for preschool through school-aged children. Written by an "apraxia mom."
  - *I Want to Be Your Friend* by Angela Baublitz (CASANA, 2011) was also written by an "apraxia mom" whose daughter has CAS. This book includes photographs of young Emma as she does normal, everyday things in addition to working with her SLP on her apraxia.
  - *Hooway for Wodney Wat* by Helen Lester (Walter Lorraine Books, 1999), a picture book for kids aged 4-8, stars a rat who can't pronounce his r's. Thanks to his speech problem, he's able to outsmart the class bully.
  - *Charlie Who Couldn't Say His Name* by Davene Fahy (Limerock Books, 2004) focuses on a little boy who has a hard time pronouncing his own name. With the help of his school SLP, he is able to overcome this obstacle.
  - *It's Okay to Be Different* by Todd Parr (Little, Brown Books for Young Readers, 2009) is not about speech and language issues per se, but it does let readers know that different is okay.
  - *Ruby Mae Has Something to Say* by David Small (Dragon Fly Books, 1999) is Little Ruby's dream of talking to the United Nations about "universal peace and understanding." At first, she's tongue-tied, but she overcomes her problem.
- Your child's school counselor may offer a group for kids who have a sibling with special needs. Look into it.
- *The Sibling Support Project* is an online resource your child(ren) may find comfort in. It's a national program with goals to promote peer support and education. Check it out at www.siblingsupport.org to see available workshops or participate in a listserv, among others.
- Ask around—your speech clinic, your parent-friends, and listservs may know of a *special sibling group in your local area.*
- Finally, refer to the previous chapters' resources and recommended readings. You may find that what helps your child with CAS cope will also help your other children.

Supporting and Educating: Extended Family and Grandparents

Grandparents care and want to help. In one of my Small Talk: All bout Apraxia groups, there was even a grandmother who attended right along with her daughter.

They both wanted to hear the information so they could both support their (grand) daughter. I was thrilled to see her support.

Like parents, grandparents worry when a child does not seem to be learning to talk according to the regular timetable. Sometimes, before a child is diagnosed with CAS, it is a grandparent who urges the parents to find out what is wrong. For example, it was my parents who urged me to get things checked out with an SLP. They continued to pester me, "So is she talking yet? Any new words?" Other grandparents may take longer to key into what is wrong, or may think their role is to reassure you that everything is all right. For example, they may tell you that "Einstein was a late talker," "She's just waiting until she can say it perfectly," or "It's no big deal."

Once you have a diagnosis, you will want to choose how to break the news to the grandparents. How you approach this may depend on whether they were the ones urging you to get an evaluation or the ones telling you that everything would be okay. Usually it is helpful to start slowly by telling them what apraxia is all about. *Give them some resources.* Print them out if your child's grandparents are not Internet savvy. Let them soak in the new information.

Follow up with them by phone or email: "Have you had a chance to read that information on apraxia yet? What did you think?" Just like you, they may have a hard time believing the diagnosis. It is not unusual for grandparents to feel stunned and have numerous questions—what does it mean, what will happen, where did it come from, and how can they help? Grandparents will likely hear terms they have never heard before and will need support and understanding just as the rest of us do. For example, "Grandma Gloria" shares: "I had never heard of apraxia. I asked a lot of questions, there were moments that my daughter seemed to be upset by all of my questions. So, I took the bull by the horns and Googled websites so I could understand the 'whys' and 'how comes'"

One mother in my Small Talk: All About Apraxia group said that she received quizzical looks when she shared her son's CAS diagnosis with her own parents. "Are you sure, honey?" her mother asked. She went on to explain that she thought her mother's response was to make her feel better: "I think my mom was probably trying to suggest that it might not be as serious as it sounds."

Another parent spoke up and said, "I had a hard time trying to explain what apraxia was to my parents. Once I finally started relating it to Uncle Bob's stroke, they totally got it." While the treatment of CAS is similar to the rehabilitation following a stroke, it's not exactly the same. True, kids with CAS need to learn how to use the motor system to articulate correctly and intelligibly, but CAS *starts* in childhood and is typically not a result of a childhood stroke. However, if you and your family have had a close connection with someone who has had a stroke, then this can prove to be a good metaphor.

Sometimes grandparents really don't "get" it, even after you've explained what CAS is all about. As one Small Talk participant relayed, "I hated it so much when my father-in-law mimicked my son's grunting. He [the grandfather] thought it was funny and would laugh, thinking he'd get my son to say something eventually. It doesn't work that way. I finally had to say something to my husband so he'd talk to his dad. It was demeaning."

In my experience, however, grandparents are much more likely to be understanding and helpful once the diagnosis has sunk in. For example, one mother told me that her parents were particularly helpful with the new diagnosis: "They would call me up out of the blue to check in. They wanted to know how speech was going. Once, they even sent me a newspaper clipping about apraxia. I thought it was really sweet."

Once the grandparents do come around, consider suggesting simple things they can do to help:

➤ Repeat and emphasize words they say in conversation with your child: "**Park…**let's go to the **park**. Can you say **park**?"
➤ Wait for a response.
➤ Practice sounds: "P makes the 'puh' sound. Can you say 'puh'?"
➤ Remind them how to praise: "That's it…you're getting it. Now try making your lips look like this." They may have to watch you and your child in action a few times to get the dialog down.

Emphasize that your child is just like any other child. Just because she can't communicate well doesn't mean she isn't as much fun to be around as their other grandchildren. Tell them what your child enjoys doing. Maybe Grandpa can take her fishing? Or Grandma can bake cookies with her? There are numerous activities they can do together that don't involve talking. Think specifically of your child's grandparents, interests, and activity level and compare them with your child. You may find that they have a lot in common!

Distinguish between difficulties speaking and difficulties understanding. Finally, remind grandparents that your child can understand almost everything, is smart, and capable. It will just take longer to hear her sweet voice. Grandparents should not talk down to your child or talk about her as if she's not there; instead, encouraging active and engaging communication is key.

Depending on your relationship with your child's grandparents, and how far away you live from them, the manner in which they can support your family through apraxia will vary. Here are some ideas to get you started:

➤ Telephone calls can prompt and encourage your child's developing speech. Keep a "question and comment" pad near the telephone so you can jot down ideas of things for Grandma and Grandpa to talk to your child about when they call. You'll likely answer the phone first, so fill them in on the list before handing the phone over to your child. My own father once confided, "When a grandchild has apraxia and lives out-of-state, it's hard to have a phone call with them. You want to hear their sweet little voice, but you can't. Grandparents miss out on that."
➤ If Internet access is available, see if your child and her grandparent(s) can exchange daily or weekly emails, or try communicating with Skype.
➤ Ask if your child's grandparents can give you some respite care: for example, a slumber party at grandma's or an outing to the movies, park, or library.
➤ Inquire if driving duty to and from speech therapy can be shared.

➤ Remember, speech therapy is important. Please do not cancel speech therapy because grandparents are coming over/will be in town.
➤ If there are opportunities for grandparents to be involved at your child's school, make sure your child's grandparents are aware of them. "My dad read a book to Emma's class and he has such a great reading voice. It made his day—and Emma's," shares a mother from my Small Talk group.
➤ Encourage grandparents to practice reading and sight words with your child.

You may or may not feel comfortable hitting up Grandma and Grandpa for financial assistance with the extra costs of CAS, but if they offer, have a few things in mind:
➤ Purchase a digital camera or video camera for the family.
➤ Assist in paying for private education or a tuition-based preschool.
➤ Help pay for the cost for testing that's not covered by insurance.
➤ Reimburse you for co-pays and therapy deductions.
➤ Make a charitable contribution to a group that offers resources or conducts research on CAS, such as CASANA/Apraxia-KIDS (www.apraxia-kids.org) or ASHA (www.asha.org).
➤ Offer a "scholarship fund" that parents can use to set up their own group for apraxia, or pay membership dues to various special need resources.
➤ Pay the tuition for a parent to attend a conference on apraxia.
➤ Help pay for family, marital, or individual therapy, if needed.
➤ Pay for a subscription to a speech journal for Mom and Dad, or a children's magazine for your grandchild.
➤ Assist in covering the costs of products, educational toys, equipment, and pricy computer software.

Grandparents need to be reminded not to focus too much time, energy, or resources on one grandchild. All grandchildren have specific and unique strengths, weaknesses, and interests.

Say That Again?! Chapter Summary

For most parents, getting a diagnosis of apraxia sends them on an emotional rollercoaster. You may have experienced even more ups and downs as you read through this chapter. As you deal with the initial diagnosis, and then move through a variety of stages in coming to terms with your child's diagnosis, it's important to keep the big picture in view: you will survive and so will your child. I hope you found some of the suggestions in the "coping corners" helpful. Please review the section on resources and recommended reading for additional support and guidance. But remember—most of all, you can help your child by taking care of you.

Read On! Recommended Resources

➤ *The Seven Stages of Motherhood: Making the Most of Your Life As Mom* by Ann Pleshette Murphy (Knopf, 2004).

➤ *Married with Special Needs Children: A Couples' Guide to Staying Connected* by Laura E. Marshak and Fran Pollack Preznant (Woodbine House, 2006) is like having a therapist nearby to assist you in your relationship.

➤ *More Than a Mom: Living a Full and Balanced Life When Your Child Has Special Needs* by Amy Baskin and Heather Fawcett (Woodbine House, 2006) is a fantastic book for maintaining your own sense of self while raising a kid with special needs.

➤ *The Mother's Guide to Self-Renewal* by Renee Peterson Trudeau (Balanced Living Press, 2008) helps you reclaim yourself with tips on relationships and self-care.

➤ If you are looking for something to tickle your funny bone, then try *Somebody's Always Hungry: Essays on Motherhood* by Julie Johnson (Nell Books, 2008).

➤ You may also appreciate *A Different Kind of Perfect: Writings by Parents on Raising a Child with Special Needs* by Cindy Dowling (Trumpeter, 2006) in which multiple families share their stories, all very eloquently written, with a focus on the stages of grief. Easy to read in short segments of time.

➤ In *The Sea Is So Wide and My Boat Is So Small: Charting a Course for the Next Generation,* Marian Wright Edelman (Hyperion, 2008) writes an inspiring letter to parents about how difficult it is to be a good parent, but how important it is to be the person you want your kids to emulate.

➤ *Things Good Mothers Know: A Celebration* by Alexandra Stoddard (Collins Living, 2009) may give you some insight and ideas on parenting.

➤ *Being the Other One: Growing Up with a Brother or Sister Who Has Special Needs,* by Kate Strohm (Shambhala, 2005).

➤ Amy Glorosio-May, the author of *My Brother Is Very Special* (Tafford, 2004) wrote the book to help her daughter understand why her little brother with CAS was going to speech therapy. It's a great book for teaching others to be sympathetic and tolerant of a child's imperfect speech, while supporting her self-esteem.

➤ Angela Baublitz, mother and author of *I Want to be Your Friend* (CASANA, 2011), wrote this book about her daughter who struggles with apraxia, but also has a lot of interests. A top pick for talking with your child—and the whole family—about our differences.

➤ *Speech Class Rules!* by Ronda Wojicki, SLP-CCC, is a children's book about speech therapy that can help a youngster accept speech therapy as a part of life.

➤ Clare B. Jones presents an honest and down-to-earth guide in *Understanding Your Special Needs Grandchild* (Specialty Press, 2001).

➤ *Grandparents* may find this article helpful: "Grandparents and Childhood Disability" by Pamela Wilson, BellaOnline's Special Needs Children's Editor. Online at www.bellaonline.com/articles.

Chapter Fourteen

. . . .

I Am More Than CAS

. . . .

Tending to
Your Child's Feelings

O f course *you* know your child is more than a diagnosis, but does your child? With speech therapy appointments, home drills, and intensive pre-schooling, it may be difficult to tease out "typical kid vs. apraxic kid." Socialization and fitting in with peers can be particularly tricky for these speech-challenged kids. Because this part of childhood is difficult, your youngster may have trouble coping or relating. He may come home in tears because the mean kids called him a name or because he wasn't accepted by the cool crowd. Of course, these types of heartbreaking scenarios can happen regardless of whether your child has CAS. Fortunately, there are things you can do to ease the hurt.

The Nuts and Bolts of This Chapter

➤ What parents can do to ensure—or at least assist with—their child's happiness

➤ How to have the "You have apraxia" discussion with your child

➤ Helping your child engage in social situations and make and keep friends

➤ Dealing with and managing bullies, aggression, and other mental health issues

➤ Helping tween girls navigate the complex social climate

➤ Exercise and recreational activities as an outlet for coping and developing friendships

Well-Being vs. Happiness

• • • • • • • • • • • • • • • • • • •

If asked their number one goal for their child, many parents would answer, "I just want him to be happy." When your child is diagnosed with CAS, however, you begin to fear that happiness may be elusive for your child—whether because he is constantly frustrated when he can't make his wishes known, because other kids might tease him, or because he may not be able to make friends. I want to help smooth this process for you.

In reality, you don't *just* want your kids to be happy, you want a lot more for them, too. Sure, you want them to achieve what most of us think of as happiness—the state of mind encompassing the ideas of contentment, love, satisfaction, joy, and pleasure. But you also care about their well-being as a whole—and happiness is only part of that. Here's what authors Aaron Cooper and Erin Keitel say you really mean when you say, "I just want my kids to be happy" in their book by the same title (Late August Press, 2008):

➤ Good physical and mental health
➤ A life of meaning
➤ A closeness with others
➤ Acts of loving kindness
➤ A sense of gratitude
➤ A sense of spirituality
➤ An optimistic outlook
➤ Gratifying pursuits
➤ A "fine" character

The book explains that happy people create gratifying and challenging goals to pursue. They get caught up in the "flow" or the "zone," which psychologists believe leads to happiness. As a parent, we can help our kids—whether or not they have CAS—get into that happiness zone by encouraging and supporting their natural talents through hobbies, classes, after school activities, and specialized camps. We can also encourage not just sports and academics at home, but respect, compassion, empathy, and courage among others.

Dr. Stanley Greenspan, M.D., offers another take on qualities needed for a happy, healthy life in his book, *Great Kids*:

1. Engagement: Relating to Others*
2. Empathy: The Ability to Care
3. Curiosity: An Inquiring Mind
4. Communication: The Transforming Power of Language*
5. Emotional Range: Passion and Balance
6. Genuine Self-Esteem: The Importance of Self-Awareness
7. Internal Discipline: Perseverance and Self-Control
8. Creativity and Vision: A Rich and Internal Life
9. Logical Thinking: Making Sense of the World
10. Moral Integrity: A Matter of Heart

I placed an asterisk next to the two qualities that made me cringe as I read through this book. It's not that I disagreed with Dr. Greenspan, but at that time I didn't feel my daughter could engage and relate to others (essential quality #1) or communicate clearly and effortlessly (essential quality #4); therefore, I felt she was doomed to become a nongreat kid. Of course, that is not at all how this list should be interpreted. Kids with CAS can and do become "great kids" in spite of their communication skills. But it's going to take extra effort on their part, as well as ours, to develop and keep those skills alive.

What Can You Do?

> *Be empathetic.* Have you ever been to a foreign country? Do you remember how nerve-wracking it was to try to communicate with the people in their own language? How stressed and isolated you felt at times? Your child may very well be feeling this same way—but in his own country, in his own language. Remind yourself and your child that he is still learning to talk and that you are going to help him.

> *Don't let him get too frustrated.* It's a fine line between having your child "reach" to say a word, or just accepting his attempt as "good enough." You can ask your child to repeat himself only so many times before you both get frustrated. Know when to stop and divert your child's attention before it all ends in tears or worse.

> *Build his self-esteem.* Everyone is good at something. Find out what it is for your child: taking care of the dog/cat, being a good friend, sports, art…. The key is to mention these traits to your child often. Of course you don't want to sound like a broken record, or you risk taking away that good feeling your child gets each time he hears it. Catch him being good: "I really like how kind you are to your little sister. That makes me feel good."

> *Be honest about his weaknesses.* Consider talking frankly about your child's difficulty with speaking: "I know sometimes it's hard for you to get the words out. It's just not fair. That's why we go see Miss Jen. She's helping you and you are doing a good job." Or, you may want to try something like this: "I am so sorry it's so hard for you to talk. If I could make it easier, I would. Do you know that everyone has something they aren't very good at? I am not good at baking and Daddy isn't very good at gardening. We all have things we struggle with. But if we work hard, we can get better."

> *Find other ways to have fun with him.* You don't always have to talk to enjoy each other's company. Look for opportunities to be together that use other skills.

Take a walk together, play tag, draw, paint, or color. Create something with Play-Doh or clay. Bake cookies. Work in the garden. Ride bikes. Explore the local library. Go to a kid-friendly movie. Go wading in a creek. These kinds of nonverbal activities strengthen your bond with your child and let him know you love and accept him, regardless of his apraxia.

➤ *Support him socially.* Your child with CAS is busy with appointments and therapy and preschool or school, but it's just as important to get him involved with activities to develop his social skills. He needs time to *just be a kid.* Make sure he has opportunities to be with other kids—playing with neighbors, hanging out at the park, attending a library story hour, or taking part in a parent-tot class. As your child gets older, consider enrolling him in a class on his own, even if his verbal skills aren't developed as much as you like. Some kids actually do better when they are on their own with peers and a facilitator/teacher.

(Some of these ideas gleaned from *A Parent's Guide to Speech-Language Disorders* by Debbie Feit.)

Parents Share...

A Glimpse of What It's Like to Have CAS

The other night I was reading *Adventures at Shelby Stables* by Julie Driscoll (Battat, 2009) to Kate at bedtime. A passage I read reminded me so much of CAS. Whether or not the author has any knowledge of CAS, I do not know. However, I was so struck by something that Lily Anna, the main character said, that I wanted to share it:

> *"Sometimes, at lunch, I'd hardly say a word—not because I didn't have anything to say. Oh no! I have lots of stuff going on in my head— lots and lots. But something happens from the point where I have a thought to where it should then come out of my mouth. It never does. And on occasion, when I do speak, I feel very awkward. I feel like running away, like one of the wild horses on my pajamas—running and running, never looking back."*

I used this passage as an opportunity to ask Kate if that's how she sometimes feels. She nodded and got a little tearful. "Not everyone has apraxia, you know," she told me. Whenever I glimpse what it must be like to have CAS, it makes me that much more determined to support my daughter, boost her self-esteem, or make sure she knows she is loved.

Do You Need to Justify Your Child's Apraxia?

This is a huge question and not to be taken lightly. Do you ever feel the need to tell others about your child's difficulty communicating? How do you bring it up? In what circumstances? Following are some suggestions to get you thinking. Remember, just as no two kids with apraxia are the same, nor are all parents. You have your own style of relating and communicating with others, so do what comes naturally.

The extent to which kids are accepted by peers (and often adults) depends partly on how parents present the situation. Therefore, we have always presented Kate as "any other kid" in social situations.

That's not to say that there have not been hurtful times. Here are a few examples:

➤ When Kate didn't readily answer questions, her friendly and well-meaning great aunt said, "What's wrong? Cat got your tongue?" At first, Kate regressed and retreated, and I felt helpless and defensive. But after I calmly explained why it was hard for Kate to talk, everyone felt better.

➤ Sitting on Santa's lap at the mall was challenging for Kate, even at almost four years of age. She couldn't tell Santa what she wanted, so I had to jump in when I saw that Santa's prompts and attempts at rephrasing the question were bringing Kate close to tears.

➤ The professional photographer was trying to get Kate to smile by having her say "stinky feet," but she was pouting instead. At the time, her /s/ blends were a challenge. Kate knew she couldn't say "stinky feet," and was looking to me for guidance.

➤ Birthday parties may cause added stress and anxiety for your and your child. Kate had a hard time at a birthday party when her peers wanted to play a game of tag. Kate wasn't sure how to play, let alone able to say, "Tag! You're it!" She was unable to ask for clarification and became tearful, clinging to my leg. Fortunately, I was there to understand what the problem was, but it didn't hurt any less.

➤ Then there's the friendly neighbor who just wants to ask your child typical getting-to-know-you types of questions: how old are you, what's your name, where do you go to school? If your kid's unable to answer these questions, the neighbor may think your kid's not friendly, hasn't been taught any social skills, or worse.

There are countless other social situations that can be problematic for a child with CAS. It's impossible to anticipate all of them. You may want to consider having a few answers in your toolbox for situations such as these. Here are a few of my favorites:

➤ "He's still learning some words, but I think he's doing a great job."
➤ "He has a hard time talking sometimes. It's called apraxia. But he's really getting better."
➤ "Sometimes his words get stuck. Try helping him out by saying, 'show me.'"

If you don't make a big deal out of it, others won't, either. Privately, you may want to talk to your child about why it's hard to get the words out. You don't have to go into detail, but you can tell him that it's hard for him to talk because he has a condition called Childhood Apraxia of Speech (you may want to shorten it to just apraxia). Remind him that apraxia is the reason he goes to speech therapy and that he's making lots of progress, and that you love him regardless.

When you acknowledge that talking is hard work, or you say to your child, "Yes, that *is* a tricky word," you are likely giving him validation and relief that you understand. Consider sharing some of your own childhood experiences with speech issues, if you had them. My husband shared with Kate that he had speech therapy in school as a kid. She brightened, "You did?!" I told her that I get nervous when I need to speak in front of a group of people, and sometimes I just don't want to be social (introverted by nature).

Parents Share...

How Other Parents Feel about this Topic

Here's a snippet of our discussion one evening during Small Talk: All About Apraxia:
"I absolutely hated when we all got together for a play date at one of those bouncy places. We showed up a little late that day because my son had speech [therapy] first. The other mothers looked at me like they wanted an explanation. I shared that he was at therapy," relates Jill, mother of 2.5-year-old Michael. "They looked at me like I was the problem. Then they looked at Michael and said, 'Why? He seems to talk fine.'" She then had to define CAS for these other mothers while supporting her son at the same time.

Another mother chimed in and said, "Yeah, it's like one big competition. I feel like I am competing with all of these other parents about whose kid is talking more or has a bigger, better vocabulary. Sometimes, I just downplay the whole thing and don't even mention it."

A third mother said, "I cringe when they ask such probing questions—when, why, how...those questions really get to me. It's like [other parents] feel like apraxia is contagious."

Another parent joked that she wished she had a card to hand out to people who ask. "If I could just shove a piece of paper under their nose about what apraxia is all about, then maybe they would stop asking so many pointed questions. I don't think people realize how sensitive this topic may be to parents [of kids with apraxia]."

Parents and Kids Cope: Talking to Your Child about CAS

● ● ● ● ● ● ● ● ● ● ●

When you talk with your child about why he has difficulty verbalizing his thoughts, feelings, and requests, try a little role-play. You'll know when the time is right. It may be after he comes inside feeling left-out when other kids were organizing a sports team or when he couldn't verbally participate in a karaoke video game. Have a little dialog ready when the time comes. It may go something like this:

PARENT (from dad's perspective): We all have things we are good at doing and not-so-good at doing. Let's see…you are really good at building things out of Legos. Your sister is really good at riding her bike. Mommy's really good at organizing. But there are some things we aren't so good at. For me, it's golf. Mommy's not very good at painting. Your sister, well, she's not very good at sharing. And you have trouble using your words.

CHILD: May or may not say much. Ask for his thoughts, anyway. Just because your child is having a difficult time communicating, doesn't mean you should avoid asking for his opinion or feelings. *Always present information to your child with apraxia as though you are expecting an answer.*

PARENT: The reason you have a hard time using your words has a special name. It's called apraxia. [Use its long formal name, Childhood Apraxia of Speech, if you don't think it will confuse your child.] You've probably heard us say that word, haven't you?

CHILD: Will likely nod his head.

PARENT: Well, apraxia is the reason we go to therapy [see Miss Jen]. She helps you use your words better. Lots of kids need to go to therapy to learn to use their words better. What do you think about that?

CHILD: Let your child answer. Be prepared to answer some questions or hear how your child doesn't want to go to therapy.

PARENT: You do know that we love you very, very much and are doing all we can to help you! End with a hug.

Sometimes kids just need to know what the big hoopla is all about. It helps to put things into words your child can understand. Doing so can validate your child's feelings and "clear the air." Of course, kids don't need to know *too* much. Avoid getting into specifics with them about adult concerns such as how much therapy costs, evaluation results, insurance issues, and your own frustration. Share those things with your child's therapist in private or with a trusted friend or your partner. If you really find yourself struggling, you might consider seeing a professional counselor.

When you have a discussion with your child about CAS and why he needs to go to therapy, he realizes how important it is to go to therapy. He may feel special and empowered. It's always best to be upfront and honest with your kids when you can.

I should point out that not everyone agrees about sharing this information with their child. A father who attended my Small Talk: All About Apraxia group said: "This may have been one of the times my wife and I argued about apraxia. I knew she was about ready to tell our son [about CAS], and I stopped her. I feared that if he got wind of this information he may start thinking that something was wrong with him; he may stop trying."

In my opinion, it all comes down to these careful considerations: is your child overly frustrated because he can't speak as well as others—or communicate his needs, wants, and desires? Do you feel he is at the point where he can understand that it's not "wrong" or "bad" if he has CAS? It could be that your child is not developmentally mature enough to understand—or care—why he can't speak well. The fact that your child sees a speech-language pathologist really is just *his* "normal."

> ### *How I Handled Telling My Daughter*
>
> You may be wondering how—or if—I told Kate about the book I was writing. She knew I spent a lot of time on the computer. She knew she was going to speech because she couldn't communicate well. I didn't really have to sit down and say, "Mommy's writing a book about why you can't talk as well as the other kids your age can." Kate's a smart cookie and pieced it all together. But we used the label "apraxia" when we talked about her speech problem. She knew she had apraxia. We never kept it a secret from her.
>
> It is important to be as honest as possible. Children sense dishonesty. Kate knew how important the book was to me—and to her. My efforts to connect with others and learn all I could about CAS in turn helped Kate and our family.

Here are some *don'ts* when talking to others about your child's apraxia:
➤ Don't share unless it is really necessary (teachers and caregivers need to know; neighbors might, strangers don't).
➤ Don't label him in front of others.
➤ Never make fun of or belittle your child's attempts to speak.
➤ Don't refer to your child as "mute" or "dumb" or "different" and don't allow others to, either
➤ Don't act like it's a big secret or that you are embarrassed by his inability to communicate well or clearly; kids pick up on that quickly.

Educating Others

Why not make a written handout about CAS? Keep these parameters in mind:

Format: Decide how you'd like to communicate this information. A plain note card with a computer print-out with CAS specifics glued on it works great and is cheap. If you want to do a little more, you can print personal calling cards by going to a site such as www.shutterfly.com or www.snapfish.com and adding information on CAS directly to the card. Or try a hybrid approach: using your home computer, make small informational tags or labels and stick them to the back of a calling/business card. Or include a blurb about CAS in your annual holiday letter or card.

What to Say: Start by giving a simple definition of CAS such as: "a motor-neurological speech disorder in which kids know what they want to say, but they can't coordinate the movements to do so." You can give a couple of specific examples: "You may have noticed that Joe has a hard time asking for what he wants—that's why he grunts and whines." Let them know that your child is seeing a speech-language pathologist/ attending preschool and is making wonderful progress! Suggest a couple ways others can help: "You can help by asking Joe to show you what he means/wants when he gets verbally frustrated. He knows what you are saying. It just takes longer for him to respond." End with something positive, "Joe is a fantastic kid and a great friend!" You may want to mention a website or book that has been particularly helpful to you. If you blog or have a website about your experience with your child's apraxia, list it.

Reaction(s) to Expect: The majority of folks will be supportive and sympathetic. Some will be very appreciative and will enjoy the opportunity to help and get a glimpse into your life. Don't be surprised, though, if you get an "Oh-sorry-I-asked" sort of response. Some people may be very surprised that you actually have a prepared answer and may be taken aback. Good for you—you are being your child's advocate! Some may see handing out informational cards as bordering on rude. But then again, who's being rude—you for giving a detailed (yet concise) answer, or strangers for asking probing questions?

Helping Your Child Make and Keep Friends

We all want and need friends. But some kids—especially those with CAS—have difficulty initiating and maintaining friendships simply because they can't communicate as easily as their peers. It can lead to hurt feelings, feelings of exclusion, isolation, and frustration. You may want to sit down with your child—regardless of his age or verbal ability—and talk about what a good friend is. Generally, a good friend is someone you enjoy being around, shares common interests, and cares about you. Friendships don't always fall into place naturally or easily. They need to be cultivated and tended to. They need maintenance.

As a parent, you may want to think about your own attitude toward friendships, status, and social structure. As a family, sit down and make a list of qualities you like in a friend on poster board or some other media. Consider doing some role play to teach social skills. Scenarios may include:

➤ How to ask a friend to play
➤ How to decide/negotiate on what to do together
➤ How to ask questions
➤ How to listen without interrupting
➤ How to be a host or hostess
➤ How to end play

Most of these skills are learned informally by modeling. For kids with CAS, they may be harder to grasp. Try going to www.modelmekids.com for ideas and inspiration. This site has videos of social behavior acted out by kids. Have your child pay close attention to body language and facial expressions. Teach your child about those concepts with specific examples you can act out at home.

Social nuances can be tricky for kids with CAS, as well. They may not "get" jokes, sarcasm, or snide remarks. It's a part of life and growing up—there will always be rude people. You can practice role play for these types of situations, too. In fact, your kids may really enjoy this type of exercise! Work also on comprehension and self-monitoring skills here. While you're at it, teach your child some kid-friendly jokes he can remember and recite in social situations. Look for a joke book at your local library.

If your child is struggling to make and keep friends despite your best efforts, consider looking for a social skills group—otherwise known as a "friendship circle," "lunch bunch," or something along those lines. Your child's preschool, day care, or church may offer something like this. If those places don't, your speech clinic likely does (or knows where to find them). These groups may be run by a SLP, a psychologist, or social worker. It's a safe environment where kids can learn social skills such as introducing oneself, taking turns in conversations, listening, asking questions, working with others, problem solving, playing "nice," and reading social cues. Some clinics offer a combination-type class in which arts and crafts or eating/dining skills are worked on together with social skills. Participants are often matched based on skills, abilities, and goals. Classes generally run for four to six weeks and may meet once or twice a week. They can be pricey. Some insurance companies may cover these groups, but it's usually an out-of-pocket fee. Call your member services folks to find out what's covered.

If you just can't afford to enroll your child in a social skills group with an SLP, you have options. If you know of other families like yours, consider pooling your resources and doing one of two things:

1. Chip in to pay for a retired or part-time SLP, special/early education teacher, or grad student to help run a similar group. To find someone who may be interested and qualified, ask at your child's speech clinic, his school, a local university's speech-language or education departments, the county health department, or placing a want ad in a local paper or community bulletin board.

2. Just start working with an interested group of dedicated parents. You can create a social skills co-op in which each family hosts the "class" at their home on a rotating basis. Each parent takes turns being the facilitator. Develop a curriculum first, make a schedule, develop your class list, and get going. The best thing about this scenario is it's free or low-cost. Again, you can gain interest by creating fliers and posting them on community bulletin boards or talking with other parents at your child's speech clinic.

When Emotional, Behavioral, and Mental Health Are Concerns

Despite your best attempts at easing your child into social situations and assisting his communication, you may still have concerns and worries about his emotional and behavioral health.

Kids with CAS may have difficulty regulating their emotions. It's hard to express them, because it's hard to talk. Kids who keep their emotions bottled up are called internalizers. They are at high risk for depression and anxiety—which can take the form of generalized anxiety disorder (GAD), obsessive-compulsive disorder (OCD), separation anxiety, social anxiety, and selective mutism in extreme cases. Those kids who "let it all out" can get very angry and frustrated, resulting in aggressive behavior and mood swings.

Having been a child and adolescent psychiatric R.N., I present this information to make you aware of the possibilities you may encounter. I also know that with the right intervention (therapy, social skills training, medication, etc.), these instances and conditions can be managed quite well.

There is no way to tell whether your child will have a mental, emotional, or behavioral health issue. However, just as I advised you to look at family history for speech- and language-related concerns, you can do the same for mental, behavioral, and emotional health and use it as a gauge. Does anyone in your family tend to be a bit unstable in any of those realms? By gathering this information now, you may be better able to identify and treat any future behavioral problems as they crop up.

Several studies have suggested that some kids with psychiatric disorders may have had undiagnosed speech-language disorders or impairments. For example, E.B. Brownlie's 2004 study in the *Journal of Abnormal Psychiatry* found that there *may* be a correlation between what she terms as "late adolescent delinquency symptoms." This is not to say that your child with apraxia is going to grow up to become a delinquent! I present this information only so you can be alert for any red flags signaling the need for help as your child grows into a more independent child. The "delinquency symptoms" Brownlie refers to are:

1. **School Functioning:** Negative school experiences, due to a variety of reasons, could lead to poor academic performance. Poor academic performance could be a sign of a learning disorder, and not delinquency.

2. **Executive Functioning:** It sounds fancy, but executive function is really best known as self-regulation. It's the cognitive ability that allows one to plan, monitor, and change one's own behavior. Executive functioning relies heavily on the ability to self-talk (talk to yourself—usually silently—about what you should and should not do). It can be assumed that our children with CAS have difficulty with self-talk; therefore they *may* have difficulty with executive functioning. If it's compromised enough, it's possible the problem is related to an attention-deficit disorder.

3. **Social Functioning:** Because hanging out with friends often involves talking with them, kids with CAS may not interact with peers as often as other kids do. They may give up, or slink to the back of the room. Even at home, kids with CAS may not be able to communicate with their parents as openly as their siblings do, causing an unnecessary rift between family members. If social functioning gets too difficult, social anxiety may develop.

4. **Empathetic Functioning:** This is a fancy term for the ability to understand and relate to the feelings of others. Brownlie calls this a child's "social competence and moral development." Oppositional Defiant Disorder (ODD) can potentially develop from a child's inability to be empathetic.

If you truly are concerned about your child's behavior, contact a child psychologist or psychiatrist. You have nothing to lose. Ask around for a recommendation.

Each of these potential concerns (learning disorders, ADHD, social anxiety, and ODD) are addressed in Appendix A.

Dealing with Teasing and Bullies

No one is immune to the "mean kids." I bet you remember who the mean kids were when you were younger. They found anything and everything to be snarky about—your shoes, your braces, your bigger-than-average nose, your academic abilities—good or bad—and athletic inability. Nowadays, kids also have to contend with cyberbullying (nasty email, texts, Facebook, My Space, and blog posts), but much has remained the same. Kids get made fun of for all sorts of reasons, sadly even for speech impediments and other special needs. It's not fair and it's not right, but it happens. As parents, we need to be equipped to help.

First of all, let's clear the air: not all teasing is bad. A lot of kids—and families, too—may engage in playful or good teasing. Everyone is having fun, laughing and smiling, and it can be seen as a sign of friendship. Kids know when this is happening because they notice the playful smiles, winks, and tone of voice. It's all about bonding and sharing a similar experience with peers.

Bad teasing, on the other hand, happens when your child is belittled, degraded, and left feeling upset. It comes in many forms: ridicule, name calling, put-downs, verbal insults, and gesturing. Other kids may make fun of your child with apraxia because he can't say words as effortlessly as his peers, or because he can't easily engage in make-believe play.

Perhaps the sting is worse if your child is being made fun of due to a speech-language issue, because it's something he can't really do much about. It hurts because it's devaluing and because your child feels unaccepted by his peers. All kids are constantly comparing themselves to their peers. It's one of the only yardsticks kids have for measuring their own skills. Remember to acknowledge that your kiddo (and other children) has things he is naturally good at and not-so-good at.

A 2010 article in the *Journal of Clinical Child and Adolescent Psychiatry* explains that kids who get teased may have an inability to pick up on and respond to nonverbal cues by their peers, plus they may find it hard to understand the social meaning, and come up with solutions for resolving a conflict, all of which have some underlying connection to speech and language.

"Today, [my son] is sixteen and a half years old and has many friends and is quite popular. This is a complete 180 from the little boy who was chronically bullied as a child. But, I won't kid you. It has taken a lot of work for him to be able to speak clearly and fluidly. I think when he was about fourteen or fifteen, his speech became pretty normal but you could still 'tell.'"

—Janice, Edmonton, Alberta

What's a Parent to Do?

➤ *Stop, look, and listen.* Give your child some time and validation while at the same time reviewing your own behavior. Has your playful parenting humor crossed the line?

➤ *Don't overreact.* When your child first reports being bullied or teased, approach it neutrally and be supportive.

➤ *Support your child.* Let your child know that if the bully/teaser makes him feel bad, he can—and should—spend time with kids who make him feel good.

That's the easy part. Here's the nitty-gritty:

1. *Teach self-talk.* We all participate in self-talk all day long. What can you teach your child to say in his mind that will take the sting out of teasing? "I'm more important than that." "That's not true—I'm good at ____." Start by listing your child's positive traits. Do this together as a family at dinner: "You are fun, smart, a great artist, creative…." Make a habit of bringing up your child's qualities and strengths often and he will begin to internalize it. Then self-talk will come easily.

2. *Ignore.* My mom used to tell me, "Make like a duck and let the teasing roll off your back." Some kids don't really know what it means to ignore. You have to define it for them. Walk away, don't make eye contact, make the bully invisible/disappear. Role play it at home—this ought to be fun and easy: "I'm going to pretend to ignore you. Let me show you how it's done" (smile).

3. *Agree with the facts.* "You're right. I am short (have a big nose, red hair)." Leave it at that. The bully will be dumbfounded.

4. *Respond with a compliment.* "I am amazed that you notice how I'm dressed every day. You are very observant." Or if the teaser notices a bad grade on your kid's math test: "You're right—I'm not loving math right now. You're good at it, maybe you can tutor me?"

5. *Visualize mean words "bouncing off."* This goes along with the adage, "I'm rubber and you're glue, whatever you say bounces off of me and sticks to you." Can you teach your child ways of "seeing" the cranky words get squashed by a sneakered foot or hit by a tennis racket?

6. **The I-message.** Start teaching your child to identify feelings at an early age by giving descriptions of them (e.g., "I can tell you are angry because your face is all red"). Next, pair the feeling words with a statement to end the offending behavior of another person. It works like this: "I feel ____ (angry) when you ____ (correct my speech). Can you please stop?" Teasing is a part of growing up, but if we start teaching our kids positive coping skills at an early age, our kids will be ready for whatever curveballs life throws at them.

(Some of the above suggestions gleaned from Judy S. Freedman's *Easing the Teasing: Helping Your Child Cope with Name-Calling, Ridicule, and Verbal Bullying.*)

Managing Your Own Child's Aggression

It may be that your child isn't the victim of some mean kid's lashing out. Your little angel may actually *be* the bully. What's going on? Your child may be hitting, punching, screaming, and throwing tantrums at home and school because he gets frustrated with his communication skills. Some kids may be cognizant of these behaviors: "I am getting frustrated because I can't communicate my ideas well, so I'm going to scream." But most kids aren't introspective enough to understand their poor reaction in a social situation.

Kids who are less efficient at using and understanding language may be more likely to deal with frustration inappropriately. That's not to say that poor communication and frustration are the *only* reasons a child becomes aggressive. There is often more than one reason for a negative behavior. I urge you to explore the situation in depth with a child psychologist, psychiatrist, or psychiatric nurse practitioner if you are truly concerned. In the meantime, here are some suggestions for managing your child's aggressive tendencies at home:

➤ *Take a break.* Encourage your child to "take a break" (this word choice often works better than "time out") when you notice your child getting revved up.

➤ *Make a "no hitting" rule.* Tell your child that there will be no hitting at home or school, even if someone hits him first. Remind him that there are consequences for hitting (time out or removal of privileges). Suggest alternatives to hitting another person: hitting a pillow, pounding on clay, stomping on the floor.

➤ *If your child does hit,* help him make apologies. Don't allow him to go on as though nothing happened. Accept an approximation of "I'm sorry," if your child has a hard time getting those words out (due to apraxia or stubbornness). When kids learn from their mistakes, they are learning consequences from action.

➤ *Help your child identify feelings.* You may want to do this when he is not angry or frustrated. Once children have a better grasp of what they are feeling, they can better manage it. Feelings of anger are often masked as sadness, frustration, or fear. Describe those feelings to your child. Act them out together. Talk about other feelings, too: loneliness, jealousy, and happiness, to name a few.

➤ *Help your child identify cues about feelings.* For example, when someone gets angry, he may get a red face, tense his muscles, scowl or groan, breathe faster, and have a pounding heart. How does your body respond? How does that compare with your body's response to happiness?

➤ *Tell him it's okay to be angry.* Recognize that we all get angry sometimes; it's what we do with anger that makes it "good" or "bad."

➤ *Teach problem solving skills.* Identify that you are angry. Count to 10 or take a deep breath. Walk away if you need to. Think about what you can do: ignore or talk to the person in nice words about why you are feeling angry.

➤ *Allow your child to make choices at home.* In other words, pick your battles. When kids are given appropriate choices, they feel a sense of ownership and empowerment.

➤ *Model good anger management skills at home.* Children learn what they see. If they see you get angry and throw things or hit others, they will think it's OK for them to do the same. If they see you taking a deep breath, walking away, and later explaining what made you angry, they will be more likely to follow your good example.

➤ *Develop a behavior management system.* It sounds fancy, but all you need to do is make a chart on poster board or on your computer. Make a column on the left-hand side with behavior you expect and on the right side make lots of columns for the stickers your child earns for doing the good behavior. Once your child reaches a pre-determined number of stickers on his "sticker chart," he earns a prize. Your child's chart may look something like this (those asterisks* are stickers/stars):

No Hitting	*	*	*		
Use all of your words	*	*			
Share toys	*	*			
Clean up	*	*			

"Catch" your child being good. You can start a program like this without any hard and fast rules. Just say, "Let's keep track of how well you can use *all* of your words. Each time I notice you doing a good job, I will give you a sticker on your chart. It will be fun to see how many stickers you can collect. We'll try the same thing for not hitting, sharing, and cleaning up. What do you say?" It may be enough of a reward to just do the stickers, especially for a younger child. But if your kiddo is older, try attaching a prize for adhering to the behavior plan. "Once you get 25 stickers, you can ____." Remember, not all prizes have to be tangible or cost money. One-on-one time with a parent, a trip to the park, or a bike ride can still be a major incentive. If it's not, keep prizes manageable for your family. Look to the dollar section at many stores, take your child out for ice cream, get a subscription to a children's magazine, a new book, etc. Just be sure the prize is something your child actually likes and wants.

For more information on this topic, check out the website of the National Association of School Psychologists at www.nasponline.org. Click the "families" button at the top of the page, and you will find a variety of articles and resources for your particular concern.

Special Concerns for Girls

Girls have an intricate world incorporating play and socialization. Not being able to speak as well as their peers can definitely put a crimp in their ability to get along with other girls.

When Kate was about three, she tried really hard to fit in with the neighborhood girls, who were just about the same age. It saddened me to see just how discriminating these other little girls were. Kate couldn't keep up with them verbally and was left behind. She often came running back to me in tears because she was frustrated and discouraged in trying to play with them. And let's face it, girls play by communicating with one another. Little girls playing dollhouse, babies, tea party, and other typical girl-style play use words to differentiate roles and routines. For example, "You be the mommy. I'll be the daddy." Or, "Here's your tea, Mr. Bear, and here's your cookie, Miss Bunny." Kate ended up feeling more aligned with the little boys in our neighborhood. She would run and jump, kick, and ride bikes with them. It was easier for her because she didn't have to communicate as much verbally. The boys accepted her and helped her along. Until, of course, they got "too big" and developed the "girls are yucky" view.

At five years, Kate was speaking better, but still struggling to keep up with her female peers. We continued to work with her through role play and modeling. It made my day—and hers—when a group of little girls rang our doorbell one afternoon and asked her to play. In fact, according to a 2009 study of the perceptions of children with speech-language concerns, "making friends and having them come 'round to see me" is one of the best indicators of a good quality of life for kids with expressive communication delays.

What's a Parent to Do?
➤ *Accept your daughter for who she is.* If she wants to play with boys, who cares? If she enjoys hopping around the driveway instead of playing dolls, let her. Once you learn what type of play drives your daughter, stock your toy collection and garage with products you know she'll like. Jump ropes, scooters, sidewalk

chalk, and balance boards have all been winners for us, as were Thomas the Train toys, movies, and books.

➤ *Offer to host 1:1 play dates with other girls.* Often, when girls are together in a group, things are intense. Try having just one other neighborhood or school girl over at a time. It will be a lot easier to bond and develop friendships than if your daughter is competing with lots of other Chatty Cathies. Often, girls with apraxia feel more comfortable with younger, typically speaking girls. When Kate was five, she often connected best with her three-year-old sister's friends. Having a play date with a younger girl is okay. Their speech abilities may be right on target.

➤ *Practice Role-Playing.* During family time at home, practice what to do when your daughter is in the company of other girls. "I know you have been invited to Alexis's sleepover this weekend. The other girls might want to talk about their American Girl dolls, nail polish, and their favorite music. What can you add to conversations like this? Let's practice. I'll be McKenzie and you just be yourself, okay?" Knowing your daughter and the current girl culture will help you both at these times.

➤ *Ask your daughter for ideas.* Parents get used to feeling like they have to always be the answer person. Try going to your daughter and voicing your concern about her friendships (but use caution with this—don't be accusatory, or you'll risk putting her on the defense). Try this, "Hey, I noticed it's hard for you to break into the Sophia-McKenzie-Emma group next door. What are your ideas?" You may get an earful!

Special Concerns for Boys

Each gender has its own challenges in dealing with friendships. Boys, by nature, are more activity-driven than verbally-driven. As a result, they may not have to deal with as many of the difficult friend situations that confront girls. But they have their own unique concerns. A boy with CAS may appear more immature than his peers because he sounds younger than he really is. Boys may gradually begin to exclude him from their play because he seems like "a baby." Of course, you know differently, so help set the record straight. Losing your temper won't help. Instead, keep a close eye on the group of boys. When you see your son being "babied" by the others, step in. Redirect the group by offering an activity that is more appealing to your son, and may get the other boys to stop the babying and engage in something else.

You may also see older girls take your son under their wings and play the role of nurturing big sister. Personally, I see this as a "good thing," but being overly nurturing or treating your son as though he is "too young" is not. Use your best judgment; if it feels wrong, it probably is.

Most of the girl strategies above can be applied to your son as well. Continue on for tips developed for both boys and girls.

Social Pointers for Both Girls and Boys

➤ *Find ways to build self-esteem.* It can be heartbreaking to see your little one struggle with same-sex friendships. Remember that children need reminders of what they do well often. For example, "You are awesome at riding your scooter!" Tell your child that he is a fun, likeable kid with lots of energy.

➤ *Get your child involved in same-sex sports.* Soccer, gymnastics, martial arts, baseball/softball, or T-ball "just for girls" or "just for boys" may be the ticket to help your child feel included and successful. One mom in my "Small Talk: All About Apraxia" group mentioned that she didn't think she was ready for extra-curricular activities, but her 3.5-year-old daughter with CAS proved her wrong:

> *"I just wasn't 'there' yet. I had a lot of anxiety over having her in a gymnastics class, even though the class was designed for three-year-olds. I was afraid she wouldn't be able to communicate and need me. But she did great. She had no problems whatsoever. No one even knew she had apraxia. I should have done it sooner for Lila's sake."*

➤ *Consider coaching a youth sports team.* If your kiddo loves soccer, why not volunteer to be the coach? Sure, it's added time and effort on your part, but you'll get to know the other children and their parents, and help *your* child at the same time. It may help develop lifelong friendships. The same goes for becoming a Girl Scout leader or Den Mother or Scout Master.

➤ *Help "coach" social situations.* You don't want to become known as a hovering parent, but if you stumble upon a potential social situation for your son or daughter (at the park, library, neighborhood), provide a few pointers before sending your child into the midst of it all. You may feel more comfortable doing it *with* your child (he'll see your model, and that is a good thing). For example, "Hi girls! This is Kate. Can she play with you?" Stay within earshot so you can help your child along if he gets stuck.

➤ *Encourage others to engage in active play.* If you are hosting a play date, or you see your child struggling with a group of friends, jump in and try to engage the other kids in the type of play where your child is more likely to shine.

➤ *Speaking of current kid culture,* you'll want to try extra hard to know what's in, what's out, and what's coming up. Your child may not know how to say some of the things that are cool (fads, foods, activities, text lingo, clothing, toys, etc.). Learn what they are (ask other parents, teachers, or librarians in the children's department) and practice with him. If it's "supersonic strawberry shakes" at Shakes R Us, then practice saying those words with him until he gets it just right. If the name of a current tween pop star is tough to say, practice that.

Exercise and Extracurricular Activities to Help Your Child Thrive

Since we've talked about kids with CAS needing vestibular stimulation to awaken the communication center (Chapters 7 and 9), it should be no surprise that exercise has multiple benefits. Aside from ensuring that your child doesn't develop weight or health issues from inactivity, exercise boosts verbal skills and serves as a coping device.

What's a Parent to Do?

➤ *Encourage physical activity.* Sometimes you have to turn off the TV and say, "We're going outside and we're going to play catch." Your child might grumble, but soon you'll both be having a good time. While you're tossing the ball around, practice some target speech sounds or words.

➤ *Limit screen time.* I'm not just talking television here, but computers, iPhones, and hand-held video games. Do what feels right for your family, but the American Academy of Pediatrics recommends no more than two hours a day of screen time for a child aged two to ten years.

➤ *Consider having your child* earn *screen time.* For every 2 minutes of outside/ active time, you child can "earn" 1 minute of screen time. So, if your child rides his bike for 30 minutes, he can play Nintendo DS for 15 minutes. See "Managing Your Child's Aggression" section, above, for ideas on behavior modification and sticker charts.

➤ *Get your child involved in a noncompetitive sport.* Not all sports need to be about peer competition. What about those that encourage self-directed competition and goal setting? Swimming, martial arts, gymnastics, and yoga are all examples your child may enjoy.

➤ *Check out your local park district or community education department.* Many states and counties have a special recreation association. If your child is dealing with profound apraxia and has other special needs, there are services and programs designed especially for him. Many of these programs offer modifications and adaptations (adapted equipment, communication tools/aids, physical assistance, behavioral management, and even 1:1 staffing). Your park district may offer dance, soccer, gymnastics, cheerleading, golf, or tennis with accommodations. Refer to Appendix C for additional resources and information.

➤ *Get involved with your child's physical life.* Consider becoming a coach for the team your child is on. Or sit on the sidelines and cheer him on. Learn the rules of the game. You could also join a program advisory committee and share thoughts, concerns, and ideas with coaches, staff, and folks in the community. Ask first at your park district or Chamber of Commerce.

➤ *Be a role model.* You know that kids learn what they see. If they see you actively engaged in physical exercise, they will be more likely to accept it as a normal, healthy, and smart choice for managing stress, weight, and maintaining a healthy lifestyle.

Balance It Out with Relaxation

Of course, life isn't all about running marathons and going to speech therapy. Kids need downtime, too. In fact, in the study about the perceptions of children with speech and language concerns about their lives (Markham, 2009), relaxation was one

Parents Share...

The Benefits of Yoga

We found that Kate responded well to yoga. Your child might, too. Yoga helps calm the mind, strengthen muscles, improve flexibility and concentration, and help manage feelings of frustration and anger. Plus, it's adorable to see your little one in a downward dog position! If you are looking for a program that fits your child, call around to local yoga studios and fitness centers. Ask if they have a kids' yoga class or a parent-child yoga class. Other ways to fit yoga-like activities into your child's life are:
- ➤ Wii Fit—yoga programs
- ➤ Balance boards and balancing games
- ➤ *Calm Classroom: Early Childhood Edition*—a book and audio CD designed for teachers to use in their preschool classrooms. When Kate came home talking about this CD she listened to in class, I was curious. I ended up purchasing it online and using it at home. It helps kids develop "self-awareness, inner calm, and mental focus." Look for it at www.lusterpublications.com.
- ➤ *Yoga to Go for Kids* by Nancy Wile, Ed.D.—an award-winning DVD that allows kids to practice yoga on their own, or with friends and family. Yoga and smoothie play date, anyone?

important key for a "good" quality of life. Kids of all ages related to the notion of relaxation and discussed the ways in which they achieve it. Kids were asked which activities they did to relax that made their lives "better and happier." Here's a sampling of how these kids responded (all of the kids in this study had a speech/language/communication need; more than half—62 percent—had an "expressive language delay"):

➤ "Riding around on my [quad] bike."

➤ "My computer game calms me down."

➤ "I like listening to music…laying down and reflecting…that's what makes me relax."

➤ "Coming home at the end of the day and being with my family…   that relaxes me… ."

Say That Again?! Chapter Summary

As parents, we'll do just about anything to help our kids become happy, well-adjusted kids. Of course, there is no magic bullet or formula to ensure this happens, but there are things we can do to help. Kids with apraxia may have a harder time fitting in with their peers, managing emotions, and navigating the often harsh cultural climate of teenager-hood. There is hope—and skills you can equip your child with—the cornerstone being improved self-esteem and self-concept.

If problems arise and you feel as if you can't manage on your own, there are professionals who can assist you and your child. Please seek guidance when you feel you are stumbling. There is often nothing to lose by having a concern examined and evaluated in more detail. In the best case, you get skills and advice to manage the situation better than you did before. In the worst case, you get peace of mind. It's win-win, if you ask me. The bottom line is: kids with apraxia just want to be accepted, to have friends, and not be labeled as "special."

Read On! Recommended Resources

➤ *I Just Want My Kids to be Happy: Why You Shouldn't Say It or Think It, and What You Should Do Instead* by Aaron Cooper and Eric Keitel (Late August Press, 2008), as referenced earlier in this chapter.

➤ *Great Kids: Helping Your Baby and Child Develop the 10 Essential Qualities for a Healthy, Happy Life* by Stanley I. Greenspan, M.D. (DA Capo Press, 2007), as referenced earlier in this chapter.

➤ The Annie E. Casey Foundation produces the annual *Kids Count* report, which provides state-by-state data on key indicators of children's well-being. However, it is not specific to speech, language, and communication disorders. Available at: www.kidscount.org/sld/compare.jsp.

➤ The Federal Interagency Forum on Child & Family Statistics releases an annual report entitled *America's Children: Key National Indicators of Well Being.* Visit their website at www.childstats.gov for more information.

➤ *What Is Friendship: Games & Activities to Help Children to Understand Friendship* by Pamela Day (Jessica Kingsley Publishers, 2009) is a nice resource with reproducible pages for teaching kids aged 7 to 10 about friendship.

➤ *Connecting with Others: Lessons for Teaching Social and Emotional Competence* by Dr. Rita Coombs-Richardson (Research Press, 1997) is a nice resource to help your child learn the difference between aggressive and assertive skills, self-concept, and socialization.

➤ If your child is dealing with sensory and cognitive processing concerns, you may find some relief and resource in *Fuzzy Buzzy Groups for Children with Developmental and Sensory Processing Difficulties* by Fiona Brownlee and Lindsay Munro. It's an easy-to-follow guide to helping kids interact with peers in a fun, relaxed way.

➤ The Social Thinking website (www.socialthinking.com) doesn't target CAS specifically, but has books, products, and other resources you can use to help your kid consider the points-of-view of other people.

➤ *Creative Coping Skills for Children: Emotional Support through Arts and Crafts Activities* by Bonnie Thomas (Jessica Kingsley Publishers, 2009) is a great resource for parents who want to help their children cope in fun, easy, and creative ways.

➤ *Helping Children Cope with Change, Stress and Anxiety: A Photocopiable Activities Book* by Debrorah M. Plummer (Jessica Kingsley Publishers, 2010) is full of ideas and activities to use with kids.

➤ A couple of resources you and your child may find helpful when planning a play date: *What to Expect at a Play Date* (a children's book) by Heidi Murkoff (Harper Festival, 2001); *How to Be a Friend* by Laurie Krasny Brown and Marc Brown, the husband-wife team of the "Arthur" series (Little, Brown & Co, 1998), and *Let's Talk about Playing with Others* by Joy Berry (Gold Star Publishers, 1999).

➤ Working on potty training your less verbal child? May I suggest *The Potty Journey: Guide to Toilet Training Children with Special Needs, Including*

Autism and Related Disorders by Judith A. Coucouvanis (Autism Asperger Publishing Co., 2008).

➤ Children sometimes respond well to picture books in which others struggle to be accepted. Try *Ruby in Her Own Time* by Jonathan Emmett (Scholastic, 2007) and *Leo the Late Bloomer* by Robert Kraus (Harper Collins, 1994).

➤ Consider *making your own story* about a child who struggles to fit in. A couple of tips: don't use your child's own name, keep the text simple, allow your child to participate in the "publication" of this title by illustrating or helping to write the text. For ideas and inspiration, read about *Social Stories* at www.thegraycenter. org or in *The New Social Story Book* by Carol Gray (Future Horizons, 2010). The book has at least 150 examples of social situations your child(ren) may need a little brushing up on. Note: a lot of the literature on Social Stories suggests using them with kids on the autism spectrum. Autism and apraxia are not the same thing! However, the concept of Social Stories can be applied to *all* children.

➤ If you are looking for *movies* that may give your child the message that he's okay regardless of his abilities, without being too obvious about it, consider these titles:
  - *The Trumpet of the Swan* (a book by E.B. White turned movie) depicts a swan with no voice. Out of desperation, the father steals a trumpet as an instrument for the child to express himself. It's a heartwarming approach to finding alternative ways of finding ones' voice. Watch it first before showing it to your child.
  - Another E.B. White creation: *Charlotte's Web,* a kid-friendly movie (or book) that will show your child that it's not always easy to speak. It's especially touching when Wilbur finds his voice and begins singing and dancing to the song, "I can talk, I can talk!"
  - *The Tangerine Bear* presents a little bear whose smile is stamped on upside-down in a factory mishap. It's a heartwarming Christmas-themed story about appearances and appreciation.
  - *Annabelle's Wish* is a holiday book turned television special (released on DVD in 2000). Young Billy, who has been mute since being in a barn fire when he was younger, learns Santa grants the animals the gift of voice on Christmas Eve….a star-studded cast, including Rue McClanahan and Randy Travis, among others.

➤ For more ideas on how to create behavioral management programs and charts, as well as a good listing of prizes/rewards, read *How to Behave So Your Children Will, Too* by Sal Severe (Viking Penguin, 2002).

➤ For your physically aggressive and explosive child, you may find some good problem-solving techniques in these titles by Ross Greene: *The Explosive Child* (Harper-Collins, 2005) and *Treating the Explosive Child: The Collaborative Problem-Solving Approach,* with J. Stuart Ablon (Guilford Press, 2006).

➤ *SOS! Help for Parents* by Lynn Clark (Parents Press, 2005) offers great advice and problem-solving tips on dealing with behavior.

➤ *1-2-3 Magic: Effective Discipline for Children 2-12* by Thomas Phelan (Parent Magic, 2004) was the "gold standard" when I was working as an R.N. in a child/adolescent treatment program. The message is simple, yet powerful and effective.

➤ Great children's books to read with your child on feelings, including anger:
  - *When Sofia Gets Really Really Angry* by Molly Bang (Scholastic, 1999).
  - *Today I Feel Silly: And Other Moods That Make My Day* by Jamie Lee Curtis (Harper-Collins, 1998).
  - *No Hitting!* by Karen Katz (Grosset & Dunlap, 2004).
  - *Hands Are Not for Hitting* by Marine Agassi (Free Spirit Publishing, 2004).
  - *When I'm Feeling* Series by Tracey Moroney (Brighter Child, 2005). This series has a lot of titles/feelings from happy to scared and jealous.
  - *Let's Talk about Feeling Angry* by Joy Berry (Scholastic, 1996). Ms. Berry has a huge collection of books that may be of interest to you and your children, some with audio CDs.

➤ *Easing the Teasing: Helping Your Child Cope with Name-Calling, Ridicule, & Verbal Bullying* by Judy Freedman (McGraw-Hill, 2002) is a great no-nonsense approach to dealing with teasing, building friendships, and developing self-esteem.

➤ For older kids who need some tips on staying safe online read: *Cyberbullying: Activities to Help Children and Teens to Stay Safe in a Texting, Twittering, Social Networking World,* by Vanessa Rogers (Jessica Kingsley Publishers, 2010).

➤ An online article by Andrea Sachs on girls and bullying, "How to Bully-proof Young Girls": www.time.com/time/health/article/0,8599,2013184,00.html.

➤ More help for girls who are being bullied: *Little Girls Can Be Mean: Four Steps to Bully Proof Girls in the Early Grades* (St. Martin's Press, 2010) by Michelle Anthony and Reyna Lindert.

➤ *Why Doesn't Anyone Like Me: Guide to Raising Socially Confident Kids* by Hara Estroff Marano (Quill-William Morrow, 1998) takes a good look at popularity, social competence, and bullies.

➤ *Helping Your Angry Child: A Workbook for You and Your Family* by Darlyne Gaynor Nemeth, Kelly Paulk Ray, and Maydel Morin Schexnader (New Harbinger Publications, 2003) is packed with worksheets and engaging activities that may help you and your child understand and manage anger better.

➤ *Last Child in the Woods: Saving our Children from Nature Deficit Disorder* by Richard Louv (Algonquin Books, 2008) is a nice book for folks who value the benefits of fresh air, the environment, open-ended play, and outdoor recreation. It's about encouraging your kids to be unplugged and inquisitive.

➤ A resource for helping your kids relax during tense times: *Deeno's Dream Journeys in the Big Blue Bubble: A Relaxation Programme to Help Children Manage Their Emotions* by Julia Langensiepen (Jessica Kingsley Publishers, 2010).

Chapter Fifteen

· · · · · · · · · · · · · ·

Resolving Apraxia

· · · · · · · · · · · · ·

Where Do We Go from Here?

*"In watching my son become more and more self-aware as he approaches adulthood,
I no longer worry about his speech impeding his future.
His own desire and persistence to overcome has added the final polish he needed
to blast this issue right out of his life."*
—Janice, mother of son with history of CAS

I know you are asking, *"Will my kid ever be able to talk?"* For most children, the simple answer is *yes* (we just can't predict when). Whether or not a child will be a talker depends on the severity of the CAS and whether she received appropriate, early, intense, and frequent speech therapy. It also depends on the child's temperament and personality—some children are just more talkative and outgoing than others.

However, as parents of a child with CAS, we want to hear, *"Your child will be an exceptional communicator! Just give her this magic pill every day and she will be spitting out oratories next year."* The thing with CAS is that it is a dynamic disorder; it changes over time. Some say it will be with your child forever, but to a lesser degree—"once apraxic, always apraxic." Others say it goes away completely and you'd never be able to pick out the adult who had childhood apraxia of speech as a youngster.

This chapter will cover the idea of "resolving apraxia" and shows readers how a child with CAS looks and sounds once she grows up. Believe it or not, most nonprofessionals won't be able to detect that your child once had a childhood speech disorder.

The Nuts and Bolts of This Chapter

➤ Our personal experience with resolving apraxia

➤ The debate over "resolving," "resolved," and "always apraxic"

➤ Why and when children have relapses, and what to do about them

➤ The *potential* ongoing academic and social struggles of a child/teen with apraxia

➤ What to do when your child no longer wants to go to speech therapy

➤ Tips, advice, and suggestions on sending your child with resolving apraxia to college

➤ Of course, lots of at-home tips for you to use right away

Let's get right down to it. First, I want to congratulate you as a parent for having gotten this far on this journey, or book, or whatever made you crack open this chapter. Chances are if you've made it this far, you've made it through the thick of it. You have found hope. You are probably *hearing* hope from your child. It comes in bits and pieces. It comes in peaks and valleys. Give yourself a pat on the back and your child a big hug. You both deserve it.

Here's a little story I think you will appreciate. One weekend, my hugely supportive husband sent me away on a "writer's retreat"—a quick jaunt down the road to the hotel for which I had a coupon. I checked in and began the invigorating task of writing some of the last chapters of this book. I called home around dinnertime to hear the chatter and clatter of my happy family. Yes, I said *chatter*. Kate was 5 years, 3 months of age at the time. She had been diagnosed as "resolving" since 4 years, 6 months. That summer evening phone call made me smile through tears of pride. Why? I heard Kate shout from the background, "Mom sure has been working on that book for a long time!"

Kate, my little sweetheart with CAS, said a twelve-word sentence about the book I was writing on the very motor-speech condition she had. *While* I was writing about it. Talk about coming full circle, so to speak!

She can talk! She can talk! Which reminds me—watch *Charlotte's Web* and focus in on the part in which Wilbur "gets" his voice and can communicate with the other farmyard animals. I think this must be how our kids with CAS feel. Trust me, you'll get teary-eyed watching this movie, especially if your kiddo is parked on your lap.

Tell Me More: Families Share Their Experiences with Resolving CAS

I can tell you all about our story, but that gets boring after awhile. Plus, you want to know how other families got through the childhood apraxia journey as well. Every

One Christmas, Kate received a book, *Knuffle Bunny*, written by Mo Willems. I hated it. It was hard for me to read to her. In it, little Trixie misplaces her lovey and tries to tell her daddy where to find it. She uses words like, "Aggle, flabble, klabble…wumpy, and flappy." I can see the pain in young Trixie's face just as I saw it in Kate's. Only Kate was much older than the character in the book. The story ends when Trixie says her first words, "Knuffle Bunny." I used to hope and pray that it was as simple as really wanting something badly enough (e.g., the lovey) to get those words out. Mo Willems actually wrote a sequel to this story, *Knuffle Bunny Too*. It begins with the words, "By now Trixie was really using her words… ." Again, I secretly hated the book. I wanted *my* kid to be using her words. But she wasn't. Not like Trixie was, anyway.

Why I am I telling you this story? Well, in the first book, you see how Trixie's daddy is working so hard to try and understand his little girl, but can't. Everyone gets frustrated. In the sequel, Trixie is jabbering away and you know…it's a little bit empowering. You can look at these two books as "apraxia" (*Knuffle Bunny: A Cautionary Tale*) and "resolved apraxia" (*Knuffle Bunny Too*). With appropriate treatment and support, your child will hopefully be jabbering up a storm by the time this tale is all said and done.

child is different. Every case of CAS is unique and dynamic as well. Here are what some "apraxia parents" had to say about the experience of getting to the point where they could say, "She's talking!"

Amy, mother of son with a history of CAS, dismissed from speech therapy at 5.5 years and currently 12 years old, shares this:

"People who meet my son are shocked to hear that he had almost four years of intensive speech therapy as a child. Only his teachers notice his fine motor skill planning problems—his handwriting is terrible! Most people see my son as a charismatic, loveable young man, as long as catching/hitting a ball or complex motor planning isn't involved. He's like the absent-minded professor—much to offer but quirky."

Says Lori regarding her twelve-year-old son with a history of CAS:

"My son Kevin is resolved and I believe it happened because he has a motor plan for all sounds. The last sound to come in for him was the /r/ sound when he was in sixth grade. We are just working on articulation. He still has slight vowel distortions, but otherwise he is doing great!"

One mom indicated that they were in speech therapy for nearly two years before they saw any significant results, but her son was making progress [slowly]. She felt that age 5.5 years was when he *really* made significant gains in speech. "At 15 years old, he stutters when stressed," but for the most part, she indicates, no one would ever know.

Another mom, also of a teenage son with a history of CAS, told me that he speaks sloppily, mumbles, or talks in shortened phrases when he isn't "trying."

My thought: aren't all teenagers—especially boys—like that? But seriously, when children go through significant growth spurts during adolescence, it may take some time, or perhaps some additional speech-language therapy, to help them reorganize their motor plans to match this significant change in structure.

The Differences Between Resolved, Resolving, and "Always Apraxic"

As mentioned in the Introduction, some professionals believe that apraxia never completely goes away, even though the person may learn to talk so well that ordinary listeners do not detect anything wrong with her speech. Others use the term "resolved" to indicate that the symptoms of CAS have "worked themselves out" with therapy and lots of work from the child and her family. Still others may talk about CAS "resolving," meaning, "it's on the way out, but it's never really completely gone."

Personally, I like the word "recovered" best. To me, it means there is no gray, no blurring, no nebulous blob hanging around you or your child any more. It means apraxia is gone. Done. Never coming back. It is very clear-cut. But not all kids with CAS may reach this stage. There is no magical age at which kids can be declared "resolved/recovered," because that depends on the quality and amount of therapy they receive, plus the severity of the disorder. For example, if a child with "mild apraxia" was identified as "likely apraxic" at a very early age—say two years—and she had quality 1:1 therapy two or three times a week, she would "resolve" in a shorter amount of time than a child who was diagnosed with profound CAS at age three and received poor, intermittent therapy.

While there really aren't any specific guidelines or criteria from the American Speech-Language-Hearing Association (ASHA) for determining who should receive the "resolved apraxia" diagnosis, there are some general characteristics SLPs and parents of children with apraxia can keep in mind. They are:

> ➤ *Consider the severity of the disorder.* If your child was diagnosed with mild apraxia, then it may be more likely that the disorder will resolve in less time and with less effort. Of course, there are various degrees of severity ranging from mild to moderate to severe to profound. You can ask your SLP where your child's diagnosis likely falls.

> ➤ *CAS no longer interferes with your child's daily life or her functioning.* This means your child can ask for what she needs intelligibly without the use of prompts, cues, or gesticulating (using hands to communicate).

> ➤ *Others can understand what your child is saying to a reasonable degree.* Folks are no longer saying, "Huh? Can you say that again?"

➤ *Most folks cannot tell that she had a previous speech/language problem.* In other words, they think little to nothing of a speech-related quirk your child may exhibit.
➤ *Your child has learned and used coping and accommodation skills such as self-monitoring.*
➤ *The biggest and best indicator of "apraxia recovery" is that your child's articulation and speech are considered age-appropriate.* Your SLP will tell you when your child has reached that level. When you hear this, it's time to celebrate!

Keep in mind, though, that some SLPs won't say that your child's CAS has "resolved." Instead, they may say something like Rhonda Banford, MAT, CCC-SLP, does: "Resolved is not a term I use in my practice. Instead, I choose to say that the child no longer has difficulty with the motor aspects of forming words or sentences."

Ms. Banford may sound like she is splitting hairs, but really she is not. Just because a child no longer struggles with the motor aspects of speaking does not necessarily mean that her speech and language skills are now normal. Remember how CAS is a motor-speech disorder? Well, it also affects other aspects of expressive language, including:

➤ Syntax (grammar)
➤ Morphology (meaningful word segments. For example, "cats" has two morphemes or segments—cat + s.)
➤ Both syntax and morphology have to do with the structure of the sentence, the length of utterance, and how complex it is. Problems with syntax and morphology are "language" disorders (whereas CAS is a "speech" disorder).

How Motivated Is Your Child to Make Progress?

Children with CAS are motivated to improve their speech by various factors. These include:

➤ the child's unique temperament and personality
➤ her intent and willingness to communicate
➤ her opportunities to practice at home
➤ how supportive the family environment is
➤ how engaged and proactive the parents are
➤ whether the child is given an effective carrot...*a what?!* A "carrot" is a unique motivator your child responds to. You'll learn what this is by trial and error. Examples may include: verbal praise from parents (siblings or therapist), a sticker on a chart, a lollipop, extra video game time, a special time with mom or dad, or just feeling that her needs and feelings are getting heard.

When you add in these characteristics of morphology and syntax, the whole equation gets more complicated. Your child may be able to initiate sounds, imitate sounds, speak spontaneously, and even say multisyllabic words, but she still trips over syntax and morphology (involving the rules of language). Is that part of apraxia? Some folks say "yes," and others don't. CAS is a motor-speech disorder, so why do children with CAS often have language disorders? Could it be that children with CAS have not had opportunities to practice morphology and syntax? Once children can *say* the words, they need to learn the rules of language by receiving feedback on their use of language.

Is Your Child "Resolving/Recovering?"

Hearing that your child's CAS is resolving is a fantastic stepping stone to the "resolved/recovered" status. You're almost there. Now you know you will *both* get there.

Again, there are no hard and fast rules for declaring a child's CAS is "resolving," but here's a little cheat sheet:

➤ *Your child has started to mature in a social and emotional sense.* Try not to confuse this with physical maturity. Your child may still look like a child, but she can greet and connect with peers in an age-appropriate manner. She can control her emotions in a more "mature" way—fewer outbursts and temper tantrums because she can now communicate these in words. For example, Jane, mother of six-year-old Abby, shares this:

> *"Sometimes, I will try to hurry [my daughter] along by completing her sentence or prompting her as she struggles to find the 'right' word. But Abby will come back and say, 'Mom, you are being rude. I haven't gotten all of my words out yet!'"*

➤ *Mild issues may still remain.* Try not to scrutinize your child's speech so much. You may have been trained to look for perfection in her communication, but really—how many five-year-olds have absolutely perfect articulation? Many children are developing their speech sounds until around age eight.

➤ *CAS is "below the surface."* There will be times when your child stumbles or gropes for words. This happens to *all* of us, right? When you can see or hear your child struggling with speech just once or twice a day instead of *most* of the time, then it's likely that her CAS is resolving.

➤ *Your child is learning and beginning to use coping and accommodation skills.* Talk with your SLP about this. Is she teaching your child to self-monitor? What does your SLP suggest your child should be doing? For us, it was "Stop. Think. Slow down." However, your child must be ready to do this important step.

➤ *Your child's speech, or lack thereof, no longer stands out.* By the time your child reaches the "resolving" status, folks are no longer asking or commenting on her speech.

➤ *Your child's CAS is no longer slowing her down, or preventing her (or your family) from doing what you want to do.* Sign her up for a soccer team, allow her to attend a birthday party without a chaperone/translator, let her order her own food at McDonald's, because she can do it!

> *"I picked my son up from a weeklong specialized comedy improv camp and I don't think I've ever heard him speak so easily before. He was very well spoken, his grammar was excellent, and there were no 'bumps' in his word finding whatsoever. On the way home, he told me that he purposefully chose workshops that were tougher for him speech-wise. He took on prominent positions in improv sketches—something he used to not do because he felt his speech would fail him at a crucial moment. He always worries about his speech a little. However, he told me that not one person at the camp noticed any speech issues whatsoever. This gave him a lot of confidence."*
> —Mark's mother

➤ *You can look back at the journey and say, "We're really making progress!"* Think back to where you and your child began (I'd recommend journaling or marking small accomplishments on a calendar early on) and celebrating them together. When you can honestly say, "It's going to be okay," you know you've reached the resolving status. And if you're not there just yet, don't lose hope.

> *"Right now, we are dealing with what remains, not apraxia per se, but common co-morbid things like fine motor struggles and distractibility. I am not sure if any other struggles will be presented to us, but I do know that Allison is a smart, spunky little girl who can talk like any other kid and has a real future. For that, I am eternally thankful."*
> — Susan, mother of Ally, 7 years old with resolving CAS

What Can You Do at Home?

When you are in the "resolving/recovering" mode, you might want a few pointers to boost your child's progress. Just keep in mind that it's not a race, and everyone develops at her own pace. Please don't push your child into something she's not yet ready to do.

Use simple and nonthreatening techniques. Find opportunities for success. The grocery store, school, the library, the park provide endless opportunities for your child to communicate with success. Look at Chapter 9 for ideas. Remember to modify these ideas for your child's current communication level.

For example, when your daughter says something spontaneously, praise her. Saying a word or phrase she has heard dozens of times (but was previously unable to say) is a big step for a child with CAS. She has likely been mentally practicing and developing these neuropathways for quite some time. Now she spontaneously says the word(s) for the first time. Hooray! Acknowledge and honor this step.

Engage your child in play. When she's hard at work playing, get down to her level and talk to her about what's going on. You might say, "What's GI Joe doing now? Who's the good guy? Who's the bad guy?" If your child doesn't respond well to questions, you could make general statements as in, "Oh, look what GI Joe is doing. He is driving in his truck." Just be a good verbal role model. Try making it more about play than about communication. You don't even have to make eye contact, if your child is not good at eye contact. You'd be surprised what might "pop out" of your child's mouth when she doesn't think you are quizzing her on speech sounds, words, or phrases.

Take a Two-Pronged Approach

Let's say your child's CAS is "resolving." The battle is half over. Now it's time to start working on her phonological skills *at the same time* you continue to work on her motor-speech skills. See Chapter 12 on phonological awareness to find some activities you and your child can do together at home.

"Once Apraxic, Always Apraxic"

We've repeated this comment several times, but what does it really mean? As you may recall, CAS may run in the family (immediate or close relatives may have a history of speech impairments or disorders). So, even if your child is considered "recovered" from CAS, she may still have the genetic predisposition for the disorder. And the bigger question is, "will there be a relapse?" (We'll get to that later.) The short answer—and the good news—is *she will probably NOT always demonstrate apraxia of speech if she is recovered.*

According to Rhonda Banford, CCC-SLP, "If your child's apraxia is mild enough, and their therapy is intensive and appropriate, then one can expect a child with CAS to become a proficient-enough speaker that no one would know their past struggles." She explains, however, that the situation is different if your child has another condition besides CAS: "We can't just tell a parent of a child who has apraxia *and* autism, for example, that the child will speak just fine one day. Parents need to understand that if CAS is the child's *only* disorder, there's a good chance that with proper therapy, she will seem perfectly normal to everyone who knows her. If the child has CAS *and* other disorders, it is far less likely. Unfortunately, the other disorders affect how well the child will progress with the apraxia therapy, so it is likely she will make progress, but she may never get to the same stage as the child without other disorders."

So why even bother with the label "resolving apraxia?" It helps to describe your child's progress in terms of her speech. It also helps you remember her recovery. And it helps you keep an eye on potential problems that may crop up in the future (see the section on "Remnants and Relapse" later in this chapter). You can say "resolving apraxia" and have it mean "a child with a history of CAS who has fully intelligible—but not perfect—speech."

When should you let go of the label? Some folks hang on to the apraxia label for years. What's the benefit, you wonder? First, the label can help the child/young adult get the services that may be needed at school or in a postsecondary institution). Some folks may like the secondary gain they receive from the attention or concern of others. Others may not have recovered enough to drop the label. Parents may still be working on a sense of closure from the intense parenting they went through during the "apraxic years"—shuffling therapy appointments, participating in home practice, and learning about the disorder. It may be hard for parents to "let go" of that identity even though they are happy apraxia no longer plagues their child.

Can Childhood Apraxia of Speech Evolve into Something Else?

Some parents and SLPs will tell you that CAS doesn't really "resolve," meaning go away completely, but may *evolve* into something else.

You may hear something like I did: "We don't think Kate has apraxia any more. In fact, I am not sure if she ever did. Who diagnosed her? She might have a slight phonological disorder, but that's all." I was taken aback when I heard this from the school IEP team. I was beyond certain that Kate had CAS. It was more likely that Kate was presenting—*at that time*—like a child with a phonological disorder.

Other parents have told me about hearing similar statements from professionals. These professionals indicated that the children who had previously had CAS had evolved into having moderate articulation disorders or mild phonological disorders or even auditory processing disorders.

If you are wondering if your child's CAS is evolving vs. resolving, find an SLP who can help you sort this all out—preferably one who has been trained specifically in the treatment of motor speech disorders.

Remnants, Relapse, and Resistant Residuals

Your child may have gotten to the point where she has intelligible speech and can pretty much communicate like any other Clara, Emma, and Grant. But now you find yourself concerned about what might be "remnants" of apraxia. What are they? What do they mean? And, what can you do about them?

Parents Ask…

Are there tests to determine if CAS is resolving?

Researchers Edythe Strand, Ph.D., CCC-SLP, and Rebecca McCauley, Ph.D., CCC-SLP, examined assessment tools that were developed to help with diagnosis of speech-motor problems: Preschool and school-age versions of the *Apraxia Profile*, the *Kaufmann Speech Praxis Test for Children*, the *Oral Speech Mechanism Screening Examination*—3rd edition, *Screening Test for Developmental Apraxia of Speech*—2nd edition, *Verbal Dyspraxia Profile*, and the *Verbal Motor Production Assessment for Children*. Their results were published in the *American Journal of Speech-Language Pathology* in 2008. Drs. Strand and McCauley found that these tools varied widely in what they assess. They concluded that an SLP may choose to use these tools to help determine if a child is progressing, but it is best to use them in conjunction with keen observation.

Diane Bahr, MS, CCC-SLP, uses a list of CAS characteristics to observe her clients' speech motor-planning concerns. The list is based on information found in the speech-language pathology literature. She assesses progress by looking at the percentage of change in her clients' skills over time. Another speech-language pathologist, Ruth Stoeckel, Ph.D., CCC-SLP, indicates that sometimes the best way for families to determine whether their children are progressing is to look at data specific to what their child is working on and ask if the progress is significant to them. Doing so is going to help you look back on the experience of CAS and feel proud that your child has come as far as she has!

First, let's identify what the remnants *might* be:

➤ Fine motor delay (difficulties with handwriting, handling utensils or scissors), as *some* children with CAS also have limb apraxia.

➤ Mild sensory symptoms (mouthing nonfood items, sensitivity to loud noise, touch, or smell, poor hand-eye coordination and tracking), as *some* children with CAS also have sensory processing disorders.

➤ Lack of organization, especially in upper grades, as coursework becomes more difficult and students have multiple teachers and classrooms.

➤ Inattention to detail, especially in instances in which your child is asked to describe objects or events in an open-ended way. Speech production requires great attention to detail and sequencing. For example, your child may have problems answering questions such as, "What did you do at day camp today?" You may have to ask very specific questions instead.

➤ The inability to verbally sequence information in a logical manner: "First we did some free play, and then had Circle Time, and after that we went on a hike and made a craft."

➤ Prosody issues—difficulties with speech rate, rhythm, inflection, syllables, and breath control.

If these signs and symptoms are apraxia lingering, mention them to your child's SLP, teacher, or school psychologist. It's not the end of the world. All of these issues can improve with a little work and assistance. You may want to add an occupational therapist (OT) to the treatment team, if you haven't already. An OT can help your child with fine motor skills such as handling utensils and handwriting. The OT can also assist with sequencing and organizational issues. An educational psychologist might also be a helpful resource. Give your insurance company a call and find out what will and will not be paid by your insurance. (See Appendix B.)

The reasons children may have these remnants varies from child to child. Your child may still chew on toys, for example, because she has a sensory processing disorder, or perhaps the act of chewing helps her attend/focus/concentrate. Or maybe your child hasn't matured in some social or emotional sense. Could it be that she has found some unique way to compensate for her speech issues? For example, if chewing is a comfort to your child, it may be something you and your child learn to modify over time. You'll likely need to provide your kiddo with appropriate items to chew (gum, licorice, oral-motor "toys"). Be sure you also suggest a socially appropriate time to use them. If you need to find appropriate mouth toys for your child, consider:

➤ Therapy Shoppe (www.therapyshoppe.com)
➤ Pocketful of Therapy (www.pfot.com)
➤ Super Duper Publications (www.superduperinc.com)
➤ LinguiSystems (www.linguisystems.com)

Remember, CAS is an ever-changing, dynamic disorder that presents itself differently as it progresses. It looks different in every child.

Word Study: "Remnant," "residual," "lingering symptomology," and "after effects" are all terms you may hear when professionals talk about your child's history of CAS. Just keep this in the back of your mind should you need to assess these concerns in greater detail someday.

Relapse and Backsliding

"Relapse," "backsliding," "slipping," or "downward spiral" might be ways to describe the phenomenon of CAS showing its ugly face after you thought everything was all fine and well. It may happen once or twice or even more along your journey. Don't worry. Just get right back in the saddle, and get the help you and your child need.

Here is our experience. Kate was doing great. She was in an intense preschool program five days per week. Her IEP had been discontinued because her testing and her classroom teacher indicated she was "doing well." We signed off and agreed to continue with private speech therapy. Three weeks later, her private SLP also thought her CAS was resolving. I ran out and purchased the Razor scooter Kate had been wanting for months, and we all went out for dinner to celebrate. Six months later, we were back at the speech clinic. It's not that they were wrong. It's not that Kate stopped trying. It's just that something started to change. Here are some reasons a relapse might occur:

➤ *The motor plans/gestures/programs were never established to the extent they needed to be in the first place.* That is, after all, one of the hypotheses that SLP researchers have suggested to explain "the whys" of apraxia. What it may mean for your child at this point is simply *strengthening* those motor plans with increased speech practice.

➤ *The linguistic complexity of what the child is trying to say has increased beyond her capability, creating a greater linguistic load.* That is, when your child was saying simpler sentences, her speech skills seemed adequate, but now that her language skills have increased (knows more vocabulary, wants to express more complex thoughts) her speech skills simply "can't keep up."

Parents Ask...

What's a linguistic load?

The linguistic load can be defined as the complexity of what is being communicated verbally. This includes the difficulty of movements of the articulators (tongue, palate, jaw, teeth, lips) from one place to the next and how much planning/programming is required to get the thoughts out verbally. (Tongue twisters, for example, have a high linguistic load.)

➤ *She may have an incorrect underlying representation of the word.* Simply put, she internalized the word wrong. Here are some funny examples from speech-language pathologist Rhonda Banford: "A couple of kids with apraxia really thought you read a 'boot' and not a 'book.' Another child insisted that the Star Wars character was 'Hand' Solo and not 'Han' Solo. Still yet another child was sure we ate 'state' and not 'steak,' and was insisting *I* was saying it incorrectly!"

➤ *She may also have actual muscle weakness.* The fancy term for this is "dysarthria." That is, the child's speech suffers because she has some underlying muscle weakness.

As you are reading this, I know you have questions. First, of all—yes, it is possible that kids with CAS also have dysarthria. That is, they can correctly recognize a sound and can move the articulators (the parts of the mouth and vocal cords) to make that sound, but the words still don't sound "right." Dysarthria is a muscle function concern related to muscle weakness, which has to do with muscle tension/tone.

Here's your take-away message: If your child has trouble planning speech movements *and* her speech sounds slurred/distorted, then it's likely she has both apraxia *and* dysarthria. Only your SLP can make that determination. If you have concerns, bring it up at your next therapy session.

Some folks become goofy and incoherent when mentally exhausted. In fact, you may be one of them! Does this mean that you also have apraxia? Perhaps you, too, were once a child with CAS? We all slip up when we are tired—some more than others—and it's actually pretty normal. When it comes to our kids with CAS, you can use this "slip-up method" as a gauge that your child is mentally taxed and would benefit from some "down time."

A mother in my Small Talk: All About Apraxia group described how her daughter relapsed when she became ill. She said:

> *"When Lila got sick a few weeks ago, we noticed some major regression. It was then that I realized how much effort it takes for her to talk. This is hard work for these kiddos."*

Coping with Relapse

If you are concerned that your child is relapsing, try not to worry or blame the therapist, yourself, or your child. Sit back and reevaluate the situation. ***Try your very best to be objective.*** You can start by documenting the behaviors/speech patterns you are seeing that lead you to question your child's progress. Again, I strongly recommend keeping track of successes and pitfalls on a daily calendar.

Give yourself a little time to think about what's going on (you might make a deadline and stick with it—say a week) and then take action. Call the speech clinic or the school and ask for a reevaluation or follow-up appointment. Tell them specifically why you are concerned. They will likely honor your request. Hopefully, with a little "brush up" therapy, your child will be back on track. If you don't succeed with the speech clinic or school, consider getting a second opinion.

The Social Animal: Your Child's Social Group

As a parent, you know that at some point your child will connect more with her peers than with you. It's only normal and a part of growing up. Allow it. You may have been your child's translator, but eventually you'll want to start letting her learn and discover the world, even though she may struggle at times. Here are some tips for making the social experience for your child (and yourself!) a little easier:

➤ ***Know your child's interests.*** Find something your child is good at doing and enjoys. Sign her up and get her involved. Here are some activities your child may want to pursue: Suzuki violin, swim team, gymnastics, soccer, or band. These activities require concentration, practice, and persistence. Plus, it will place her into positions to interact with others where talking isn't always the focus.

➤ ***Get to know your child's friends.*** It sounds simple, but you'll need to make an effort to do this. There's a fine line between getting to know your child's friends and hovering. If they come to the house, greet them. Call them by name and learn at least one or two interesting things about each child. Then remember to ask them about their interests the next time you see them.

➤ *Get to know the parents of your child's friends.* Your child picks up behaviors and values from you (good or bad), right? This also happens with friends. If you have a sense of where these other children are "coming from" (their parents, their home), you'll have a better sense of the children with whom your child is associating. You don't have to become best friends with their parents, but get to know them in a social setting or two. Exchange periodic emails, or invite them to stay for a play date.

➤ *Have some "cool" things at your house that other kids will enjoy and associate with your home.* It doesn't really matter what it is; just make sure it's safe and kid-friendly. Examples include a pet, a swing set, a nice assortment of Legos, or a popular book series. Of course, don't run out and buy something specifically for this purpose. Make sure it's something you and your family value and will use as well.

➤ *Your child may still stumble on certain words or phrases, or struggle to find the right word from time to time.* Other kids may find this funny. Some kids can be mean. Teach your child a few coping skills, just in case. For examples, please refer back to Chapter 14.

➤ *Kids can be very patient.* They may take your child under their wing and help her out. They may prompt your child (they may not realize they're doing this) so your child can communicate more effectively. It's a sweet and touching blessing for your child to have a friend like this!

➤ *Let your child know what you think about her friends.* You don't have to draw any attention to this method. Just say something like, "I really like Megan. I think you two get along nicely. I like how she helps you out when you get stuck." Your child will begin to internalize that and will begin to seek out other like-minded friends. She will also see that you are paying attention to her friendships as well.

➤ *Finally, it's not important that your child have a ton of BFFs.* It's quality, not quantity that matters.

Please refer to Chapter 14 for more ideas in helping your child cope with CAS.

Wanting to Quit Therapy

At some point, your little sweetie, who has been all too compliant in the speech therapy rigmarole, is likely to rebel. She won't want to go to speech anymore. You may have to poke, prod, and cajole her to get her into the car and to the clinic.

Kate once asked me in an exasperated voice, "Doesn't speech have a drive-through?" She was serious, but I died laughing.

Kids get tired of speech therapy, just as you get tired of driving them there, communicating with the therapist, paying the bill, and drilling your child at home. But you know your child needs to continue to receive the benefits of speech therapy. And sometimes, we have to continue to do things we aren't so keen on doing.

What's a Parent to Do?

➤ *Sympathize with her.* "I know you don't really want to go to speech [therapy] today, but it's really important."

➤ *Remind her of her progress.* "But you have come so far. Just think, when we first started seeing Ms. Diane, you couldn't say all of the things you can say now. Isn't it fun to be able to talk?" You may even consider showing your child some old progress reports or charts if you have them.

➤ *Ask this tough question: "Are you okay if you aren't speaking as clearly—or as well—as some of your friends?"* This is a particularly important question to ask if you (and your child's therapist) really don't think your child is ready to end therapy but your child is. Often, kids will want to quit therapy when therapy is interfering with more fun and interesting activities. They may also want to quit when they perceive the work as "too hard." This is where you and your SLP simplify tasks, so your child can feel successful.

➤ *Reward her with a treat.* Think of some positive reinforcement that will get your kiddo to therapy without struggle. It may work to have a "prize box" of trinkets stowed in your car. After therapy is over, offer her a choice from the prize box. Head over to the local park after a session or take her out for ice cream. It could even be as simple as allowing her to stay up a half-hour later than usual on therapy days or providing extra video game time. You'll know what works best for your child and your family.

➤ *Talk to your child's SLP.* Maybe your child really *is* ready to stop therapy. Bring this up with your SLP; perhaps some readjustment can help. Some children participate more readily at a different time of day, a different day of the week, or in a shorter session. Perhaps group therapy with other socially and age- and diagnosis-matched kids would be more ideal. Your child may also do better if she assists in therapy planning—get her ideas for a more fun, effective session. Of course, your SLP must be willing to do this.

"We ended private speech therapy just after he turned ten when the therapist told me she was having a hard time coming up with new goals."
—mother of Matt with resolving CAS and PDD-NOS.

➤ **Go ahead, end therapy.** I am not saying this to be defiant. It really might be time, or your child may just need a break. After talking with your child's therapist, your child, and your spouse/significant other, you may come to the conclusion that it's time to move on or take a break. It's not the end of the world if you end therapy for a period of time. You can always go back.

➤ **Go back to therapy if you have to.** We were discharged from therapy at one point with the understanding that we monitor Kate's progress (or problems) for several months. We were encouraged to call and come back to the clinic if we had any concerns. And, we did. Kate went right back once we saw a bit of regression. It was no big deal, and it was the appropriate thing to do.

How Does the End of Therapy Look?

Every situation and child is different, of course. So are speech clinics and SLPs, for that matter. Here's what you might expect:

A periodic formal testing period. Your child's SLP will likely want to do a formal test to assess her progress. This will probably be done over the course of a couple of sessions. Your SLP will compare past assessment scores with "now" assessment scores, too.

➤ **A sit-down results session with you and your significant other.** If your child is speaking at "developmentally appropriate" levels, then it will likely be recommended that therapy end.

➤ **Give yourself, your child, and the SLP a little bit of warning.** After you have heard the good news, you might want to give your child one more session to bring things to closure. After all, she has likely developed a pretty close relationship with the SLP and needs some time to say good-bye. You might, too.

➤ **Mark your calendar and prepare for the final day.** Kate's therapy sessions ended when she was entering full-day kindergarten. She would be in school until nearly 4 p.m. (after the bus ride home). We just couldn't imagine tacking on yet another "to-do" at the end of a long, busy day. Since she was speaking at "developmentally appropriate" levels at this point, it made the decision easier.

➤ *Celebrate and recognize a job well done (for both your child and your therapist).* Kate drew a picture for her therapist of a kindergarten classroom and signed her name. I added a personal note, "Thanks for helping me prepare for school. I'm all ready because of you." I included a gift card to a coffee shop. We hugged our SLP and said "thank you." We were told to call or email with any questions, whatsoever. Here are some other ideas:

- Some clinics provide families and kids with a certificate of completion. If they don't, consider making your own. It really *is* a big accomplishment.
- Take your child out for dinner at a special restaurant.
- Bake cookies for the therapist.
- Give your therapist a therapy-related toy, book, or game for his or her practice.
- Donate a subscription to the speech clinic waiting room in your child's name.

➤ Make sure that your child knows how proud and happy you are of her accomplishments!

Parents Cope with the End of an Era

Now what? Your child isn't going to therapy several times a week and you have all of this free time….What are you going to do now? You have just spent a huge portion of your life trucking your kid to and from speech therapy. Your calendar was always booked on Monday afternoons and Thursday mornings for speech therapy. You'd think you'd be jumping for joy now that you have these "windows" of time open again. Instead, you may feel lost and directionless. Give yourself time to adjust. Slowly you can start adding in some new activities. If your child is not otherwise engaged, maybe you can use this time to enroll her in a class or sport. Maybe you can make this an opportunity to arrange a standing play date for your child with a friend.

Just be prepared for an adjustment period for you and your child. While the end of therapy is something you both wanted, it can still be a time of transition.

One mother I spoke with talked about the transition from speech therapy to no speech therapy:

"I did not find the adjustment hard at all. I was very proud of how far my daughter had come. It just seems like when time in my schedule opens up, something else comes in to fill it—it wasn't hard with three kids! It seems as kids grow, they have more opportunities for activities. [My daughter] did join Girl Scouts, so it is just a different kind of busy."

"I do remember feeling anxious about letting go and saying "Okay, this is over," commented Vicki on how it felt when her son, Evan, ended therapy.

A mother named Karyn relates, "I didn't think I would miss taking [my son] to therapy but I did. [Speech Therapy] was also my therapeutic social hour with the other moms whose kids were there at the same time. I learned the most from those other moms, and together we got through all the drama that comes from being a mom of a child with special needs."

And just who do they tell? How does one share the "news" with others?
"I told my Mom. I told all my friends. I told my mother-in-law. They were so happy. While they have been so supportive over the years, none of

How We Celebrated My Child's Discharge from Speech Therapy

Kate Welder, founder of the website Apraxia Speaks (www.apraxiaspeaks.com) and author of ebook *Apraxia Explained*, says:
"By all means, a small family celebration is in order. It could be something simple such as cooking your child's favorite meal or going to their favorite restaurant. We have always made home movies of our children since birth. With Josie, we often filmed her "talking" on the movie, gathering these over a period of a few years. When we interviewed her for her graduation [from speech], it made a lasting tribute to her progress."

Another mother was less sentimental:
"There was no big party or event to mark the end of this important and critical piece to [my son's] development…it just happened. Maybe to be compared to any kind of transition that just happens—from childhood to adolescence, from reading to not reading, from breastfeeding to not—it just comes to an end and you have to kind of squint to remember how that came about."

"I'm a card-maker so I made the therapist a pack of greeting cards as a good-bye/thank you," says one mom of a child who was dismissed from speech therapy at age 10. I love the personal touch of her thank you for providing such a personal service: the gift of speech.

Finally, you will hear the emotional sentimentality as this mother shares her experience hearing from her child's long-time physician that things were okay:
"I can distinctly remember the real 'end' moment for me. At her follow-up last year, we finally heard the words that we have been waiting years to hear. [The developmental pediatrician] said, 'Congratulations, [your daughter] presents as a typical child her age. She looks great.' I cried. Then I let it sink in, I really tried to be present in the moment. Then I cried some more. We hugged [our daughter] and told her we were so proud of her. At that moment, that was the perfect thing."

them really understood the enormity of the moment. Unless you have been there, you have no idea. My husband and I still cry when we think about it," relates Susan, after ending speech therapy for her daughter, now 7 years old.

On a personal note, I made preschool graduation announcements for Kate and mailed them to our close friends and family. I started with something along the lines of, "Preschool Graduation?! Really?!" I typed up a little blurb on the computer, complete with cute fonts and colors about Kate's struggle with CAS, along with information about the intense preschool she attended five days a week. I wasn't expecting anything in return—other than a sense of closure for me. But I was floored with the response Kate got—cards and small gifts came her way. It was a sweet way to end her "speech preschool," and send her on to mainstream kindergarten.

Middle Grades and Beyond

While I cannot say for certainty that your child will be speaking normally by middle school, note that Childhood Apraxia of Speech is called a *childhood* speech disorder for a reason. It may be that you are really beginning to see that your child will overcome her CAS. Continue to keep an eye on your child's progress and look for any concerns that may crop up as your child enters the middle grades of elementary school, middle school, and into high school. If you do start to see concerns, you know there are resources available to help you and your child. Seek them out when or if it's appropriate. After a quick "refresher," your child may be back to performing at her top!

Some adolescents with a history of CAS really do not like the fact that the descriptor "childhood" is even part of the moniker. For example, you may hear your adolescent say something like, "I don't have childhood apraxia of speech any more. I am *not* a child!" This can become a touchy subject.

Instead, tweens and adolescents could explain their variable speech to friends or teachers as: "I used to have a childhood speech disorder when I was younger. It's better now, but sometimes I still have trouble with certain words or phrases, especially when I am tired or stressed."

Linda, the mother of a teenager previously diagnosed with CAS, described her daughter's lingering difficulties this way:

"My daughter is sixteen and definitely has resolving apraxia. She is easily understood by strangers. However, her apraxia still has subtle impact. Last year, she was an honor roll student, yet we went round and round with her science teacher, who complained that my daughter raised her hand without having an answer ready. She could not understand that my daughter needed a few moments to figure out how to turn the words in her brain into spoken words with the unfamiliar science vocabulary."

Another mother, Suzanne, mentioned this about her daughter's resolving CAS:

"I also recognize that the end may not always be the end. I am confident in Allison's ability to communicate; her speech is perfect nowadays. I am confident that she has a bright future…I am incredibly optimistic; but I also know that with neurological differences, there may be additional surprises. She has come so very far, though, that I know that we can tackle anything that comes our way. Allison will have a great life. I believe that this experience has made her better, harder working, more empathetic."

Sending Your Young Adult to College

At this point, your child will probably be talking like any other college student. (Provided she had "pure" apraxia of speech, without any added disabilities.) You may be able to detect slight variations in her speech because you've been there since the beginning. By the time your child reaches college age, she will have learned to accommodate and self-correct little errors in her speech. She will know that when she gets tired, she isn't as eloquent in her communication. She probably realizes that when she's stressed, she makes mistakes in her speech. Your child has come a long way and overcome some significant obstacles.

Be aware that if she still has disabilities that entitled her to special education or accommodations in high school, she may or may not qualify for accommodations in college. The Individuals with Disabilities Education Act (IDEA) discussed in Chapter 11 does not cover college students. Your child may, however, qualify as a student with disabilities under Section 504 of the Rehabilitation Act of 1973 or the Americans with Disabilities Act (ADA). She will need to submit official reports of psychological and educational testing to the college after admittance (if she chooses to disclose her disability to the school). Students who qualify for Section 504 or ADA supports can receive extended time on tests, note-taking assistance, access to text-to-speech software, and other types of accommodations, depending on their needs. For more information on rights and supports for college-bound kids, you may want to start with the Wrightslaw flyer "Help for College Students with Disabilities" at: www.wrightslaw.com/flyers/college.504.pdf

If your child is college-bound, buckle down, read those college admission guides, and help your child prepare for the ACT and SAT. Start thinking about scholarships. However, ***every child is different.*** Not all children with CAS will go to college, based on many variables (academic ability, financial resources, interest, other co-occurring conditions, etc.).

Say That Again?! Chapter Summary

We covered resolving and recovering from CAS, we shared some reasons for relapse and possible solutions, then we moved into the big question of when or if it's appropriate to end therapy, and how to determine when it's time to move on. We discussed potential problems and concerns as children move into higher grade levels at school (understanding and communicating complex multisyllabic words, among others). We briefly touched on the college years and beyond.

Please don't be overwhelmed. If you already are, then it's time to take a deep breath, and remember *your child will likely get over her difficulty with verbal communication.* I know that at times, it feels doubtful. It may reassure you to look back at the beginning of this chapter where other parents commented on how well their children are doing, or the "ah-ha" moments in which everything just fell into place.

Read On! Recommended Resources

➤ The "Family Start Guide" on the CASANA/Apraxia-KIDS website has some valuable information for you to consider as you seek information on *resolving CAS*: www.apraxia-KIDS.org.

➤ For information on the *difference between an articulation disorder and a phonological disorder,* look at this page by Keri Spielvogle, M.C.D., CCC-SLP: www.superduperinc.com/handouts/pdf/45-ArticVSPhonology.pdf.

➤ The American Speech-Language-Hearing Association (ASHA) has good information on *articulation and phonological disorders* at: www.asha.org/public/speech/disorders/SpeechSoundDisorders.htm.

➤ You can find additional information on *dysarthria* from:
   ● the U.S. National Library of Medicine: www.ncbi.nlm.nih.gov/pubmedhealth/PMH0004947/
   ● The American Speech-Language-Hearing Association (ASHA): www.asha.org/public/speech/disorders/dysarthria.htm
   ● The Mayo Clinic: www.mayoclinic.com/health/dysarthria/DS01175

➤ If you want to *hear and see children with a history of CAS* speak (and sing!), go to www.Youtube.com and type "apraxia" in the search field. You're sure to get several hits.

➤ *What Color is Your Parachute for Teens: Discovering Yourself, Defining Your Future* by Carol Christen and Richard N. Bolles (Ten Speed Press, 2010) is a spin on the adult version of the book that combines suggestions on finding one's passion with discussions of high-interest jobs in the 21st century.

➤ For students with disabilities who are ready to *transition from high school to college*, check out The Department of Education's brochure, "Students with Disabilities Preparing for Postsecondary Education: Know Your Rights and Responsibilities": http://www2.ed.gov/about/offices/list/ocr/transition.html.

➤ AHEAD (www.ahead.org) has some helpful resources for *students with disabilities headed off to college.*

Chapter Sixteen

• • • • • • • • • • • • •

Shaking Your Groove Thing

• • • • • • • • • • • • •

Networking, Advocating,
and Resources

"There isn't a single book out there for parents on apraxia," I complained to my daughter's SLP. "I know," Ms. Jen replied. "There's not much out there."

I went on to explain that I just wanted a book, a *real-life* book, I could hold in my hands and read and go back to refer to if I needed. I wanted a comprehensive guide that would start at the beginning and cover the definition of apraxia, what caused it (even if it was just a bunch of theories—I didn't care—I wanted something, *anything*), and what I could do about it. Most of all, I wanted something I could relate to.

Ms. Jen listened like any good therapist or friend would do. When I was done with my wish list, another therapist chimed in, "Sounds like it's a job for you."

"What?!" I shook my head in confusion and disbelief. I hadn't even noticed Sylvia—another SLP—walk into the room.

"It sounds like the job is yours. Write a book about apraxia," she repeated with utmost certainty.

I went home that evening and suggested the idea of writing a book about apraxia to my husband.

"Why not?" he countered.

"I don't know anything about it, that's why. Remember, it's *me* who needs the book?"

"Well, make it a little research project," he suggested. "You'll learn something in the process."

After a few more rounds of rebuttals and excuses (I didn't have time, not to mention that I'd never written a book before), he convinced me to do it.

> **The Nuts and Bolts of This Chapter**
>
> ➤ How to become an advocate for your child and why you are the best person.
> ➤ How you can network, advocate, and seek resources *all along* your child's journey with CAS; it doesn't have to come at the end of the journey.
> ➤ How to "navigate the field" to find your way out of the woods.
> ➤ Starting and establishing your own support group on apraxia.
> ➤ National and local organizations devoted to CAS; reputable online resources

And so, the networking, advocating, and resource-getting began. I'm not going to fool you—it wasn't easy. There were days I wanted to claw my eyeballs out and delete everything about CAS from my computer. But I didn't. You are reading the fruits of my labor. I did it for you and for your little ones with CAS. I did it for me. And most of all, I did it for Kate. And you know what? I am so glad I did.

You're the Best, Mom and Dad: What YOU Have to Offer

I know what a big job it is to raise kids. There's a lot to think about, take care of, organize, delegate, pay for, and understand. Not to mention the morals and values you hope to instill, the lessons you want to teach, and fun you so desire for your family. Why on earth would you want to add one more thing to your growing list of to-do's? Because you love your child. It's as simple as that. No one else can love and care for your child as much as you do. Not only do you *love* your child to the moon and back, but you also *know* your child inside and out. *You are the best, Mom and Dad.*

But you can't just hear that your child has apraxia on Tuesday and then go out and tell everyone you know about it on Wednesday. You need time. You need understanding. You may need to shed a few tears. You may need to talk to a few trusted friends about it. You may need to do a little reading on CAS first. You may need to see your child make some progress in speech therapy. Everyone has a different gauge as to what needs to happen before they are ready to move into the world of advocacy.

Think for a minute about what you might need before you reach out. Now jot it down.

What Are You Good At? Identifying Your Strengths and Weaknesses

Part of being a good advocate for your child is determining what you are good at doing. I bet you already have a good sense of your strengths and weaknesses. If not, just ask your spouse or significant other—I am sure you'll get an earful (especially if you ask about your weaknesses)!

Now, make a list of your strengths and weaknesses.

Need some prompts? Think of things you naturally love to do, are particularly skilled at, have a strong interest in, or would like to learn more about. You'll know what you're weak at if it's something you often have to ask for assistance to complete, have failed at before, or hear complaints about (from friends, your spouse, or coworkers).

Now, take a look at your list. Is there anything that stands out? Something you might be able to apply to the world of apraxia?

Why You Should Network, Advocate, and Look for Resources

Besides helping your child, you will be helping others along their journeys when you advocate, network, and seek out resources. You say you aren't the "helping kind?" You are concerned that you don't have the time or knowledge to put into all of this "work?" Well, here are a few more reasons to convince you:

➤ You will recognize your own expertise.
➤ You will become more informed as a consumer.
➤ You will be able to ask the "right" professionals well-phrased questions.
➤ You will be able to give praise and credit to those in the field who deserve it.
➤ You will feel empowered.
➤ You will develop your own personal support team.
➤ You will be able to document your child's progress better.
➤ You will communicate more effectively with your child's SLP.
➤ You will control your emotions and feelings better when you under-stand more.
➤ *You can teach your child to become his or her own advocate!*

Networking, Advocating, and Seeking Resources Along the Journey

Let's take a look at the grief cycle one last time. It may seem a stretch, but you actually need to work through these stages of grief in order to be an effective advocate for your child. Read on to see how this cycle can affect you as a parent and as an advocate.

Denial: You'll know you're here when you resist taking your child to the speech clinic or the pediatrician because you don't want to hear what you fear they'll say. You know you are here when you insist on a second opinion because "they don't know what they're talking about, anyway."

Anger: You'll know you're here when you hate the sound of your neighbor's chatty two-year-old talking a mile-a-minute when your four-year-old is still grunting. You'll know you're here when your friend brings you this book and you feel like throwing it at her after shouting a few obscenities her way.

Bargaining: You'll know you're here when you say to your husband, "I suppose if you hadn't been late-to-talk, Gavin wouldn't have this problem either." You'll know you're here when you say a little prayer, "Please—I'll give up coffee/shopping/Facebook if you just make my baby talk."

Depression: You'll know you're here when you can barely get out of bed because facing yet another day with your nonverbal kiddo makes you want to be ill. You'll know you're here when you cry more than you smile or eat more (or less) than you should or scream and fuss most of the time.

Acceptance: You'll know you're here when you are ready to make a difference in the apraxia world. You'll know you're here when you can smile and say, "My daughter has apraxia, too."

Parents Share...

Moving from Denial and Bargaining to Acceptance

Vicki, whose son Evan is recovering from CAS, says this:

"I have had to let go of a lot of things in this journey—letting go of the early dreams, of the expectations, of the benchmarks I thought for sure we would make if only we worked hard enough. Letting go has allowed me to be quite okay with where my son is at and who he is. I am much freer to accept him and love him all the more for being so special. I try not to let myself be my own worst enemy wishing we had done more....We did a lot and he came a long ways from the frustrated little three-year-old who was so angry that he could not even get anyone to know he wanted a drink of water to a young man of twenty-one who shows great compassion for any small child or animal that seems to live out in the margin where he has so often found himself to be."

In looking over this list, it may appear as though the only time to be an advocate is when you are at the acceptance stage. Well, yes and no. Perhaps the acceptance stage is the best time to be a really effective and positive advocate. That doesn't mean that you can't do little things along the entire journey. Even when you are lounging in bed and crying yourself to sleep, you can be networking. Even when you are complaining to your spouse or partner that it was his or her "bad" gene that gave your son apraxia, you can be looking for resources. Let's break it down with some hard-core suggestions.

Join a Support Group for Childhood Apraxia of Speech

I'm talking about a real-live support group that offers face-to-face communication and support for you and other parents and caregivers of children with apraxia. There may be one in your area. It's a great opportunity to get together with like-minded parents seeking support, education, and socialization. The benefit here is that you can form deep and meaningful relationships with parents who know *just where you are*—emotionally and psychologically.

Some of the parents may have been in your shoes a few years ago and can help you make sense of your child's newly diagnosed state; they can give you good "been-there-done-that" advice. Other members may be new to the game. You will be able to "repay" them with your expertise and advice. You may even find a lifelong friend in the group

If anything, membership in a group like this is validation that **you are not in this alone.**

How to Find a Group?

For starters, you can go right to your child's speech clinic and ask them. They may have a name or contact information for a parent from their practice. If they don't and you still want the connection, you may consider starting your own group (see "Wanna Get Something Started?" in this chapter). Head to the Apraxia-KIDS website (www.apraxia-kids.org). From there, go to "Learn about Apraxia," then "Library," then "Resources & Support." At last check, this site was set up to show support groups by state. Click on your state to see if there is a group in your area. The caveat here is that group facilitators need to "register" their group with Apraxia-Kids, so not every available group in your area will appear here. You may have to get creative (keep reading). Apraxia-KIDS and CASANA will be discussed later in this chapter, too.

By the way, a support group specifically on CAS may be a rare find. If you can't find something just for apraxia in your area, consider joining a general support group for speech-language disorders.

What If Groups Aren't Your Thing?

If a support group isn't your style, or you're just not into starting one of your own (it's a big task and not to be taken lightly), you can still make a difference and find a little understanding for yourself.

Blog On: Nowadays you don't have to be a Pulitzer prize-winning writer to get your thoughts out there. Try blogging. Anyone can do it. It's easy. Check out various free sites for starting your own blog such as www.wordpress.com or www.blogspot.

com (just to mention a couple) and start blogging. You can control how you want the site set up (usually), how often you write, what you write about, and how it's distributed. Sure, it's a bit overwhelming at first, but you never know when someone might stumble upon your blog and find comfort and wisdom in your words.

Start a Website: The next step up from blogging is to start a website on apraxia. Kate Welder, mother of Josie, did just that. At the time of her daughter's diagnosis in 2004, she was eager to connect with other parents also struggling with CAS. But she lived in a remote area of North Dakota. After several years, she launched her website, *Apraxia Speaks: Hope and Help for Parents of Children with Verbal Apraxia of Speech.* You can access her site at www.apraxiaspeaks.com. In 2010, Ms. Welder released an ebook, *Apraxia Explained: A Parent's Guide to Unlocking Their Child's Voice.* Her book can be purchased through her website. You'll also find stories of success and information, from toilet training to speech therapy, among others. Want to start your own website? Take a look at Site Build It—a build-you-own web business—at www.sitebuildit.com.

Another special-needs mom, Dawn Villarreal of Naperville, Illinois, started an online special needs resource website, *One Place for Special Needs* (www.oneplace-forspecialneeds.com), after it *dawned* (yes, pun intended) on her that her individual experiences with autism were likely universal. Her site is comprehensive—not all about autism and not just about resources in Illinois, either. One Place for Special Needs covers many special needs, including Childhood Apraxia of Speech.

Join Online Discussion Boards and Groups: There are a couple of "big name" groups dedicated specifically to apraxia. They are discussed in greater detail in the next section. For now, I will mention their names briefly and how to get connected to their online groups.

➤ **Apraxia-KIDS** has an online discussion board (a.k.a. listserv) where you can participate in online conversations on CAS. This message board consists of a large network of parents and professionals (many SLPs, among others) who post daily on issues concerning apraxia. You can post questions, thoughts, comments, success stories, or requests for resources or simply support. This site is moderated and professional. You can opt to receive email notices each time a post is made to the listserv, or you can receive the "digest" version. When you first learn of your child's diagnosis of apraxia, you may feel more comfortable being a "lurker" on the site. Posting questions or responding to them may be too intimidating at first. Once you get a grasp on your understanding of the way it works, your feelings, and knowledge of apraxia, you'll feel more at ease with the process. Information about the Apraxia-KIDS listserv can be found by visiting www.apraxia-kids.org and clicking on the "eCommunity" button on the left-hand side of the page. From there, choose "join apraxia-kids email group list." There you will see links for learning more about the listserv, its purpose, rules of conduct, and how to subscribe to the listserv. Otherwise, you can do so directly by following these steps:

1. Send an email message to: listserv@listserv.syr.edu.
2. Leave the subject line blank.
3. In the message area write: Subscribe Apraxia-kids (your first name) (your last name).
4. Example: subscribe apraxia-kids Jane Doe.

My First Encounter with Apraxia-KIDS

Apraxia-KIDS was the *very first* resource I was told to seek out. With that in mind, I found it somewhat overwhelming. My first experience on the listserv brought posts from parents asking about alternative communication devices (ACC), reading difficulties, and IEPs. Yikes! In all honesty, my first glance left me scared and intimidated. While that is certainly *not* the intention of the Apraxia-KIDS listserv, I walked away from that first session thinking my daughter would never read or speak normally, and that she would have an IEP all through school. I didn't know any differently at that time as a newbie "apraxia mom."

I tell you this not to discourage you from checking out and joining the listserv, but to prepare you for a first impression. As time went on, I found that the Apraxia-Kids listserv gave me lots to think about and consider and that I didn't need to do everything the day I read about it. Instead, I would jot down suggested websites or books and file them away in Kate's binder for when I might need them in the future.

➤ **CHERAB** is an organization on communication delays and disorders with neurological underpinnings. It has a Yahoo groups communication tool for parents and professionals to join. Just go to their website at www.cherab.org and click on "join group." You will be directed to a registration page. Afterwards, you can begin receiving and sending discussion points on questions, concerns, resources, and success stories on your journey with CAS. More on CHERAB in the next section, "Wanna Get Something Started?"

➤ **Chicagoland Apraxia Network** counts over 400 families in the Chicagoland area as members. Headed up by "apraxia mom" Holly Olmsted-Hickey, this network has been providing information and education to parents and caregivers of children with apraxia for over twelve years. Through their online message board and face-to-face meetings in the Chicago area, the group provides great information and camaraderie on therapy approaches, IEPs, specialists, and raising a child with apraxia.

Interested in joining the e-group? Look for it at
http://groups.yahoo.com/group/windycityapraxia.

➤ **SPEAK**, St. Louis Parent Extension for Apraxic Kids, is a support service
for language disorders in children focused in the St. Louis metro area.
They have an online discussion group you can join by going to
http://health.groups.yahoo.com/group/speakgroup.

➤ **Speechville Express** has a message board you can join at www.speech-
ville.com. Speechville Express is more than just a message board, though.
You'll find information and resources on aphasia, articulation disorders,
phonological disorders, dysarthria, SLI (specific language impairments),
and stuttering, to name a few. They also have tips on starting your own
support group, as well as making connections for existing groups.

➤ **Apraxia-KIDS Canada** is an up-and-coming group in a similar vein as
Apraxia-KIDS/CASANA. This is a virtual group of parents who have
children with CAS. It's a place to ask questions, contribute to discussions, and get information on childhood apraxia. You'll also find Cana-
dian-specific supports and resources. To join the group, you may send
an email to apraxia.kids.canada@groups.facebook.com.

➤ **The Ontario Association for Families of Children with Communication Disorders (OAFCCD)**, www.oafccd.com. While this organization
has been around since 1992, it is currently taking a more active role
in developing outreach for families affected by CAS. The chapter of
OAFCCD dedicated to childhood apraxia of speech is "SPEAKING OUT-
Apraxia," which provides participants the opportunity for networking
and offers presentations to enhance their lives. Interested participants
can connect at speakingout.apraxia@yahoo.ca.

➤ **Ottawa Parents of Children with Apraxia (OPCA):** A parent support
group organized to support families dealing with childhood apraxia of
speech (CAS). Parent meetings are held every other month and family activity days held on a regular basis. For more information, send an
email to Ottawa.apraxia@gmail.com or join the Facebook group at "Ottawa Parents of Children with Apraxia."

There are many other groups and organizations that provide similar services.
This list is not meant to be all-inclusive. Start asking locally, and you just may be surprised what you'll find in your region.

How They Got Connected with Other "Apraxia Parents"

Here's how it worked for one participant in Small Talk: All About Apraxia:
"I was just hanging out around my son's school when I casually mentioned that my son had a speech disorder. A woman overhead me and said hers did, too. We got to talking and learned that both of our sons had apraxia. I went home and 'friended' her on Facebook."

It worked this way for me: I was at the library when I bumped into a mom I had seen there before. We got to chatting about preschools and I mentioned that Kate was attending the public school district's preschool. She cocked an eyebrow. I said, "She has a speech disorder," not wanting to get into the specifics of CAS. The other mother perked up: "Oh, really? We have apraxia." Needless to say, we've been friends ever since.

It's amazing how small the world really becomes when you start chatting and learning about others. So, look for excuses to strike up a conversation.

Wanna Get Something Started?

No Support Group? No Problem. Start something of your own! Of course, every group starts small and grows bigger. It's up to you to determine where and how it happens. You may not even *want* a large group. But you *do* want something that matters to you and others who have a stake in CAS.

➤ *Start small.* Gather a few "apraxia" parents and meet at a coffee shop. Sip a cup of Joe while you chat about apraxia (I know, sounds kind of ironic). You may already know these parents from your child's speech clinic. Perhaps you've sat in the waiting room together or have bumped into one another as you were coming or going. Or post a note on a community bulletin board, "WANTED: Individuals or families affected by Childhood Apraxia of Speech to participate in small discussion/support group." Try posting something like that at your child's speech clinic or asking your SLP to help you connect with other like-minded parents.

➤ *Grow a little bigger.* Once you have a few folks to meet with on a regular basis, consider expanding your circle. You can reach out to schools, speech clinics, physicians' offices, libraries, places of worship, online message boards, and local nonprofit organizations. You'll want to market your group well. Send letters, make phone calls, connect online, and show up in person.

➤ *Set some guidelines.* You'll likely want to have a set of bylaws or rules for your group. Determine how many participants you'd like, where you'll meet, how often you'll meet, how long the meetings will be, what the topics will be, if there will be a facilitator/leader (and how that person is chosen, what their duties are), and who will help organize and maintain the group. Confidentiality is important. Since everyone will likely be sharing private and potentially emotional information about a minor child, you'll want to keep your discussions just between the group participants.

➤ *Keep it warm, welcoming, and helpful.* Groups need to be supportive, while being educational and social. Make it an event folks *want* to attend. Have fun, provide snacks and encouragement. Let others know this group is about helping others cope with their apraxia journey.

➤ *Know when it's time to let go.* Whether you're a participant or core leader, you'll want to gauge when it's the best time for you to move on. Leaders and facilitators get burned out just like the rest of us. It may be time to give control to another member. The worst thing you can do for yourself and your group is to continue when you are burned out.

➤ *Start a local nonprofit organization.* This is a huge task and certainly not for everyone. But you could do it if you really wanted to. Here's what Rebecca Christiansen, Executive Director of Celebrate Differences: Celebrating the Abilities of Those with Disabilities in Oswego, IL, did. Ms. Christiansen, a nurse, was shocked to find that healthcare providers do not present a child with special needs in a positive light. While her son has Down syndrome, not apraxia, she saw quickly that a child with special needs is more the same than "different." Celebrate Differences aims to help local parents with education workshops, finding information on local resources, and provide a library of resource materials. You can access their website at www.celebratedifferences.com.

My Road to Advocacy

As described above, I felt compelled to write this book because there wasn't anything specific enough out there for me. I joined a listserv or two. I started blogging about CAS and parenting on Wordpress, www.leslie4kids.wordpress.com, *Practical Parenting with a Twist.* I started a *Small Talk: All About Apraxia* education group series, originally facilitated through the speech clinic where Kate received speech therapy. The owner of the clinic agreed that it would be a worthwhile endeavor. My goal was to connect other parents and caregivers together once a week for five weeks. Each meeting had a specific topic and guided discussion. In the end, I hoped these parents would continue to call upon one another for resources, support, and maybe even play dates! Much of what is in this book was presented in a condensed—fast-paced—version during those in-person sessions.

Parents Share...

What Do Folks Want from a Support Group?

Here's what some of the participants in my Small Talk: All About Apraxia series had to say:

➤ "I found that I loved the session on resources and networking. Not only was there so much out there that I didn't know about, it was presented in such a fun, you-can-do-it manner that really made me feel empowered."

➤ "I was really looking for support and to share my experiences with apraxia. Talking with other women—moms of kids with apraxia—was so helpful."

➤ "The group really met my expectations. I received so much information and knowledge that I otherwise would not have received."

➤ "Being with other parents struggling with apraxia was a wonderful learning experience. We can all learn from others."

➤ "Support and friendship was big to me. I really felt isolated in this whole apraxia thing. I didn't know anyone else with apraxia until this group."

The Big Names in Apraxia Support

There are a few large apraxia organizations out there. We have alluded to them earlier in this chapter because there are elements of these big organizations that you may like to have a little affiliation with—like their message board, for example. The big names you will hear along your apraxia journey are Apraxia-KIDS/CASANA and The CHERAB Organization. These groups both seek to educate, inform, and assist families, professionals, and kids who are struggling with CAS. Over time, you may develop a distinct preference for one over the other. Much of your feelings on these two groups will be influenced by your understanding of what CAS is, what your stance is on the theories that caused it, how it can be best remediated, and your overall aims of how you'd like to help your child.

There is no "right" or "wrong" organization for families of children with CAS. It's subjective and individual. Whatever you lean towards is right for you and your child.

CHERAB Organization: Started by "apraxia mom" Lisa Geng in conjunction with her husband, Glenn, and educational consultant Cheryl Bennett Johnson, CHERAB (which stands for Communication Help, Education, Research, Apraxia Base) strives to increase awareness of communication delays and disorders. CHERAB is a worldwide nonprofit organization seeking to bring education and understanding to neurologically-based speech concerns. The organization ties parents, along with medical, research, media, and educational professionals, to one endeavor in an effort to develop more effective treatment strategies and prevention of neurologically-based speech disorders. To join them in their efforts and gain valuable information on helping your own little angel, you can visit the CHERAB organization at www.cherab.org or join the listserv at www.cherabfoundation.org/about.

Apraxia-KIDS: Sharon Gretz, Executive Director of CASANA, started Apraxia-KIDS in 1997, back when the Internet and email were just becoming available to most folks. Ms. Gretz was frustrated with the lack of educational information for parents who had children diagnosed with apraxia. She started the first parent support group in Pittsburgh, PA, and started networking with local apraxia experts. Today, Apraxia-KIDS falls under the umbrella of CASANA (Childhood Apraxia of Speech Association of North America)—a larger organization that was "born" thanks to the contributions of the Hendrix family and other parent activists. It became a nonprofit 501 (c) (3) public charity in 2000. CASANA/Apraxia-KIDS has much to offer, including:

➤ Parent and professional message boards (often known as a listserv);
➤ Social media site on Facebook and Twitter;
➤ Online newsletter and helpdesk;
➤ Parent and professional workshops and conferences;
➤ An apraxia treatment research fund for collecting monies to help pinpoint the best treatment methods for kids with apraxia;
➤ Information on how to "Walk for Apraxia."

A Word of Caution

Everyone copes and learns differently. Don't feel like you have to knock yourself out and write books and blogs, and start a nonprofit after reading this chapter. You'll want to cherry-pick your favorite activities based on your skills, interest, time, and financial resources. But I encourage you to do something—big or small—it all makes a difference.

Final Bits of Wisdom

Have you ever heard or sung this early childhood jingle: "Smooth road, smooth road…bumpy road, bumpy road, rough road, rough road, whoops! Pothole!" When you play this game with a toddler, you seat him on your outstretched legs near your knees, usually facing you. You hold his hands and move your legs side to side during the "smooth road" part. When the road gets "bumpy," you wiggle your knees to give your child a little bounce, a little *more* for a "rough" patch, and then the grand finale is when you "pop" your child up in the air with extended arms for the "pothole" effect. Kids die with laughter and you see the twinkle in their eye as they ask for more.

Where am I going with this? Yep. It's an analogy for your journey with apraxia. There will be smooth sailing times. There will be bumps along the road. And it will be rough at times, too. On really, really bad days, you will hit a pothole (or two).

But then, your child will look at you with bright, engaging eyes, he'll whisper or sign "I love you," and it will renew your efforts to give him what he needs. Again. You'll do it because you love your child.

Say That Again?! Chapter Summary

This chapter is all about how you—mom, dad, or anyone else raising or caring for a child with CAS—can help. It is about empowering yourself and your child to be the best you can be and finding—or creating—the resources that matter to you. We covered in-person and online support groups, websites, blogs, and nonprofit organizations, but most of all, we talked about you. *You* are the best person to help *your* child. *Your little person depends on you for his or her success.*

Read On! Recommended Resources

➤ *The Parent You Want to Be: Who You Are Matters More Than What You Do* by Drs. Les and Leslie Parrott (Zondervan, 2007) is a very readable book that explains how to cultivate the traits you most desire for your children.

➤ *Know Your Parenting Personality: How to Use the Enneagram to Become the Best Parent You Can Be* by Janet Levine (Wiley, 2003) is another book that may help you determine your strengths and weaknesses as you look at ways you can help advocate for your child.

➤ *MotherStyles: Using Personality Type to Discover Your Parenting Strengths* by Janet Penley and Diane Eble (Da Capo Press, 2006) may be of interest to mothers who want to identify their strengths when navigating the road of advocacy.

➤ *Special Needs Advocacy Resource Book* by Rich Weinfield and Michelle Davis (Prufock Press, 2008) covers how to work with schools to achieve optimal learning situations and accommodations for their child, from IEPs to 504 Plans.

➤ Your local community may hold a *special education community services fair* offering speakers, services, and exhibitors. Ask at your school district or speech clinic for more information.

➤ Browse through the *archives of the Apraxia-Kids listserv/messageboard* by going to www.apraxia-kids.org, clicking on "eCommunity," and following the link for "join apraxia-kids email group list." Once there, you will see a menu of services. Click on "participate in messageboard," which will direct you to all of the messages ever posted on a particular topic, in alphabetical order.

➤ For more information about the **CHERAB** organization, contact them at P.O. Box 8524, Port St. Lucie, FL 34952-8524. Phone: 772-335-5135.

➤ *"How You Can Help Your Child Learn to Be a Good Self Advocate"* is available on the website of the Pacer Center at: www.pacer.org/parent/php/PHP-c95.pdf. Also check out the Pacer Center's long list of free handouts on a variety of advocacy and special education topics: www.pacer.org/publications/specedrights.asp.

➤ You and your older child may want to check out *Kids as Self-Advocates* for articles, resources, and a forum where kids and young adults with a variety of special-needs meet in cyberspace to discuss their concerns: www.fvkasa.org.

References

Chapter 1

Goddard, Sally. *Reflexes, Learning, and Behavior: A Window into the Child's Mind, a Non-Invasive Approach to Solving Learning and Behavior Problems.* Eugene, Oregon: Fern Ridge Press, 2002.

Hall, Penny, Jordan, Linda, and Robin, Donald. *Developmental Apraxia of Speech: Theory and Clinical Practice.* 2nd ed. Austin, TX: Pro-Ed, 2007.

Hamaguchi, Patricia. *Childhood Speech, Language, and Listening Problems: What Every Parent Should Know.* 2nd ed. New York, NY: John Wiley and Sons, 2001.

Koballa, Joyce. "Conference Held to Discuss Speech Disorder." *Herald Standard*, August 26, 2010.

Lewis, B.A., Freebairin, L.A., Hansen, A.J., Iyengar, S.K., and Taylor, H.G. (2004). "School-age Follow-up of Children with Childhood Apraxia of Speech." *Language, Speech, and Hearing Services in Schools 35*:122-40.

McCauley, Rebecca. "Childhood Apraxia of Speech: An Overview & Assessment Considerations." Retrieved from www.speechpathology.com on July 27, 2011.

Vossbeck, Kelli and Meredith, Amy. "Diagnostic Criteria for CAS: A Survey Study." 2008 Convention Handout. Retrieved from www.asha.org on July 17, 2011.

Weitzman, Elaine. "A Closer Look at the Late Talker Study: Why Parents Should Beware of a 'Wait and See' Approach." Retrieved from www.hanen.org on July 17, 2011.

Chapter 2

Caruso, Anthony, and Strand, Edythe. *Clinical Management of Motor Speech Disorders in Children.* New York, NY: Thieme, 1999.

Doughtery, Dorothy. *Teach Me How to Say it Right: Helping Your Child with Articulation Disorders.* Oakland, CA: New Harbinger, 2005.

Eliot, Lise. *What's Going on in There? How the Brain and Mind Develop in the First Five Years of Life.* Minneapolis: Bantam, 1999.

Feit, Debbie. *A Parent's Guide to Speech and Language Problems.* New York, NY: McGraw-Hill, 2007.

Hamaguchi, Patricia McAleer. *Childhood Speech, Language & Listening Problems: What Every Parent Should Know.* 3rd ed. Hoboken, NJ: Wiley, 2010.

Owens, Robert E., Jr. *Language Development: An Introduction.* 8th ed. Upper Saddle River, NJ: Allyn & Bacon, 2011.

Pulvermuller, F., and Fadiga, L. "Active Perception: Sensorimotor Circuits as a Cortical Basis for Language." *Nature Reviews in Neuroscience 11* (May 2010).

Rousey, Carol G. *A Practical Guide to Helping Children with Speech and Language Problems: For Parents and Teachers Only.* Springfield, IL: Charles G. Thomas, 1984.

Schetz, Katherine, and Cassell, Stuart Kent. *Talking Together: A Parent's Guide to the Development, Enrichment and Problems of Speech and Language.* Blacksburg, VA: Pocahontas Press, 1994.

Chapter 3

Childhood Apraxia of Speech Association of North America (CASANA). 416 Lincoln Ave., Pittsburgh, PA 15209. www.Apraxia-Kids.org.

Feit, Debbie. *A Parent's Guide to Speech and Language Problems.* New York, NY: McGraw-Hill, 2007.

Hamaguchi, Patricia McAleer. *Childhood Speech, Language & Listening Problems: What Every Parent Should Know.* 3rd ed. Hoboken, NJ: Wiley, 2010.

Chapter 4

Feit, Debbie. *A Parent's Guide to Speech and Language Problems.* New York, NY: McGraw-Hill, 2007.

Kumin, Libby. "You Said It Just Yesterday, Why Not Now? Developmental Apraxia of Speech in Children and Adults with Down Syndrome." *Disability Solutions 2,* no. 2 (Nov./Dec.2002).

McCauley, Rebecca J. *Assessment of Language Disorders in Children.* Hillsdale, NJ: Lawrence Erlbaum Associates, 2001.

McCauley, Rebecca J. *Assessment of Speech-language Disorders in Children.* London: Psychology Press, 2000.

Chapter 5

Boh, Andrea, Csiacsek, Emily, Duginske, Rachel, Meath, Theresa (student researchers), and Carpenter, Linda, Ph.D. (faculty collaborator and mentor). "Counseling Parents of Children with CAS." Poster Presentation at ASHA Conference. 2008.

Craniofacial Society of Great Britain and Ireland webpage. Information on Muriel Morley ("Honorary and Life Members"). Retrieved from www.craniofacialsociety.org.uk/info/honmems.html on March 25, 2011.

Duffy, J. *Motor Speech Disorders.* St. Louis: Mosby, 1995.

Hall, Penelope K., Jordan, Linda, and Robin, Donald. *Developmental Apraxia of Speech: Theory and Clinical Practice.* 2nd Edition. Austin, TX: Pro-Ed Publishers, 2007.

Hickman, Lori. "Prognosis for Apraxia: What Does the Future Hold?" Article available on the Apraxia-KIDS website: www.apraxia-kids.org. (Type Lori Hickman in the search box.)

Morley, Muriel. *The Development and Disorders of Speech in Childhood.* London: E & S Livingstone, Ltd., 1957.

Strand, E.A. "Assessment and Treatment of Childhood Apraxia of Speech." Presentation at CASANA conference. February 19-20, 2010.

Strand, E.A., and McCauley, R.J. "Differential Diagnosis of Severe Speech Impairment in Young Children." *The ASHA Leader 13,* no. 10 (Aug. 12, 2008): 10-13.

Strohm, Kate. *Being the Other One: Growing Up with a Brother or Sister Who Has Special Needs.* Boston: Shambhala, 2005.

Velleman, Shelley. *Childhood Apraxia of Speech Resource Guide.* Albany, NY: Delmar Publishing, 2003.

Chapter 6

"About Potocki-Lupski Syndrome." Baylor College of Medicine Dept. of Molecular and Human Genetics. Retrieved from www.bcm.edu/genetics/potocki_lupskindex.cfm? PMID =10628 on July 30, 2011.

American Speech-Language-Hearing Association. "Childhood Apraxia of Speech" [Technical Report]. (2007). Retrieved from www.asha.org/policy on September 24, 2011.

American Journal of Medical Genetics 146A, no. 17 (July 31, 2008): 2227-33. http://onlinelibrary.wiley.com/journal/10.1002/(ISSN)1552-4833/homepage/ProductInformation.html

Bridgeman, Elizabeth, and Snowling, Maggie. "The Perception of Phoneme Sequence: A Comparison of Dyspraxic and Normal Children." *British Journal of Disorders of Communication 23* (1988): 245-52.

Fish, Margaret. *Here's How to Treat Childhood Apraxia of Speech.* San Diego, CA: Plural Publishing, 2010.

Guenther, Frank H. "Cortical Interactions Underlying the Production of Speech Sounds." *Journal of Communication Disorders 39* (2006): 350-65.

Hurst, J.A., Baraitser, M., Auger, E., Graham, F, and Norell S. "An Extended Family with a Dominantly Inherited Speech Disorder." *Developmental Medical Child Neurology 32,* no.4 (April 1990): 352-5.

Jakielski, K., Marquardt, T., and Davis, B. "Developmental Apraxia of Speech: Information for Parents." Retrieved www.apraxia-KIDS.org on September 24, 2011.

Kumin, Libby. *Early Communication Skills for Children with Down Syndrome: A Guide for Parents and Professionals.* 2nd ed. Bethesda, MD: Woodbine House, 2003.

Kumin, Libby. "You Said it Just Yesterday, Why Not Now: Developmental Apraxia of Speech in Children and Adults with Down Syndrome." *Disability Solutions 2,* no. 2 (Nov./Dec. 2002).

Lewis, Barbara, Freebarin, Lisa A., Hansen, Amy, Taylor, Gerry, Ivengar, Sudha, and Shriberg, Lawrence. "Family Pedigrees of Children with Suspected Childhood Apraxia of Speech." *Journal of Communication Disorders 37,* no. 2 (March/April 2004): 157-75.

Maassen, Ben. "Issues Contrasting Adult Acquired versus Developmental Apraxia of Speech." *Seminars in Speech and Language 23* (2002): 257–66.

Nelson, C. Donald, Waggoner, D., Tuerck, J., Donnell, G., and Buist, N. (1991). "Verbal Dyspraxia in Treated Galactosemia." *Pediatrics, 88,* no. 2: 346-50.

Rosenbek J., and Wertz R. A Review of Fifty Cases of Developmental Apraxia of Speech. *Language, Speech, and Hearing Services in Schools 5* (1972): 207-24.

Shriberg, Lawrence, Ph.D., CCC-SLP. "What Do Researchers Know about Genetics and CAS?" Retrieved from www.apraxia-kids.org "library" on August 7, 2011.

Strand, E.A. *Childhood Apraxia of Speech: Description, Definitions, and Underlying Neurologic Factors.* Paper presented at the Childhood Apraxia of Speech Association of North America (CASANA) National Conference on Childhood Apraxia of Speech, July 2009.

Chapter 7

Bahr, Diane. *Nobody Ever Told Me (or My Mother) That!: Everything from Bottles to Breastfeeding to Healthy Speech Development.* Arlington, TX: Sensory World, 2010.

Cole, Kevin, Maddox, Mary, Notari-Syverson, A., and Lim, Y.S. *Language is the Key: Video Programs for Building Language and Literacy in Early Childhood.* Seattle, WA: Washington Learning Systems, 2006.

Drake, Martha. *Just for Kids: Apraxia.* East Moline, IL: LinguiSystems, 1999.

George, Karen. "Treatment of Childhood Apraxia of Speech by Chicago Therapy." www.chicagospeechtherapy.com/treatment-of-childhood-apraxia-of-speech-by-chicago-speech-therapy. Retrieved April 27, 2011.

Hall, Penelope K., Jordan, Linda, and Robin, Donald. *Developmental Apraxia of Speech: Theory and Clinical Practice.* 2nd ed. Austin, TX: Pro-Ed Publishers, 2007.

Hammer, David. *Treatment Strategies for Childhood Apraxia of Speech with David Hammer.* Pittsburgh, PA: Children's Hospital of Pittsburgh, 2006.

Helfrich-Miller, Ph.D., Kathleen. Information on Melodic Intonation Therapy (MIT) acquired from email correspondence on Sept. 13, 2011.

Kent, Ray D. "Theory in the Balance." *Perspectives on Speech Science and Orofacial Disorders 18* (July 2008): 15-21.

Marshalla, Pam. *Becoming Verbal with Childhood Apraxia: New Insights on Piaget for Today's Therapy*. Kirkland, WA: Marshalla Speech and Language, 2007.

McCaffrey, P. "The Neuroscience on the Web Series: Dysarthria vs. Apraxia: A Comparison." (2001). www.csuchico.edu/~pmcca/syllabi/SPPA342/342unit.15.html.

McCauley, Rebecca J. and Fey, Marc E. *Treatment of Language Disorders in Children*. Baltimore, MD: Paul H. Brookes Publishing, 2006.

Strand, Edythe and Caruso, Anthony. *Clinical Management of Motor Speech Disorders in Children*. New York, NY: Thieme, 1999.

Strode, Robin and Chamberlin, Catherine. *Easy Does It for Apraxia-Preschool*. East Moline, IL: LinguiSystems, 1994

Velleman, Shelley. *Childhood Apraxia of Speech Resource Guide*. Clifton Park, NY: Delmar Publishing, 2003.

Chapter 8

American Speech-Language-Hearing Association, Working Group in AIT. "Auditory Integration Training." www.asha.org/docs/html/TR2004-00260.html.

Cuthbert, S.C. and Barras, M. "Developmental Delay Syndromes: Psychometric Testing Before and After Chiropractic Treatment of 157 Children. *Journal of Manipulative Physiological Therapy 32*, no. 8 (2009): 660-9.

Feit, Debbie. *Parent's Guide to Understanding Speech and Language Disorders*. New York, NY: McGraw-Hill, 2007.

Fish, Dee. *Here's How to Treat Childhood Apraxia of Speech*. San Diego: Plural Publishing, 2010.

Goddard, Sally. *Reflexes, Learning, and Behavior: A Window into the Child's Mind: A Non-Invasive Approach to Solving Learning and Behavior Problems*. Eugene, OR: Fern Ridge Press, 2002.

Kaplan, Melvin. *Seeing Through New Eyes: Changing the Lives of Children with Autism, Asperger's Syndrome and Other Developmental Disabilities through Vision Therapy*. Philadelphia: Jessica Kingsley Publishers, 2008.

Kranowitz, Carol Stock and Miller, Lucy Jane. *The Out of Sync Child*. Rev. ed. New York, NY: Perigee Trade, 2006.

Morris, M.D., Claudia, of Oakland Children's Hospital. Interview and quote from email reprinted with permission granted on April 23, 2011.

Morris, Claudia R. and Agin, Marilyn C. "Syndrome of Allergy, Apraxia, and Malabsorption: Characterization of a Neurodevelopmental Phenotype that Responds to Omega 3 and Vitamin E Supplementation." *Alternative Therapies,* Volume 15, no. 4 (July/August 2009).

Rutek, Donna. "Animal-friendly Therapy: Contact with Horses Has Profound Effect on Kids with Disabilities." *Chicago Tribune,* June 2, 1999.

Sena Moore, Kimberly. "Music, Rhythm, and Their Potential Benefits for Childhood Apraxia of Speech." Published online at PediaStaff, May 28, 2010. www.pediastaff.com/blog/music-rhythm-and-their-potential-benefits-for-childhood-apraxia-of-speech-647.

"What Is Music Therapy?" Retrieved from www.neurosong.com on April 27, 2011.

Chapter 9

Bahr, Diane. *Oral Motor Assessment and Treatment: Ages and Stages.* Upper Saddle River, NJ: Allyn and Bacon, 2001.

DeThorne, Laura S. et al. "When 'Simon Says' Doesn't Work: Alternatives to Imitation for Facilitating Early Speech Development." *American Journal of Speech-Language Pathology 18,* no. 2 (May 1, 2009): 133-45

Doughtery, Dorothey, P. *Teach Me How to Say it Right: Helping Your Child with Articulation Disorders.* Oakland, CA: New Harbinger Publications, 2005.

Fish, Margaret. *Here's How to Treat Childhood Apraxia of Speech.* San Diego, CA: Plural Publishing, 2010.

Osby, Jasmine. "Company Helps Students Learn by Playing Games." *St. Louis Post-Dispatch,* August 20, 2010.

Schetz, Katherine and Cassell, Stuart Kent. *Talking Together: A Parent's Guide to the Development, Enrichment and Problems of Speech and Language.* Blacksburg, VA: Pocahontas Press, 1994.

Schwartz, Sue. *The New Language of Toys: Teaching Communication Skills to Children with Special Needs, a Guide for Parents.* 3rd ed. Bethesda, MD: Woodbine House, 2004.

Chapter 10

Caspari, Susan S., Strand, Edythe A., Kotagal, Suresh, and Bergqvist, Christina. "Obstructive Sleep Apnea, Seizures, and Childhood Apraxia of Speech." Pediatric Neurology: *Science Direct.* Vol. 38, Issue 6, pp. 422-425.

Doheny, Kathleen. "Can't Sleep? Adjust the Temperature." *WedMD.* www.webmd.com/a-to-z-guides/features/cant-sleep-adjust-the-temperature. Retrieved on July 25, 2011.

Haiken, Melanie. "5 Foods to Help You Sleep." *Yahoo Health.* http://health.yahoo.net/caring/5-foods-that-help-you-sleep. Retrieved on Feb. 3, 2011.

Hiss, Tony. *The Experience of Place: A New Way of Looking At and Dealing With Our Radically Changing Cities and Countryside.* New York, NY: Vintage, 1991.

Mindell, Jodi, Ph.D. Quote from personal correspondence used with permission.

Mosheim, Jason. "Apraxia and Obstructive Sleep Apnea: Is There a Link?" *Advance for Speech-Language Pathologists and Audiologists.* Vol. 18, Issue 10, p 6. Retrieved from http://speech-language-pathology-audiology.advanceweb.com/Editorial/Content.

Chapter 11
Anderson, Winifred, Chitwood, Stephen, Hayden, Deirdre, and Takemoto, Cheri. *Negotiating the Special Education Maze: A Guide for Parents and Teachers.* 4th ed. Bethesda, MD: Woodbine House, 2008.

Dwight, Valle. "Getting Off to the Right Start: Ten Tips to Make Sure Your Child's IEP Is Ready to Go on Day One." Great Schools website: www.greatschools.org/special-education/legal-rights/IEP-day-pne.gs?content=2866. Retrieved September 11, 2010.

Encyclopedia on Early Childhood Development. www.child-encyclopedia.com/en-ca/home.html.

Wrightslaw. "Do You Know Who Is Providing Your Child's Speech Language Therapy?" Wright's Law Blog. www.wrightslaw.com/blog/?p=129. Jan. 29, 2009.

Chapter 12
Al Otaiba, S., Puranik, C., Ziolkowski, R., and Montgomery, T. (2009). "Effectiveness of Early Phonological Awareness Interventions for Students with Speech or Language Impairments." *Journal of Special Education 43*: 107-28

Bourdreau, D.M. and Hedberg, N.L. "A Comparison of Early Literacy Skills in Children with Specific Speech Language Impairment and Their Typically Developing Peers." *American Journal of Speech-Language Pathology 8* (1999): 249-60.

Catts, H. W. (1993). "The Relationship between Speech-Language Impairments and Reading Disabilities." *Journal of Speech & Hearing Research 36* (1993): 948-58.

Catts, H. W., Fey, M. E., Zhang, X. Y., and Tomblin, J. B. "Estimating the Risk of Future Reading Difficulties in Kindergarten Children: A Research-based Model and Its Clinical Implementation." *Language Speech and Hearing Services in Schools 32* (2001): 38-50.

Catts, H. W., Fey, M. E., Zhang, X., and Tomblin, J. B. "Language Basis of Reading and Reading Disabilities: Evidence from a Longitudinal Investigation." *Scientific Studies of Reading 3* (1999): 331-62.

Gillon, Gail. *Phonological Awareness: From Research to Practice.* New York, NY: Guilford Press, 2004.

Larrivee, L. and Catts, H. "Early Reading Achievement in Children with Expressive Phonological Disorders." *American Journal of Speech-Language Pathology 8* (1999): 118-28.

Liberman, Alvin M., Cooper, Franklin S., Shankweiler, Donald P., and Studdert-Kennedy, Michael. "Perception and the Speech Code." *Psychological Review 74,* (1967): 431–61.

Lewis, B. A., Freebairn, L. A., and Taylor, H. G. "Academic Outcomes in Children with Histories of Speech Sound Disorders." *Journal of Communication Disorders 33, no. 1* (2000): 11-30.

McNeill, Brigid, Gillon, Gail, and Dodd, Barbara. "Effectiveness of an Integrated Phonological Awareness Approach for Children with Childhood Apraxia of Speech (CAS)." *International Journal of Language & Communication Disorders 44,* no. 2 (2009): 175-92.

Meier, Daniel R. *The Young Child's Memory for Words.* New York, NY: Teachers College Press, 2004.

Rvachew, Susan. "Phonological Processing and Reading in Children with Speech-sound Disorders." *American Journal of Speech-Language Pathology 16* (2007): 260-70.

Stackhouse, Joy. *Persisting Speech Difficulties in Children: Children's Speech and Literacy Difficulties.* Hoboken, NJ: Wiley and Sons, 2006.

Chapter 13

Baskin, Amy and Fawcett, Heather. *More Than a Mom: Living a Full and Balanced Life When Your Child Has Special Needs.* Bethesda, MD: Woodbine House, 2006.

Feit, Debbie. *The Parent's Guide to Speech and Language Problems.* New York, NY: McGraw-Hill, 2007.

Marshak, Laura E. and Prezant, Fran. *Married with Special Needs Children: A Couples' Guide to Keeping Connected.* Bethesda, MD: Woodbine House, 2007.

Michael, Rudolph, Rosanowski, Frank, Eysholdt, Ulrich, and Kummer, Peter. "Anxiety and Depression in Mothers of Speech Impaired Children." *International Journal of Pediatric Otorhinolaryngology 67* (2003): 1337-41.

Murphy, Ann Pleshette. *The Seven Stages of Motherhood: Making the Most of Your Life As Mom.* New York, NY: Knopf, 2004.

Chapter 14

Freedman, Judy. *Easing the Teasing: Helping Your Child Cope with Name-Calling, Ridicule, & Verbal Bullying.* Chicago: Contemporary Books, 2002.

Markham, C., van Laar, D., Gibbard, D., and Dean, T. "Children with Speech, Language, and Communication Needs: Their Perceptions of Their Quality of Life." *International Journal of Language and Communication Disorders 44,* no. 5 (Sept./Oct. 2009): 748-68.

Nixon, Robin. "Studies Reveal Why Children Get Bullied and Rejected." LiveScience.com. February 2, 2010.

Sparrow, Joshua. "When Children Hit." *Scholastic Parent and Child.* October 2008.

Chapter 15

Ashmore, Jean. "Transitioning from High School to College—Students with Disabilities." Disability Blog. Retrieved from http://usodep.blogs.govdelivery.com on September 7, 2010.

Bahr, Diane. *Oral Motor Assessment and Treatment: Ages and Stages.* Upper Saddle River, NJ: Allyn & Bacon, 2000.

Jakielski, Kathy J. "Will My Child with CAS Ever Achieve Normal Speech?" Apraxia-Kids.org Family Start Guide. www.apraxia-kids.org. Retrieved August 3, 2010.

McCauley, Rebecca and Strand, Edythe. "A Review of Standardized Tests of Nonverbal Oral and Speech Motor Performance in Children." *American Journal of Speech-Pathology 17* (February 2008): 81-91.

Wright, Pam and Pete. *From Emotions to Advocacy: The Special Education Survival Guide.* Hartfield, VA: Harbor House Law Press, 2004.

Appendices

Eliot, Lisa. *What's Going on in There: How the Brain and Mind Develop in the First Five Years of Life.* New York, NY: Bantam, 1999.

"Facts for Families: The Depressed Child." *The American Academy of Child & Adolescent Psychiatry.* Retrieved from www.aacap.org/cs/root/facts_for_families/the_depressed_child on March 19, 2011.

Feit, Debbie. *A Parent's Guide to Speech and Language Problems.* New York, NY: McGraw-Hill, 2007.

Hamaguchi, Patricia McAleer. *Childhood Speech, Language & Listening Problems: What Every Parent Should Know.* Hoboken, NJ: Wiley, 2001.

Hesketh, A., Dima, E., and Nelson, V. "Teaching Phoneme Awareness to Pre-literate Children with Speech Disorders." *International Journal of Language and Communicative Disorders 42,* no. 3 (May-June 2007): 21-71.

Kuhl, Patricia, et al. (2003) "Foreign-language Experience in Infancy: Effects of Short-term Exposure and Social Interaction on Phonetic Learning." *Proceedings of the National Academy of Sciences of the United States of America 100,* no. 15 :9096-101.

Mahoneab, E., et al. "A Preliminary Neuroimaging Study of Preschool Children with ADHD." *The Clinical Neuropsychologist* (June 9, 2011):1009-1028.

Newmeyer, Amy, et al. "Results of the Sensory Profile in Children with Suspected Childhood Apraxia of Speech." *Physical & Occupational Therapy in Pediatrics 29,* no. 2 (2009): 205-20.

Nijland, Lian. "Speech Perception in Children with Speech Output Disorders." *Clinical Linguistics & Phonetics 23,* no. 3 (2009): 222–239.

Puranik, C., Petscher, Y., Al Otaiba, S., Catts, H. W., and Lonigan, C. "Development of Oral Reading Fluency in Children with Speech or Language Impairments: A Growth Curve Analysis." *Journal of Learning Disabilities 41* (2008): 545-60

Sensory Processing Foundation. Online articles on SPD. Retrieved from www.spdfoundation.net on March 19, 2011.

Sharma, M., Purdy, S., and Kelly, A. "Comorbidity of Auditory Processing, Language, and Reading Disorders." *Journal of Speech, Language, and Hearing Research 52* (2009): 706-22.

Smith, S., Scott, K., Roberts, J., and Locke, J. "Disabled Readers' Performance on Tasks of Phonological Processing, Rapid Naming, and Letter Knowledge Before and After Kindergarten." *Journal of Learning Disabilities Research & Practice* 23, no. 3 (2008): 113.

Squires, Jane, Bricker, Diane, et al. *Ages & Stages Questionnaire (ASQ)*.3rd ed. Baltimore, MD: Paul Brookes Publishing, 2009.

Vail, Tracy. "Similarities and Differences in Young Children with Autism and Those Children with Apraxia of Speech." Retrieved from www.apraxia-kids.org on Oct. 1, 2011.

Appendix A

•   •   •   •   •   •   •   •   •   •   •

A Guide to the
Most-Asked-About Conditions
in Relation to CAS

•   •   •   •   •   •   •   •   •   •   •   •   •   •

Because of its neurological underpinnings, Childhood Apraxia of Speech is rarely found alone. This question and answer guide provides an overview of some of the most common conditions associated with CAS. *Your child may or may not have these conditions or symptoms.* Bear in mind, however, that many of them become more apparent over time, as conditions and demands on the child increase or change. Refer back to this appendix if you begin to have concerns.

Auditory Processing Disorder (APD)
• •

APD, which is also known as Central Auditory Processing Disorder (CAPD), is not well defined just yet. In fact, the jury is still out on whether it is a *central* (nervous system) issue, or "just" an auditory processing issue. Some folks refer to it as "central deafness." Others compare it to dyslexia, calling it "dyslexia of the ear." Still others wonder if it really exists. Generally, auditory processing is what we do with the sounds we hear. Kids who struggle with APD have a hard time organizing the information they hear, so their speech is often affected. Think of it this way: your child's brain doesn't "know" how to listen. Why it *may* be associated with CAS: In a 2009 study on the sensory profile, the group of children with suspected apraxia had significant differences from same-age peers in auditory processing, as well as visual processing and multisensory processing.

In a basic sense, kids with APD hear sounds, but they can't make sense of what they are hearing (it may look like a receptive language disorder). Clinicians and practitioners indicate that there may be subtypes of APD. According to the authors of *The Mislabeled Child* (see references at the end of this chapter) the seven subtypes are: background noise, discrimination, prosody, localization, delayed processing, memory, and hypersensitivity.

Causes: The number one theory is that there is a familial tendency. Others indicate a contributing factor may be chronic ear infections as a young child. If kids are missing sounds due to an ear infection(s), then that may lead to a processing problem like APD. Another theory is that it has to do with neuromaturational development—that is, the child's auditory perception is somehow delayed or immature.

Red flags that a child may have (C)APD:
➤ At around 18 months, your child has delayed jibberish speech patterns (is not making the normal sing-song sounds mimicking speech).
➤ Your older child has difficulty with rhyming words and articulation, and frequently says "huh?" or "what?" or asks speakers to slow down.
➤ Your child has a decreased attention span, inability to concentrate, difficulty following directions, and is easily distracted. Of course, these symptoms overlap with ADHD and childhood in general.
➤ Your child is sensitive to sound, or has a sensory integration disorder (SID).
➤ Your child has poor pre-reading skills (difficulty matching sounds with letters or rhyming).
➤ Your child has relatively poor social skills.

Bear in mind that APD has nothing to do with IQ, although some kids with APD have some other developmental disability that *may* affect overall intelligence.

Diagnosis: Only an audiologist trained in APD can diagnose this condition. The SCAN (**S**creening Test for **A**uditory **P**rocessing Disorders) test is the "gold standard" screening tool for APD.

Treatment: Based on various diagnostic tests (electrophysiologic and behavioral measures done in a sound room with earphones and an audiometer), the audiologist will determine which treatment(s) is right for your child. Therapy treatments and tools may include:
➤ Auditory Training (AT)
➤ Auditory-based computer programs such as *Fast ForWord Learning Programs* and *Earobics*
➤ FM Trainers
➤ Multisensory reading programs like Lindamood-Bell and the Orton-Gillingham Methods

➤ Modified listening programs such as Auditory Integration Program (AIT)
➤ Speech therapy and occupational therapy, with a focus on sounds/words, rhymes, and body language awareness.

How can I help a child with APD?

➤ Make sure the child is seated close to the speaker/teacher so he can see and hear well.
➤ Minimize background noise (turn off fans and heaters, attempt to control road noise and classmate chatter, consider asking the teacher to use a microphone).
➤ Decrease visual distractions (streamline the space so there is less chance of verbal confusion).
➤ Improve acoustics (carpeting and wall hangings help).
➤ Simplify language you use around your child—avoid metaphors and abstract references.

For more information on APD:

➤ American Speech-Language-Hearing Association: www.asha.org/public/hearing/disorders/understand-apd-child.htm
➤ Auditory Processing Disorders: Classroom Accommodations and Modifications Checklist for APD: http://aitinstitute.org/auditory_processing_classroom_modifications.htm
➤ Dr. Maxine Young's website: www.maxineyoungcentral.com
➤ Karen Foli's book, *Like Sound Through Water: A Mother's Journey Through Auditory Processing Disorder* (Pocket Books, 2002).
➤ *The Sound of Hope* by Rosie O'Donnell and Lois Lam Heyman (Ballantine, 2010)

ADHD/ADD

● ● ● ● ● ● ● ●

Attention deficit disorder, with or without hyperactivity, is a common syndrome that can result in a variety of academic, social, and behavioral problems. Parents often notice these problems beginning in early childhood and continuing into teen and adult years. Kids with attention concerns can have difficulty in working up to their academic potential, as well as lack of follow-through, distractibility, impulsivity, and/or forgetfulness. Why it *may* be associated with CAS: Researchers from the Kennedy Krieger Institute in Baltimore found that the region of the brain responsible for cognitive and motor control was smaller in preschool children with symptoms of ADHD. Since CAS is a motor-neurological speech disorder, this *may* account for the correlation.

Red flags that a child may have ADHD:

➤ Challenges with following through and completing schoolwork or chores

➤ Difficulty organizing himself, tasks, paperwork, and materials
➤ Making careless mistakes: lack of attention to details
➤ Easily distracted
➤ Forgetful
➤ Blurting out answers, interrupting others often
➤ Restless/fidgety, acting as if "driven by a motor"
➤ Difficulty carrying out simple three-step directions, even ones that are part of the household routine
➤ Difficulties working up to academic potential
➤ Interpersonal clashes due to inability to meet expectations
➤ Impulsive

This list is not exhaustive, nor is it diagnostic! Many of these "red flags" are common in young children anyway. A trained professional (see below) can help tease out what is due to ADHD or ADD or just "typical kid" behavior.

Diagnosis: A neuropsychological evaluation needs to be conducted. This battery of tests includes a medical history, structured questionnaires, as well as many assessment tests looking at attention, concentration, learning, processing speed, perceptual organizational skills, encoding of rote input, among others. *The Vanderbilt Attention Deficit/Hyperactivity Disorder Parent Rating Scale* (VADPRS)—also a teacher version of this test, the *Vanderbilt Teacher-Behavior Evaluation Scale* (VTBES)—and the *Conners Rating Scales, Revised* **(CRS-R)** are the most commonly used screening tests.

Many factors must converge before a formal diagnosis can be made (not usually before age 6). There is not one magic assessment tool that will tell you, "Yes, your child has ADD (ADHD)." You'll want to complete testing if you have strong concerns, a teacher (or other service provider such as your child's SLP) has concerns, or if ADHD runs in your family. The earlier ADD/ADHD is confirmed, the better your child's chances of school success.

Any of these professionals are considered qualified to diagnosis ADHD:
➤ Child/adolescent psychiatrist—an M.D. who can prescribe medication
➤ Child/adolescent psychologist (a Ph.D. or Psy.D.)—can't prescribe medication, but can provide counseling and may be less expensive than psychiatrists
➤ Pediatrician - an M.D. who is familiar with your child, but may lack the skills and specific knowledge to make a formal ADHD diagnosis
➤ Pediatric neurologist
➤ Psychiatric nurse practitioner (they often work in collaboration with a medical practice)

Treatment: The MTA study (multimodal treatment of ADHD, funded by the NIMH) indicated that the best treatment is stimulant medication. Medication helps control symptoms—but is not a cure. Children/adolescents on stimulant medications need careful monitoring by a physician. The "best" treatment is often a combination (medication plus therapy) approach. Some parents supplement their child's treatment with behavioral modification programs (designed with a psychologist), social skills training, or occupational therapy.

How can I help a child with ADD or ADHD?
- Model good time and organizational management yourself.
- Develop and stick with household/school routines.
- Establish clear and reasonable expectations.
- Improve your communication style so that kids are clear as to what is expected.
- Use clocks and timers to create tangible parameters for completing a task.
- Design a place for quiet reflection at home and school.
- Pursue a 504 plan or IEP at school if your child could benefit from accommodations such as extended time, small group testing, use of a calculator, note taking assistance, etc.

For more information on ADHD:
- CHADD (formerly Children and Adolescents with ADD): www.chadd.org
- The National Resource Center for ADHD: www.help4adhd.org
- *Identifying and Treating ADHD: A Resource for Home and School:* http://www2.ed.gov/teachers/needs/speced/adhd/adhd-resource-pt1.pdf
- The Multimodal Treatment of ADHD (MTA) study: www.nimh.nih.gov/trials/practical/mta/multimodal-treatment-of-attention-deficit-hyperactivity-disorder-mta-study.shtml
- *ADDitude Magazine*: www.ADDitudeMag.com
- *Raising Your Spirited Child* by Mary Sheedy Kurcinka
- *Understanding Girls with AD/HD* by Kathleen Nadeau, Ellen Littman, and Patricia Quinn
- You and your child may enjoy reading *Houdini's Gift* by Jeanne Gehret in which a child with ADHD convinces his parents he can care for a pet by staying on top of his chores.
- Drs. Stasi and Dodzik of North Shore Pediatric Therapy offer a free e-book that covers ADHD—*Neurodevelopment of Children: 4 Common Childhood Disorders*: www.NSPT4kids.com

Autism Spectrum Disorder (ASD)

Autism and apraxia are both neurological disorders, but they are completely different in nature. However, the same child can have both autism and CAS. Just as with CAS, autism runs on a continuum (spectrum). Therefore, kids can have mild to profound symptoms. Kids with autism have impaired communication, social, and emotional skills, whereas kids with CAS have impaired speech skills and may have impairments in gross and fine motor skills. Why ASD *may* be associated with CAS: Because of their neurological underpinnings, ASD and apraxia are sometimes found together. Children with ASD have trouble with social and communication skills, which sometimes overlap into the apraxia diagnosis.

Red flags that a child may have ASD:

➤ Facial expressions tend to be unanimated; smiles often not related to social interactions
➤ Not readily making eye contact and seeming to look beyond others
➤ Not responding to name when called
➤ Delayed or nonexistent waving, pointing, or other basic communicative gestures
➤ Using another person's hand as a tool (e.g., taking his mother's hand to open door)
➤ Delays in speech or using speech for noncommunicative purposes (repeating dialog from a TV show to himself). Sometimes child develops speech on a normal timetable, but talks excessively about his special interests without noticing others' cues that they are bored.
➤ Difficulty imitating others' actions
➤ Not playing in a typical manner (performing the same action over and over, such as spinning the wheels on toy cars or placing toys in a line)
➤ Having little or no interest in reciprocal play with others

Diagnosis: The "best" diagnosis for an autism spectrum disorder (autism) is given by a child/adolescent psychiatrist or pediatric neurologist. Some child/adolescent psychologists specialize in autism spectrum disorders, and may be involved with assessment.

Your pediatrician may give you a screening tool. Examples of such screening tools are the *CHAT (Checklist of Autism in Toddlers)* or the *M-CHAT (Modified Checklist of Autism in Toddlers)*, the *STAT (Screening Tool for Autism in Two-year olds)*, or the *SCQ (Social Communication Questionnaire)*. After a series of screenings, a child who is considered a "concern" for autism should be given a complete evaluation by a multidisciplinary team.

Treatment: There is no one treatment that is "best" for ASD, although it is essential to begin early intervention once the disorder has been properly identified. Parents often advocate for intensive ABA (applied behavior analysis) treatment, which involves breaking tasks down into small steps, "errorless learning," and frequently reinforcing or rewarding the child for progress. Therapies that can help include: behavioral, communication, occupational therapy, physical therapy, and social play. In elementary school and beyond, most children with ASD benefit from special education services and accommodations provided either in the regular classroom or in a specialized setting that allows the child to best learn up to his abilities. Medication may help a child with ASD for symptomatic treatment. For example, a child who is aggressive may benefit from an antipsychotic, and kids who have difficulty with inattention and hyperactivity may benefit from a stimulant. Children with ASD may not respond to medications in the same manner as a "typically developing" child. Medication administration should be carefully monitored by a treating physician.

How can I help a child with ASD?

Allow your child to select the type of play he engages in. Do not insist that he try to talk. Give him a slow introduction to sounds, events, and experiences, and gentle encouragement to verbalize. Educate yourself about how to reinforce the behaviors you want to see, as well as the optimal methods and placements for educating children with autism.

Where can I learn more?

➤ Autism Society of America: www.autism-society.org (800-328-8476)
➤ *Not My Boy: A Father, A Son, and One Family's Journey with Autism,* a memoir about raising a son with autism written by former NFL quarterback Rodney Peete
➤ For dozens of different perspectives on what it's like to have a child with an ASD, try *Gravity Pulls You In,* a collection of essays edited by Vicki Forman and Kyra Anderson.
➤ *The Everyday Advocate: Standing Up for Your Child with Autism* by Areva Martin, a step-by-step guidebook with lots of personal stories
➤ *Dancing with Max: A Mother and Son Who Broke Free (Zondervan, 2010),* by Emily Colson, may be a nice resource to turn to for hope and thought-provoking insight
➤ For information on a variety of issues related to raising a child with autism, contact Woodbine House (www.woodbinehouse.com; 800-843-7323). Publications include *Right from the Start: Behavioral Intervention for Young Children with Autism; Jumpstarting Communication Skills in Children with Autism; Reaching Out, Joining In: Teaching Social Skills to Young Children with Autism; and Autism 24/7: A Family Guide to Learning at Home and in the Community.*

Anxiety Disorders

"Anxiety" is a broad umbrella covering many specific disorders, such as generalized anxiety disorder (GAD), separation anxiety disorder, specific phobias, selective mutism, and obsessive compulsive disorder (OCD). Different types of anxiety disorders have different symptoms, but generally these kids worry excessively over a variety of events—their health, academics, athletics, friends, world events, what will happen if they do/don't do something, or family matters. Why it *may* be associated with CAS: Sometimes kids with CAS can become anxious or unsure in situations in which speaking and socializing is a large part of the event.

Red flags that a child may have an anxiety disorder:
Constant feeling of being "keyed-up" or "on edge"
➤ Restlessness
➤ Easily fatigued
➤ Decreased concentration
➤ Increased irritability
➤ Muscular tension
➤ Poor sleep/sleep concern
➤ In the case of OCD, repeated actions that seem senseless or excessive to an outside observer (such as frequent hand washing or needing to arrange items "just so")

Diagnosis: It is best to have a full assessment and evaluation conducted by a child/adolescent psychologist (Ph.D. or Psy.D.) or child/adolescent psychiatrist (M.D.). It's difficult to diagnose kids with an anxiety disorder because it is often accompanied with disruptive behavior, which may overlap with symptoms consistent with ADHD or oppositional defiant disorder (ODD). In addition, childhood anxiety shares some characteristics with some autism spectrum disorders, learning disorders, bipolar disorder, and depression. Mental health specialists are likely to administer a screening tool such as the *Hamilton Anxiety Rating Scale* or the *Beck Anxiety Inventory* to help determine cause, type, and severity.

Treatment: Several different approaches to therapy may be used for childhood anxiety. Exposure response prevention treatment is highly evidence-based, especially in cases of OCD. Cognitive behavioral therapy (CBT) can be effective for children. In addition, it is helpful to teach children about anxiety, its symptoms, and nonmedical ways of managing it. In some cases, medication may help manage symptoms.

How can I help a child with an anxiety disorder?
Both parents and teachers can help children recognize symptoms of impending anxiety, as well as ways to change those anxious thoughts into more positive ones (reframing). In addition, teachers and parents ought to provide positive reinforcement for kid's continued success in school and home matters.

For more information about childhood anxiety:
➤ *Freeing Your Child from Anxiety: Powerful, Practical Solutions to Overcome Your Child's Fears, Worries, and Phobias* by Tamar Ellsas Chansky
➤ *Helping Your Anxious Child: A Step-by-Step Guide for Parents* by Ronald M. Rapee, Ann Wignall, Susan H. Spence, and Vanessa Cobham
➤ *Childhood Anxiety Network:* www.childanxiety.net/index.htm
➤ *University of Maryland Medical Center* has some good information on anxiety: www.umm.edu/patiented/articles/what_will_confirm_a_diagnosis_of_an_anxiety_

➤ disorder_000028_5.htm
➤ Childhood anxiety disorders are covered in the free e-book, *Neurodevelopment of Children: 4 Common Childhood Disorders,* by Drs. Stasi and Dodzik: www.NSPT4kids.com.

Childhood Depression

Depression is a disorder involving several neurotransmitters within the brain. Although it is a real concern, affecting 5 percent of children and adolescents, it is very treatable. It tends to run in families, so if there is a tendency for depression in your family, be aware that it *could* affect your child. Significant life events (loss, stress) can contribute to depression, as can chronic illness. Why it *may* be associated with CAS: Kids who lack social connections may be more likely to be depressed than their more socially-connected peers.

Red flags that a child may have depression:
➤ Sadness, tearfulness, crying
➤ Decreased interest in typical activities
➤ Feelings of hopelessness and helplessness
➤ Decreased energy
➤ Social isolation
➤ Irritability, anger
➤ Decreased self-esteem
➤ Psychosomatic complaints (frequent complaints of headaches or tummy aches)
➤ Major change in eating or sleeping behavior (increased or decreased weight)
➤ Destructive behavior/ "acting out"
Be aware that this list is not exhaustive, nor is it diagnostic!

Diagnosis: A qualified mental health professional makes the official diagnosis of childhood depression. An evaluation by a child/adolescent psychiatrist (M.D.) is imperative. Psychologists (Ph.D. or Psy.D.) can provide counseling. Generally, children who have five or more of the above "red flags" for two or more weeks are considered depressed. If you are concerned about your child and depression, early intervention by a qualified profession is needed. They will provide screening tools (such as the *Beck Depression Inventory*) to determine cause and severity, and to develop a treatment plan.

Treatment: Comprehensive family and/or individual therapy in conjunction with an antidepressant is often the treatment for childhood depression. Talk with your prescribing physician for guidance and supervision of a medication regimen.

How can I help with childhood depression?

It may not be apparent to you that your child is struggling with depression since it is often masked by other symptoms such as anger, irritability, or destructive behavior. Ask your child if he is sad or unhappy. Doing so will often give you additional insight if he is exhibiting these nontypical symptoms of depression. Providing emotional support, building self-esteem, and assisting with medication monitoring are important ways others can help a child with depression.

For more information on depression:
➤ *KidsHealth,* a comprehensive site on various topics, including depression, for parents, kids, and teens: http://kidshealth.org/parent/emotions/feelings/understanding_depression.html#
➤ The American Academy of Child & Adolescent Psychiatry has a nice "for parents page": www.aacap.org/cs/root/facts_for_families/the_depressed_child
➤ Childhood depression is covered in Drs. Stasi's and Dodzik's free e-book, *Neurodevelopment of Children: 4 Common Childhood Disorders:* www.NSPT4kids.com
➤ *Helping Your Depressed Child: A Step-by-Step Guide for Parents* by Martha Underwood Barnard

Neurodevelopmental Delay (NDD)

A Neurodevelopmental Delay is a complex of various disabilities and delays that overlap with one another. A neurodevelopmental delay is an omission or arrest of an early developmental stage of a child. It is difficult to pinpoint any one cause, but may be due to a combination of developmental and environmental factors that delay the neurodevelopment of the child. Many of the symptoms of NDD overlap with the diagnostic categories of dyslexia, (dys)apraxia, and ADD, as well as a dysfunction of attention, motor, and perception (DAMP). For example, 80 percent of kids with dyslexia have some symptoms of (dys)apraxia and up to 80 percent of kids with (dys)apraxia have some problems in common with dyslexia (especially balance, orientation, and motor skills—or lack thereof). Why it *may* be associated with CAS: If a child is delayed in a variety of neurological areas, speech and language may be affected as well, including the possibility of having CAS.

Red flags that a child may have NDD:
➤ Attention and focus problems on a specific task
➤ Poor balance, orientation, and motor skills (difficulty learning to ride a bicycle)
➤ Poor body awareness (proprioception)
➤ Poor hand-eye coordination, inability to sit still and remain silent

- ➤ Mixed laterality (no true preference for handedness, foot, eye, or ear beyond the age of eight years)
- ➤ Difficulty learning to read and write
- ➤ Poor speech and articulation problems
- ➤ Travel sickness beyond puberty

This list is not exhaustive, nor is it diagnostic!

Diagnosis: If you are concerned that your child has a neurodevelopmental delay (NDD), then, chances are, your child's pediatrician has seen some red flags as well. Concerns are often noticed during a well-child exam. Visiting a developmental pediatrician, pediatric neurologist, or a pediatric psychiatrist may be the next step in a diagnosis.

Children need a full neurological assessment and evaluation, testing for reflexes, balance skills, and central nervous system (CNS) maturity levels, in addition to other recommended testing. A screening tool developed by the Institute for Neuro-Physiological Psychology can be found at www.inpp.org.uk/questions/index.php. This questionnaire was published in the *British Journal of Occupational Therapy in* October 1998.

Treatment: Generally, the treatment for neurodevelopmental delay(s) is geared toward the underlying cause of the delay. If you are concerned about the possibility your child has a NDD, please consult your physician, who can advise you on professionals to consult about diagnosis and treatment.

How can I help with NDD?

Parents and teachers need to support these children academically and emotionally by monitoring homework, helping to increase the child's self-esteem, helping the child identify and implement rewards that are motivating to him, and participating in social and academic areas of the child's life. Depending on the diagnosis, you may also need to educate yourself on appropriate educational supports for your child, and seek out an IEP or 504 plan to help him succeed in school.

For more information on NDD:

- ➤ The Institute for Neuro-Physiological Psychology: www.inpp.org.uk/ndd_neuro_developmental_delay/diagnosis.php
- ➤ The Brain and Behavior Enhancement website: www.brainandbehaviour.ie/en/understanding-neuro-developmental-delay.html
- ➤ *A Mind at a Time* by Mel Levine, M.D., which covers different ways in which children learn, as well as developmental delays
- ➤ Other books you may find helpful in your journey: *A Parent's Guide to Developmental Delays* by Laurie LeComer and *How to Detect Developmental Delays and What to Do Next: A Practical Intervention for Home and School* by Mary Mountstephen

Sensory Processing Disorder (SPD)

In the recent past, this disorder was referred to as Sensory Integration Disorder. In a general sense, SPD occurs when the nervous system doesn't recognize and organize input from the senses in an appropriate and meaningful way. According to the Sensory Processing Disorder Foundation's website, between 1 in 20 kids and 1 in 6 kids are affected with SPD. As with ADHD, CAS, and autism spectrum disorders, researchers propose that SPD falls along a spectrum of severity. Why it *may* be connected to CAS: According to a 2007 study headed up by Amy Newmeyer, children with CAS had significant differences from same-age peers in a number of areas, including sensory seeking (particularly oral stimulation), emotional reactivity, and academic skills. Also, the 2007 ASHA technical document on CAS suggests that CAS may be motoric *and* sensory in nature.

Red flags that a child may have SPD:
➤ Overly sensitive to physical touch (clothing tags are very bothersome)
➤ Problems eating or sleeping
➤ Difficulty coping; prone to temper tantrums
➤ Very clumsy; "floppy"
➤ Little reaction to extreme temperatures
➤ In constant motion
➤ Often these children are referred to as being "in your face"
This list is not exhaustive, nor is it diagnostic!

Diagnosis: A multidisciplinary team (M.D., child psychologist, nurse practitioner, etc.) *may* diagnose a sensory processing disorder, but not necessarily so. An occupational therapist (OT) is also qualified to make the diagnosis. Often, a screening is performed on kids who are suspected of having SPD. This can be done in a pediatrician's office, at school, or at a private clinic. Screening tools that may be used are the *Sensory Integration & Praxis Test* (SIPT), as developed by Jean Ayres, Ph.D., OTR (for kids ages 4-8), or *The Sensory Profile.* Based on the results of the screening test, a more in-depth evaluation may be conducted, including a clinical observation and parent report measures. *(Please be warned, SPD is a controversial subject to some professionals.* Many mainstream professional organizations do not accept it as a valid diagnosis.)

Treatment: It's often recommended that children with SPD work closely with an occupational therapist (OT) who has training in and uses a sensory integration approach in his practice. Medication typically does not help.

How Can I Help with SPD?
Help build these kids' self-esteem, as they are often referred to as "klutzes" and may not make friends as easily as their typically developing peers. Good modeling

of social skills may also be helpful. Parents can ask their child's OT about a possible "sensory diet," which is an individualized plan to provide the child with the types of sensations throughout the day that can help him stay focused and organized and control his behavior.

For more information on SPD:
➤ The Sensory Processing Foundation is a website designed for parents: www.spdfoundation.net
➤ Tips, hints, and activities on creating a sensory diet at Sensory Smarts: http://sensorysmarts.com/sensory_diet_activities.html
➤ *The Sensory Processing Disorder Answer Book: Practical Answers to the Top 250 Questions Parents Ask* by Tara Delaney
➤ *Parenting a Child with Sensory Processing Disorder: A Family Guide to Understanding & Supporting Your Sensory-Sensitive Child,* by Christopher R. Auer and Susan Blumberg
➤ *S.I. FOCUS Magazine,* c/o Shannon Media, P.O. Box 821404, Dallas, TX 75382; 214- 341-9999 (www.SIfocus.com), an international, quarterly magazine

General Resources and Recommended Reading

➤ *The Well Balanced Child: Movement and Early Learning* by Sally Goddard Blythe (Hawthorn Press Early Years, 2006).

➤ *The Mislabeled Child: How Understanding Your Child's Unique Learning Style Can Open the Door to Success* by Brock Eide and Fernette Eide (Hyperion, 2006).

➤ *Different Learners: Identifying, Preventing, and Treating Your Child's Learning Problems* by Jane Healy, Ph.D. (Simon and Schuster, 2010).

Appendix B

Health Insurance

Early in our apraxia journey, I phoned our insurance company. I was driving along the back roads to work when we lived in Minnesota. I made the call on my cell phone, fearful I would lose coverage during this fateful phone call. Yes, "coverage" has multiple meanings here.

After the usual interminable hold, I got through. "I'm calling to see if speech therapy is covered for my daughter. She isn't talking much. I don't know what to do. My doctor thinks she needs to see a speech-language pathologist. Are we covered?"

"What is your policy number?"

"Uh…um," I stammered. I had no idea what my policy number was.

The member services representative sighed, "Ma'am, is the policy in your name or your husband's?"

"Uh, it's in my husband's," I responded.

"And what is his social security number?" As if I knew that off the top of my head! Somehow, I managed to muster up his social security number and provide it to the woman on the other end of the phone.

"I see your policy does cover speech therapy by a qualified speech-language pathologist if the child is found to be moderately to severely impaired in their communication, also if there is a distinct neurological or medical necessity."

"So I can take her to see this person recommended by our doctor?" I asked cautiously.

After giving the member services representative the clinic and SLP's name, I got the green-light to head to the speech clinic the next week.

I hung up the phone, biting the side of my cheek in effort to hold back tears. I called my husband. I reiterated the part about moderate to severe impairment and medical or neurological necessity. He sighed. I heard his office chair squeak. Hot tears rolled down my face.

"Honey, you don't need to cry," he reassured me. "It's covered. She'll be okay."

And she *is* okay. Speech therapy *was* covered. But it hasn't always been smooth sailing.

I know this process—the speech therapy and paying for it—can leave you feeling emotional, drained, and overwhelmed. Coverage for speech and language disorders can be tricky, to say the least. Each policy has its own set of rules and parameters, and it's helpful to know early on what they are. Here are a few pointers to keep in mind:

➤ *Understand your policy.* Get your hands on a copy of your policy. If you can't find it at home, check with your HR contact at work or call your insurance company directly for an extra copy.

➤ *Find the section on speech and language therapy.* It may be listed under headings such as "rehabilitative services," "physical and occupational therapy," "other medically necessary services," or "therapies." Read it and be sure to note any "exclusions."

➤ If you *are* covered, consider yourself "lucky," but realize this is not the end of the game. *The top 5 questions to ask:*

1. *"Are both the evaluation and ongoing therapy covered?"* You'd assume they *would* be, but stranger things have happened. Be sure you know ahead of time.

2. *"Is therapy covered for CAS?"* You will want to know what diagnostic code (ICD-9) your speech clinic is using when they submit to insurance. The ICD-9 code for CAS is 784.69. Know this early on to avoid a bill several weeks later because the clinic coded for something that your insurance company doesn't cover. If you are interested in more ICD-9 codes, refer to this website, ICD-9 Data: www.icd9data.com/2011/Volume1/default.htm.

3. *"Do you need to choose a SLP who is in-network?"* Some insurance plans require that you see providers who are in-network, others allow you to see out-of-network providers but may pay less per visit (more dollars out-of-pocket for you and often with a high deductible). Some others will allow you to go wherever you want. It depends on the plan you have.

4. *"Is there a deductible or co-pay?"* In our case, we had a $500 deductible to meet for the calendar year. "Deposits" towards this $500 accrued each time we took Kate to therapy. For example, therapy cost $140/hour. We paid that amount toward our $500 deductible each time until we hit the $500 deductible. Afterwards, insurance was billed and we were responsible for the $10 co-pay for each visit. Each plan is different; find out how yours works.

5. *"Is there a maximum number of visits per year/dollar amount paid?"* I can't over-emphasize how important it is to know this! Some insurance companies only allow a set number of visits per year. It may be as high as 100 or as few as 10. Some average around 60. Others have a yearly maximum of a pre-determined dollar amount, such as $5,000. Ask how your policy operates. Ask if there are allowances for more therapy if your SLP recommends it. Ask, too, if speech therapy falls under the same umbrella as occupational and physical therapy. We were lucky—each therapy had a $5,000 max/year.

Help! We maxed out our yearly dollar coverage!

Kate had been making lots of new speech sounds. Her SLP recommended we consider feeding therapy for her eating issues (overstuffing, "forgetting" to chew, etc.), so we added "feeding therapy" to our already busy therapy schedule. She was going to the clinic three or four times a week. We didn't think much of it until a bill came in the mail for over $1,000! I was shocked! The year wasn't over yet! I called the insurance company after I simmered down. We had reached our $5,000 max on these therapies, they told us. (Feeding and speech therapy came out of the same "pot" in our case). I was dumbfounded. Sure, I was responsible for knowing and managing our insurance, but you would think that when we got close to that $5,000 max, our insurance company would have given us a heads-up. Or that the speech clinic might have said, "Oh, by the way, a claim was denied. It may be time to cut back on therapy or check your insurance." None of that happened, nor does it typically. Learn from my mistake: keep careful track of your insurance dollars!

If you're not covered for speech therapy at all, there are a few things you can do:

➤ *Talk to your employer's HR person or department and see if they can offer another plan that has coverage.* It's your employer's choice which insurance plan they offer its employees. They may have no idea that your child needs speech therapy if you don't speak up. If you present a compelling enough case, they may back you up by finding a better-suited plan, but don't bank on this.

➤ *For help persuading your employer to switch insurance plans,* request an "Employer Insurance Packet," by visiting ASHA (www.asha.org) or calling 800-638-8255. The packet suggest ways to talk with your employer's HR person, make the case for more speech coverage, and hold a meeting with your HR department.

➤ *Look for free or reduced cost speech therapy at a local college or university.* This was the #1 suggestion we received when our insurance was maxed out and Kate still needed services. It didn't work out for us, but it may for you. Call the college's communication disorders department or program and inquire. You can also place an ad at the college indicating you are seeking the services of a student to come to your home and work with your child on speech-language concerns. Pay him or her a small fee, just as you would a tutor or babysitter. A college student isn't likely to turn down quick cash that may actually be helpful for their studies. Plus, you won't have to drive to and from the clinic, and your child has additional interaction with someone who cares.

➤ *Early intervention programs and public school-based preschools offer free or very low cost speech services.* Early intervention programs often provide therapy free of charge, or based on a sliding scale. Generally, EI will help you get your foot in the public preschool door, as well. Providing your child meets criteria set forth by the evaluation and treatment team, your child may be eligible to attend a public preschool with speech services at no additional cost to you.

➤ *Apply for financial assistance such as Medicaid.* According to Debbie Feit, author of *The Parent's Guide to Speech and Language Problems,* the Medicaid program allows for direct reimbursement to speech-language pathologists. Each state's eligibility rules vary, so do your homework by checking www.cms.hhs. gov or call the Centers for Medicare & Medicaid Services at 877-267-2323.

➤ *You may even qualify for a grant through United Healthcare Children's Foundation (UHCCF).* These grants can help families pay for children's medical expenses that are not covered, or partially covered, by a commercial healthcare plan. Qualifying families may receive up to $5,000 for services and equip-

Parents Ask...

Can I deduct [speech] therapy costs on my income tax?

Generally speaking, if you: 1) itemize deductions on your tax return, *and* 2) your medical expenses for the year exceed 7.5 percent of your adjusted gross income (AGI), then you can deduct the amount over and above that 7.5 percent. Let's say your income is $50,000. $3750 is 7.5 percent of your AGI. If you have medical expenses (to include speech therapy) of $6000 for the year, then $2250 would be deductible (6000 – 3750). Note that in 2013 and later, medical expenses may need to exceed 10 percent of your AGI to qualify. For more information on deducting medical expenses, call 800-829-1040 and ask for Publication 502, or go to: www.irs.gov/taxtopics/tc502.html.

ment such as physical, occupational, and speech therapy, counseling services, surgeries, prescriptions, and the like. Parents or legal guardians can apply for grants at www.uhccf.org.

➤ **Look for other organizations that offer financial assistance.** Go to ASHA's website (www.asha.org)—head to "information for public" in the left-hand corner, then click on "speech, language, and swallowing funding resources." You will find many organizations listed offering funding for speech-language therapy (Easter Seals, March of Dimes, Scottish Rite/RiteCare, to name a few). Each organization requires an application process, and eligibility varies, so be sure to look into each one carefully.

As you can see, there are many ways to seek financial services for your child's speech-language treatment. Please do not let money stop you from giving your child what he needs most to overcome Childhood Apraxia of Speech: frequent and intense speech therapy provided by a qualified speech-language pathologist.

Appendix C

. . . .

Summer Speech Camps and Enrichment Programs

. . . .

School's out! As a parent reading this, you may have mixed feelings about summer "vacation." While the months of not having to deal with the morning rush or nagging your child(ren) to complete their homework *is* a break, you still have things to think about, especially when it comes to your child's speech and language goals.

Your child may or may not qualify for extended school year (ESY), depending on his age and severity of apraxia. Even if he does, it's not a bad idea to supplement your child's summer with some additional speech enrichment. Keep in mind, your speech clinic *may* offer summer social skills classes or day camps as well, so be sure to ask. For example, you may find something like what Suburban Pediatric Therapies in Aurora, IL, has available: social skills training using "Model Me Kids" videos.

An ideal summer program will offer:
- a balanced program with daily opportunities for enrichment of a variety of skills, including recreation;
- engaging, kid-friendly activities;
- a safe and structured program with positive, caring, and professional role models;
- low "camper": staff ratio.

You may have to select a summer program months in advance to secure your child's spot. Consider asking these questions to help you winnow down your decisions for your child's needs, abilities, and interests:

1. Does the program have a mission? What is it?

2. How is a typical day/week organized? How will children spend their time?
3. What are the program hours and dates?
4. How does the program assess or track each child's progress? What evidence does the program have to show past results?
5. What is the typical experience of the staff members who will work with my child? Are any of them SLPs, OTs, or PTs?
6. Does the staff receive any special training?
7. What type of communication can families expect?
8. Is financial aid available? Does insurance cover any of the costs?

For more information about what makes a summer learning program successful, visit The National Summer Learning Association at www.summerlearning.org.

State-by-State Programs

Here is a list of some speech and language-based camps (day camps and overnight camps) throughout the U.S. that may be of interest to you. If any interest you, contact the camps directly to inquire about their suitability for your child and lifestyle.

Arizona
➤ *Foundations Development House*—Speech and language summer camps in Chandler and Scottsdale: www.fdhkids.com.
➤ *Kamp Talkalot*—Speech and language summer camps in Chandler and Scottsdale: www.pediatricspeech.net.

California
➤ *Building Bridges Camp*—Overnight camp in Boulder Creek for AAC users: www.bridgeschool.org/camp.html—(630) 696-7295.
➤ *Say 'n' Play Speech Camp*—Summer camp in Culver City for children with speech and language issues: www.speakla.com.
➤ *Total Education Solutions Camp*—Enrichment programs in Los Angeles, San Diego, and Sacramento for children 2-5 years with focus on speech, language, and early reading skills; specialized programs for kids between 6-12 years: www.tesidea.com—(888) 4TES-KIDS.
➤ *Square Peg Horse Camp*—Camp in San Francisco for children with special needs; includes instruction in horsemanship: www.everyonebenefits.org.
➤ *Camp Chatterbox*—Social Skills Camp in San Jose for children with social skill concerns, including CAS: www.progressivespeech.com—(408) 377-3064.

Colorado
➤ *Talking with Technology Camp*—Overnight camp in Empire for AAC users: Kovach.Tracy@tchden.org—(303) 861-6024.

District of Columbia (Washington, D.C.)

➤ *The George Washington University (GWU) Summer Apraxia Camp*—An intensive weeklong summer camp for children ages 3-10 years diagnosed with CAS or suspected CAS. Informal video pre-assessment. Camp incorporates multi-modal treatment approach in daily individual, small group, and large group therapy by graduate level clinicians supervised by a certified and licensed speech-language pathologist. Not an overnight camp. Contact camp supervisor at jkumar@gwu.edu or (202)994-7363.

Florida

➤ *The Foundation for Dreams*—Overnight camp in Sarasota for children with various disabilities: www.foundationsfordreams.org—(941) 746-5659.

Georgia

➤ *Camp Rayin*—Summer camp in Atlanta for children ages 2-6; serves all children, including those with special needs: www.rayinconnection.com.
➤ *P.R.O.M.P.T. and Play*—Intensive summer speech therapy camp in Suwanee utilizing PROMPT facilitation technique for kids ages 4-7 with CAS and dysarthria, among other conditions: www.kidscreektherapy.com—(770) 337-4387.

Illinois

➤ *Intensive Summer Language Program*—8-week summer day camp program in Chicago-Lincoln Park for children 2-12 years with speech and language concerns: jaleduc@ix.netcom.com—(312) 944-6336.
➤ *The Augustana College Center for Speech, Language and Hearing Summer Clinic*—6-week day camp program in Rock Island in the form of individual, small group, and whole group work. Groups are based on ability, for beginning communicators (ages 3-6) through teens: (309) 794-7350.

Maryland

➤ *Cue Camp Friendship*—Summer weekend camp in Buckeystown open to anyone interested in Cued Speech: www.marylandcues.org.
➤ *Speech Pathways*—Summer groups focused on social skills, early language/play, reading, writing, and art meet throughout Carroll County: www.speechpathways.net—(410) 374-0555.
➤ *Camp Littlefoot*—Day camp in Rockville for children with speech, language, perceptual motor, and/or learning issues: www.ttlc.org—(301) 738-9691 x 145.

Michigan

➤ *Communicative Disorders Clinic at the University of Michigan*—Summer day camp in Ann Arbor for language, learning, and literacy: www.languageexperts.org—(734) 764-8440.

➤ *Central Michigan University Summer Speech-Language Specialty Clinics*—Half-day sessions in Mount Pleasant for kids with communication disorders: www.cmich.edu—(989) 774-3803.

➤ *Total Education Solutions Camp*—Enrichment programs in Troy for children 2-5 years with focus on speech, language, and early reading skills. Specialized programs for kids between 6-12 years: www.tesidea.com—(888) 4TES-KIDS.

➤ *Kaufman Children's Center for Speech, Language, Sensory-Motor, and Social Connections*—Summer program in West Bloomfield for CAS, autism, social skills, Baby Signs ™, language groups: www.kidspeech.com—(248) 737-3430.

Minnesota

➤ *Camp Courage*—Overnight camp in Maple Lake for kids with speech/hearing/language disorders and AAC users; day camps also available in various areas within MN: www.couragecamps.org—(763) 520-0504.

Missouri

➤ *SCAMP (Summer Classes for Articulation & Motor Speech Progress)*—Intensive 6-week day camp in Ballwin for young children, ages 3-6 with CAS and other significant articulation or phonological delays: www.gotospeech.com—(636) 220-8200.

➤ *Fontbonne University*—Eardley Family Clinic in Clayton offers a developmental language group for 6-8 children ages 2-5 years in a 2-hour day camp setting fall, winter, and summer semesters: bmeyer@fonbonne.edu—(314) 889-1407.

➤ *Robert G. Combs Language Preschool at the University of Missouri-Columbia*—Language-rich preschool in Columbia for ages 3-5 years with a speech/language diagnosis; low clinician: student ratio: http://healthprofessions.missouri.edu/csd/preschool.php.

➤ *St. Louis University Childhood Apraxia of Speech Summer Camps*—Intensive 2-week day camp in St. Louis with a.m. and p.m. sessions for preschoolers through adolescents: www.slu.edu—(314) 977-2943.

New Hampshire

➤ *Easter Seals Camps* offered throughout the state for a variety of disabilities: (603) 740-3534 or (603) 895-1522.

New Jersey

➤ *Camp Chatterbox*—Overnight camp in Hudwich for AAC users: www.camp-chatterbox.org—(908) 301-5451.

➤ *Camp Fun and Gains*—Day camp in Montgomery for communication, social, and motor skills: www.psllcnj.com/camp_fun_and_gains—(609) 924-7080.

New York

➤ *Summer Child Language Institute: Speech-Language-Hearing Clinic*—Summer program in Brooklyn with intensive therapy, parent groups, and guest speakers: www.summeroncampus.com—(718) 488-3480.

North Carolina

➤ *The Speech Garden Summer Camp*—Camp in Charlotte for children ages 2 years through 2nd grade with mild to severe expressive or receptive language, oral motor, or articulation problems: www.speechgarden.org/summer-camp.

Ohio

➤ *Total Education Solutions Camp*—Enrichment programs in Fairlawn for children 2-5 years with focus on speech, language, and early reading skills. Specialized programs for kids between 6-12 years: www.tesidea.com—(888) 4TES-KIDS.

Pennsylvania

➤ *Lee Mar Summer Camp and School*—Special needs camp in Dresher for children and young adults with moderate learning and developmental challenges: www.leemar.com.

Tennessee

➤ *Parent Child Services Group Inc.—Summer Programs*—Summer program in Knoxville for children with speech/language, sensory, motor, or learning concerns: www.parent-childservices.com/home.htm.

➤ *Camp Livitup*—8-week day camp in Memphis for children ages 5-15 with any disability: www.ncpad.org—(901) 761-4277.

Texas

➤ *Capitol School of Austin Summer Camps*—Enriching summer learning experience in Austin for children, preschool through 3rd grade with speech, language, & learning concerns: www.capitolschool.com.

Utah

➤ *Wasatch Speech and Language Center*—Summer therapy program in Lake City for social communication skills: (801) 308-0400.

Virginia

➤ *Cue Camp*—Camp in Williamsburg that focuses on cued speech: www.nvcsa.org.

National Programs

➤ *National Cued Speech Association*—Teaches cued speech in informal camp settings throughout the U.S.: www.cuedspeech.org.sub/resources/camps.asp.

➤ *National Easter Seal Society*—Day or overnight camps for children with disabilities located throughout the U.S.: www.easterseals.com.
➤ *The Scottish Rite Mason's RiteCare Childhood Language Program*—Nationwide speech and language summer clinics: www.scottishrite.org.

International Programs

Canada
➤ *Camp Inukshuk*—Day camp in Newmarket, Ontario, for children with speech/language/communication issues: www.campinukshuk.com—(905) 954-1312.
➤ *Talking About Fun*—Summer day camp in London, Ontario, for children with speech and language issues: www.londonspeech.com.

United Kingdom
➤ *Christopher Place*—Summer camp in London for children with speech and language concerns: www.speech-lang.org.uk.

State-by-state camp guide adapted from *Special Camps Edition* of *The Apraxia-KIDS Newsletter*, edited by Dawn Klein (Volume 12, Number 1, January/February 2011). The list may be accessed at: www.apraxia-kids.org/site/c.chKMI0PIIsE/b.980831/apps/s/content.asp?ct=9119319. Reproduced with the permission of the Childhood Apraxia of Speech Association of North America.

Speech & Language Milestones

I don't want to make you feel worse by introducing you to the "typically speaking child." But I do want to present you with some facts. Read over these charts quickly, without putting much thought into it. Make a little tick mark next to the milestones your child has reached. Look at this as a quick assessment tool from your own perspective.

Keep in mind, these charts are just guidelines to development. Please don't get too "hung up" in believing that these are the absolute way things must go. No two children develop at the same rate. These charts are here for your reference, so you can see where your child meets, exceeds, or falls behind in terms of what typically developing kiddos often experience.

Birth to 3 months
- ➤ Reacts to sudden noises by crying or jerking limbs (moro reflex)
- ➤ "Knows" familiar objects (pacifier, bottle, breast) and people (parents & siblings)
- ➤ Watches objects with great interest
- ➤ Has a different type of cry for hunger vs. pain vs. boredom
- ➤ Begins to coo and make prolonged vowel sounds—"ahh"

3—6 months
- ➤ Babbles—"ba-ba-ba"
- ➤ Laughs and shows pleasure, especially when favorite things are presented

- ➤ Looks for source of sound(s) by turning head
- ➤ Knows own name and will react when she hears it
- ➤ Voice is now louder for crying and babbling

Babbling and cooing are the same thing, right? Not quite. When an infant coos, she is practicing open-throat consonants—h, k, g, and vowel sounds such as *ah* and *oo*. When she starts to babble, at around 4 months, she will add consonants made with her palate and lips (*ta, na, da, ma, pa*).

6—9 months
- ➤ Understands simple words such as "yes" and "no"
- ➤ Will look at family members upon hearing them named
- ➤ Babbling becomes singsong in nature
- ➤ Sometimes sounds as though she is saying "mama" but doesn't understand the label yet
- ➤ Reacts to facial expressions of others; will attempt to mimic them
- ➤ Attempts peek-a-boo and bye-bye gestures
- ➤ Shakes head to indicate "no"
- ➤ Uses more sounds when babbling—*da, ba, ka, pa, ma, and wa*

Babbling gets more complicated the older the baby. "Complicated" can be defined in terms of more complex syllable structure and faster consonant-vowel transitions. Complex babbling is a direct result, according to one study, of direct nonverbal contact (smiles, kisses, and touches) from those who care for the baby (2003 study at Franklin & Marshall College). For more information about infant babbling, go to: www.vocaldevelopment.com (provides good information and audio clips).

9—12 months
- ➤ Enjoys imitating simple sounds
- ➤ Begins to say "mama" and "dada" with meaning
- ➤ Understands that words stand for objects
- ➤ May "dance" to music
- ➤ Imitates common animal sounds
- ➤ Will find a toy or object when asked
- ➤ Watches and imitates others

By 12 months, the typically developing baby is mixing consonants and vowels together and is able to say *dada, baba, mama, nana,* and *papa*. She can pronounce most of the vowel sounds and about half of the consonants of her native language. Keep in mind that babies are captivated by the people in their life and their names. That is why first words are often mama and dada. Secondly, babies find the actions that their caregivers do especially enthralling—these may very well become their next spoken words.

12—18 months

➤ Understands 50-75 words
➤ Uses 3-20 "real" words consistently, even if not said clearly
➤ Will accurately point to the right place when asked where something is located
➤ Points to a few body parts when asked (eyes, nose, ears)
➤ Will babble and use nonsense words while pointing to something of interest
➤ Follows simple commands: "Put this in the toy basket."
➤ Uses words such as *all-gone, more, down, done, mine, no, mama, daddy, gimme*

Around 15 months, children understand more and more words. They are most interested (and able to say) the words that are important and meaningful, such as family members' or pets' names and the words for familiar objects like cup and ball. They may be able to use some modifiers such as "hot," and "mine." Keep in mind that a typically developing child won't be able to say much more than one word at a time. When she says "cup," she is trying to communicate a more complex idea such as: "I want my cup," "Take my cup," or "Where is my cup?"

18 months—2 years

➤ Understands about 300 words
➤ Uses about 50 words, mostly nouns
➤ Uses real words most of the time; occasionally babbles and uses jargon
➤ Shakes head yes/no to questions
➤ Will show a change in tone when asking a question: *"More?"*
➤ Follows two-step commands: "Go to the laundry room and get your shoes."
➤ Begins to use some verbs (go) and adjectives (little)
➤ Two related words to make one word (allgone)
➤ Speech often difficult to understand
➤ Tells her name when asked (but may not be very clear)
➤ May start to ask, "What's that?" (What 'at?")
➤ Wants to hear same stories over and over; may join in when singing or reading

At this point, the typically developing child can make many speech sounds, but not always use them in the correct context. She might be able to say "shh" to her stuffed animals or while singing "The Wheels on the Bus" (the mommy on the bus goes "shh, shh, shh"), but is unable to say "shoe." Why is this? It's easier to produce strings of the same sound than it is to make a quick change from sh- to –oe to form "shoe." She may even substitute a "t" sound for the "sh-" simply because it's easier.

2—3 years

➤ Understands about 900 words
➤ Can say about 500 words
➤ Speech is understandable about half the time (maybe as much as 70%)
➤ Uses eye contact appropriately

➤ Voices frustrations more with words and less with whining and crying
➤ Wants to show you everything: "Look, Mommy!"
➤ Will correctly answer questions beginning with *who, where, what* ("What goes meow?")
➤ Understands prepositions (*in, on, under, on top of*)
➤ Begins to ask yes/no questions ("Is it night-night?")
➤ Talks to self aloud when playing
➤ Begins to use function words such as *the* and *is*
➤ May use past tense verbs (*walked, jumped*), but will use some incorrectly (*runned, sleeped*)
➤ May stutter when especially excited
➤ Consistently pronounces sounds of *m, n, p, d, b, f, h, y*

3—4 years

➤ Understands about 1,200 words
➤ Uses about 800 words
➤ Speech is understandable about 70-80% of the time
➤ Begins to use "*Is*" at the beginning of a question
➤ Asks lots of questions: *"Why?" "Who is...?"*
➤ Often will ask same question many times in a row
➤ Understands time concepts such as *now, later, morning, lunchtime*
➤ Uses plurals consistently: *books, plates, blocks*
➤ Uses *are* ("The boys *are* playing") and *and* ("Davin *and* Rhys are here")
➤ Initiates conversations by making comments and observations
➤ Consistent eye contact during conversations
➤ Produces beginning, middle, and ending sounds in words
➤ Consonant blends are still difficult (bl, st, fr, cr)
➤ Uses *k* and *g* sounds correctly
➤ May lisp on *s* sounds and distort the *r* sound

4—5 years

➤ Understands 2,500-2,800 words
➤ Uses 1,500-2,000 words
➤ Understandable about 80-90% of the time
➤ Uses pronouns correctly (*I, he, she, you, them*)
➤ Uses past, present, and future tenses of verbs correctly (run, runs, running, ran, will run)
➤ Uses irregular verbs (sleep=slept, eat=ate) and irregular nouns (child=children, woman=women)
➤ Explains events from the past in detail
➤ Can describe pictures with complete sentences
➤ Understands common opposite terms: *yummy/yucky, big/little, quiet/loud*
➤ Consonant blends still difficult
➤ May mispronounce *s, r, v, l,* and *j* sounds

5—7 years: Refinement
➤ Increases vocabulary by adding new words into spontaneous speech
➤ Refines pronunciation, sentence structure, attention span for listening
➤ Retells experiences in cohesive, sequential manner
➤ Participates in group discussion; knows when it's her turn to speak
➤ Begins to learn language relationships: opposites, synonyms, classifications/categories, & associations (*peanut butter/jelly, pen/paper*)

7 years to Adolescence
➤ Language system is functional and abstract
➤ Reading, writing, speaking, and listening skills are age-appropriate
➤ Understands and uses idioms (*pain in the neck, cut it out, wear me out*)
➤ Can pronounce multisyllabic words after practice
➤ Language of a child at this stage will mimic an adult's, but with greater simplicity
➤ Masters word relationships

Information adapted from *A Parent's Guide to Speech and Language Problems* by Debbie Feit (McGraw-Hill, 2007) and *Childhood Speech, Language & Listening Problems: What Every Parent Should Know* by Patricia McAleer Hamaguchi (Wiley, 2001).

For more insight into where your child is developmentally, check with your SLP or child's school for *"HELP...at Home"* hand-outs by VORT Corporation. They are handy little guides with checklists that will give you an *idea* of where your child's abilities are, developmentally speaking. They'll also give you lots of ideas on how you can move the process along at home. They are not meant to be diagnostic in nature.

Please remember that any given child may be at a different level of the communication skills continuum. For example, you may have a three-year-old who is not doing the things she is "supposed" to be doing at the three-year-old level. If so, find out where she really is, and work from there. Trying to force your child to perform at the level where experts say she should be is just frustrating for you both. See Chapter 9 for activities you can do at home.

Research on Reading Difficulties and Speech & Language Disorders

This appendix summarizes *some* of the research I've come across related to reading difficulties in children with diagnosed speech and language disorders. Keep in mind that I am not a statistician, nor am I a speech-language pathologist. Also keep in mind that most of the researchers did not specifically study children with Childhood Apraxia of Speech. Below the summaries is a key to help you decipher acronyms and terms.

1. Phoneme awareness in pre-reading kids with a speech disorder
(Study in *International Journal of Language and CommunicativeDisorders* (Hesketh et al., May–June 2007)

Who Was Studied? 42 kids, aged 4–4 ½ years with a speech disorder.

How They Did It: RCT in which the kids were divided into two smaller groups with two different interventions. Group 1 received a "phonological awareness" intervention and Group 2 received a "Language Stimulus" intervention. Both groups were measured on: 1) alliteration awareness; 2) phoneme isolation; 3) word segmentation; and 4) phoneme addition/deletion pre- and immediately post-intervention. Using Fisher's Exact Test to compare the outcome, these kids were determined to be "improved" or "not improved."

What They Found: Kids with Speech Disorders were considered to be "significantly improved" in all measures, except alliteration awareness. The more advanced tasks (segmentation and phoneme add/delete) showed just a small number of kids who improved. The major improvement was in phoneme isolation.

Why We Should Care: Some of the kids weren't cognitively ready for the more advanced tests of phoneme awareness. Speech therapists can help kids work on these tasks.

2. Predictors of reading abilities in kids

(Study in *Journal of Learning Disabilities Research & Practice* (Smith et al., Nov. 2007)

Who Was Studied? Reading disabled kids at the beginning of kindergarten and again just before they entered 1st grade.

How They Did It: Kids were measured on knowledge of the alphabet, phonological awareness, and rapid naming skills in a pre- and post-intervention study.

What They Found: Before kindergarten, the kids with reading disabilities were easily distinguished from kids who did not have a reading disorder by their performance on letter knowledge, phonological awareness, and rapid naming skills. After kindergarten (post-intervention), researchers found that only phonological awareness remained a challenge.

Why We Should Care: Kids need a baseline assessment of reading skills, which will help identify kids at-risk. Early skills need to be taught and reinforced regularly.

3. Auditory processing & language impairment and reading disorders

(Study in *Speech Language and Hearing Research* (Sharma, Purdy & Kelly, 2009)

Who Was Studied? 68 kids suspected of auditory processing disorder with a nonverbal IQ of 80+.

How They Did It: Using the Frequent Pattern Test (FPT), these kids were assessed using auditory, language, reading, and attention/memory measures.

What They Found: 72 percent of the kids had an auditory processing disorder based on these test results. 47 percent had difficulty with auditory processing, a language impairment, and a reading disorder—which might make one question whether these disorders could be grouped into one syndrome.

Why We Should Care: Kids with auditory processing disorder often have a language impairment and a reading disability. Attention and memory may be linked. More studies are needed.

4. Speech perception in kids with speech output disorders

(Study in *Clinical Linguistics & Phonetics* (Nijland, March 2009)

Who Was Studied? Three groups of kids: one with CAS, another with phonological disorders, and a third group of kids with both CAS *and a* phonological disorder

How They Did It: Various perception tests were given to the kids in the three groups. Perception tests included: nonword auditory discrimination, word rhyming, categorical classification, and discrimination.

What They Found: Kids with phonological disorder only showed difficulty with higher-order perception problems and kids with CAS showed problems with both high- and low-order perception problems. See notes for definition and examples of high- and low-order perception.

Why We Should Care: If kids with CAS have trouble with low-order perception, this may affect the higher-order ones that are in development.

5. Oral reading fluency in kids with speech (SI) or language impairments (LI)
(Study in *Journal of Learning Disabilities* (Puranik et al., 2008)

Who Was Studied? A total of 1,991 kids with SI or LI. 1,388 of them had a Speech Impairment. 603 of them had a Language Impairment. Same group of kids followed from 1st through 3rd grade.

How They Did It: Longitudinal study in which kids were divided into two groups: 1) Speech Impairment Group, further divided into "resolved" or "persistent; as was 2) Language Impairment Group.

What They Found: A large proportion of kids with SI or LI did not meet grade-level fluency goals. Kids with SI performed better than those with LI. The lowest performing kids were those who were originally diagnosed with SI or LI and had it changed to a learning disability later. Not all kids will go on to have reading fluency issues, but those who carry the "persistent" SI or LI label often do.

Why We Should Care: Identify, monitor, and address reading fluency issues early. Those kids who were considered "resolved" at age 5 to 6 years were not at risk for developing reading difficulties; some issues did resurface once they began writing and oral reporting.

Definitions You May Find Helpful in Understanding the Studies

➤ **Higher-level Knowledge:** The ability to take apart and put words back together based on sound patterns. For example, with rhyming words like cat, bat, mat, sat, pat, kids recognize a pattern and can add a letter to the beginning of the "___ at" pattern to make a new word. So, if a kid had a higher-level perception problem, he or she wouldn't be able to do this well—or at all. (As communicated by Ruth Stoeckel, CCC-SLP, Ph.D.)

➤ **Language Impairment (LI):** A problem related to the form, content, or use of language (grammar, syntax, symantics, vocabulary, and pragmatics). Can affect gestures (as in American Sign Language) as well as spoken words. Examples of a LI can range from *1) articulation problems* such as a lisp or problems with just a few sounds to *2) phonological problems* (a problem in sound substitutions, and maybe *3) motor speech problems* such as CAS and dysarthria. If kids have a severe speech issue, it's likely they have multiple language problems.

➤ **Low-level Perception Problem:** Best described as one's basic ability to perceive small changes in sounds. It also has to do with how we move our articulators (small muscles and structures involved in speech—tongue, palate, teeth) to maintain a certain sound. For example, a child with a low-level perception problem may have trouble producing and perceiving the /l/ sound, but can identify when an adult does it correctly. Rhonda Banford, CCC-SLP, explains: "Kids with CAS may not notice when they produce speech inaccurately, because of perceptual problems. The inaccuracy may come from an inability to produce correct motor movements themselves, or motor movements that are correctly targeting incorrect words. Both scenarios can occur. As for the latter, the child may say "boot" and fully intend to say 'boot,' when, in fact, the correct word is 'book.'"

➤ **"Persistent"** can be defined as carrying the SI or LI diagnosis throughout all grade levels. Persistent is a descriptive term and not diagnostic.

➤ **RCT:** Randomized Control Study. There was a group receiving the treatment that was being studied, and a control group that did not receive the treatment (for comparison purposes). Children were randomly assigned to either the treatment or control group.

➤ **Speech Impairment (SI)/Sound System Disorder:** A problem with *how* things are said. If you remember back to Chapter 4, we talked about ASHA's current definition of CAS relating to just the time-space (spatiotemporal) sequencing of movements for sound production. ASHA acknowledges that CAS is likely related to a deficit in phonological and literacy skills as well. It's likely that CAS falls under this category.

My interpretation of these studies does not imply definitive conclusions. I urge you to seek out the studies yourself should you question the specific measures, conditions, and conclusions. This appendix is only meant to be a *summary* of the small number of research-based articles I had available at the time.

Appendix F

. . . . .

Glossary

. . . . .

Accommodation: A change made in the learning environment to help a student compensate for the effects of a disability, thereby leveling the playing field. Examples include extra time to complete a test or seating closer to the teacher. Accommodations do not change the content of what the student is expected to learn, in contrast to modifications.

ADHD: Attention deficit hyperactivity disorder. A common childhood neurological disorder in which a child has difficulty with attention, impulsivity, distractibility, and sometimes hyperactivity. When the disorder occurs without hyperactivity, may be referred to as ADD.

Anxiety: As a psychological condition, an anxiety disorder is an overwhelming sense of dread or worry that affects daily life. *Some* anxiety in life is normal and should not be confused with an anxiety disorder. Children with CAS may experience heightened levels of anxiety when asked to speak in uncertain or new situations, or when the phrase is too demanding.

Apraxia: A disorder characterized by difficulties planning movements. Someone with apraxia of speech has difficulties planning the movements needed for speech. In the U.S. the most accepted term for apraxia of speech in children is Childhood Apraxia of Speech.

Articulation: The ability to form speech sounds correctly and clearly. Sometimes abbreviated as "artic."

Articulators: The articulators for speech production are primarily the jaw, lips, and tongue.

Autism Spectrum Disorder (ASD): A developmental disorder that appears in the first three years of life and results in difficulties in social and communication skills and unusual or restricted interests.

Babbling: Can be referred to as pre-speech. It consists of relatively long strings of syllables such as ba-ba-ba, ah-ah-ah, or ee-ee-ee, or combinations of these sounds that may be used communicatively, or as solo sound-play. *See also* Conversational Babble.

Broca's Area: A part of the brain named for Pierre Paul Broca, a French physician who reported language impairments in two of his patients after an injury to the posterior inferior frontal gyrus of the brain. These two patients lost the ability to speak after their injuries, leading researchers to conclude that this area is likely responsible for speech production.

(C)APD: An acronym which stands for central auditory processing disorder. Kids who struggle with APD have a hard time organizing the information they hear receptively, and their speech is often affected. The jury is still out as to whether condition affects the central nervous system. Sometimes you will find that the disorder is referred to as "just" auditory processing disorder (APD).

CCC: Certificate of Clinical Competence, certification from the American Speech-Language-Hearing Association that a speech-language pathologist has completed a rigorous professional program including master's degree work from an accredited program and extensive supervised practice, and has also passed a national certification examination.

Comorbid, Co-occuring, or Concomitant: Two or more medical or educational conditions that exist together, although typically independent of one another.

Conversational Babble: Conversation in which tone, eye contact, and gesture strongly resemble those used in adult conversational interactions. *See also* Babbling and Expressive Jargon.

Critical Period: A period in development during which certain events must take place if they are to take place at all.

Cued Speech: A mode of communication in which hand shapes placed on the face are used to represent the sounds of a spoken language. Cueing allows users who are deaf, hard of hearing, or who have language/communication disorders to access the basic, fundamental properties of spoken languages through the use of sight.

Dysarthria: Refers to a group of motor speech disorders that are caused by central or peripheral nervous system damage that results in muscle tone differences that cause weakness, paralysis, or incoordination of the speech muscles. Dysarthria may affect respiration, phonation/voicing, articulation, and resonance.

Dyspraxia: An older term that may be used in place of apraxia. Dyspraxia can be translated to mean "difficult" (dys) "planned motor movement" (praxis).

Expressive Jargon: Babbling consisting of strings of sounds uttered with a variety of stress and intonation patterns. *See also* Conversational Babble.

Expressive Language: The use of speech, gestures, text, or other communication systems to communicate with others.

IDEA: The Individuals with Disabilities Education Act, a federal law in the United States that governs the provision of special education to qualifying children with disabilities, ages birth to 21. The law requires the provision of a free, appropriate public education in the *least restrictive environment*.

IEP: Individualized Education Program, the document setting out prescribed goals, services, educational setting, and other details related to the education of students with disabilities ages 3 to 21 under *IDEA*. The IEP document is jointly developed by teachers, therapists, parents at an IEP meeting and revised at least annually.

IFSP: Individualized Family Service Plan, the document setting out agreed-upon objectives, goals, and services for infants and toddlers with disabilities (ages birth through age two) who are receiving early intervention.

Jargon: Strings of unintelligible speech sounds produced with the intonation pattern of adult speech.

Language: A socially shared code or conventional system for representing concepts through the use of arbitrary symbols and rule-governed combinations of those symbols.

Learning Disability: A condition that results in difficulties learning in one or more specific areas (such as reading or math) that would not be expected based on the individual's overall intellectual abilities. That is, the child's performance in one or more areas of learning is notably lower than in other areas of learning.

Least Restrictive Environment: The requirement under IDEA that a child who is receiving special education services must be educated to the maximum extent possible in the regular education environment while still achieving the goals in his IEP.

Loudness: The volume of our voice from quiet to loud. You've no doubt noticed voices that "carry well." That would be an example of loudness combined with good articulation resulting in projection.

Motor Cortex: The portion of the brain's frontal cortex that plans, controls, and executes voluntary motor movements.

Motor Planning/Programming: In a speech-language pathology sense, motor planning/programming refers to the formation of a spatial (space) and temporal (time) strategy for producing a sequence of speech sounds. The "space" is within the brain, which orchestrates where the articulators need to be in order to sequence a desired string of sounds. Children with CAS have a disruption in learning and controlling the motor planning/programming process of speech.

Multidisciplinary Treatment Team: A group of professionals such as a speech-language pathologist, an occupational therapist, a physical therapist, an educator, a psychologist, and perhaps a doctor or nurse who pool their expertise to arrive at a diagnosis or treatment plan for a child. An evaluation completed by such a team can result in a more complete understanding and diagnosis of a child's strengths, weaknesses, and needs.

Neurobehavioral disorders: Behavioral problems associated with brain disorders.

Neuromuscular: Pertaining to the brain, nerves, and muscles.

Phonics: The correspondence between letters and the sounds they make. For example, the sound /k/ can be represented by *c, k, ck, ch,* or *q* spellings. Phonics also involves teaching the blending of sounds to produce approximate pronunciations of unknown words.

Phonological: Relates to the scientific study of phonology, which is concerned with the sound structures of languages.

Phonological Disorder: A range of developmental communication disorders in which sound production is affected. *See also* Speech Sound Disorder.

Phonology: The language rules that control speech sound use.

Pitch: Just as in music, the pitch of one's voice can be high or low, or in between.

Pragmatics: The rules for the use of language in social context, and in conversation, or the study of these rules.

Prosody (intonation): "The melody of speech," including syllable stress, intonation, inflection.

Rate: Refers to the overall speed at which we speak.

Receptive Language: Language comprehension; the ability to understand others' spoken or written messages or gestures.

Resolved Apraxia: A term applied to a child whose previous concerns regarding Childhood Apraxia of Speech have improved to the point that they no longer affect learning, social relationships, and general functioning. Each child resolves in his own unique time and manner. Also known as "recovering apraxia" or "resolving apraxia."

Retention: The ability to maintain a skill or information over time. *Grade retention* refers to "being held back"[in a grade level] due to the inability to master key academic skills.

Semantics: A Greek word meaning "the study of meaning." This scientific discipline is often concerned with studying the meaning of words, phrases, signs, and symbols.

Speech: The neuromuscular process of producing voice and sounds and combining them in words to communicate.

Speech or Language Impairment: One of the disability categories listed in IDEA as qualifying a child for special education services such as speech. It is defined as "a communication disorder such as stuttering, impaired articulation, language impairment, or a voice impairment that adversely affects a child's educational performance."

Speech Sound Disorder: Some professionals prefer to use the term "speech sound disorder" over phonological disorder. The reason is that the term "phonological" is so closely linked with language and reading. Calling it a "speech sound disorder" helps distinguish the two. *See also* Phonological Disorder.

Stress: Refers to the emphasis (stress) placed on certain syllables of words.

Syntactic: Relating to the rules of syntax or grammar, including the grammatical arrangement of words and phrases into sentences.

Transfer: The ability to generalize a skill to other contexts; to use a skill learned in one setting or situation in another setting or situation.

Vocal Quality: Refers to the "smoothness" of voice—describing whether it is harsh or hoarse, smooth or gravelly. Resonance also affects vocal quality (e.g., "nasal" with too much sound coming from the nose, or "denasal," in which the person sounds as if he has a cold).

Wernicke's Area: Originally identified by the Polish-German neurologist/psychiatrist, Carl Wernicke, this is the area of the brain necessary for speech comprehension. It is located in the posterior (back) section of the superior temporal gyrus in the left (dominant) cerebral hemisphere.

Advisory Board

The following individuals provided review and feedback on assigned chapters of the book. They provided many suggestions and ideas from which I made decisions about what to include in the book. These folks definitely helped round out the vast amount of information included in this book. For it is not only a village that helps raise our children, but a village of professionals who care deeply about children.

I am so very grateful to all of these individuals for the unique expertise, experience, and value that they have added to this book, as well as to the lives of *all* children they touch—both with and without apraxia. Although these highly qualified and diverse individuals have provided feedback for this book, as the author, I am responsible for the interpretation of provided feedback.

Diane Bahr, M.S., CCC-SLP, CIMI, is a certified speech-language pathologist and infant massage instructor in private practice. She has practiced speech-language pathology since 1980 and has been a feeding therapist since 1983. Her experiences include teaching graduate, undergraduate, and continuing education courses; working with children and adults who exhibit a variety of speech, language, feeding, and swallowing disorders; and publishing/presenting information and research on oral motor function, assessment, and treatment. She is the author of the textbook *Oral Motor Assessment and Treatment: Ages and Stages* (Allyn & Bacon, 2001) and a book for parents entitled *Nobody Ever Told Me (or My Mother) That!: Everything from Bottles and Breathing to Healthy Speech Development* (Sensory World, 2010).

Rhonda J. Banford, M.A.T., CCC-SLP, is a certified speech-language pathologist and early childhood special educator in private practice in Ballwin, MO. She is currently working toward certification in the field of orofacial myology. While working for her local school district as a preschool speech and language diagnostician, she became concerned about the best way to address therapy with the students who had unintelligible speech but good receptive language. She noticed that in most preschool classrooms, the students did far more listening than speaking. As such, she designed and implemented a successful intensive speech classroom for unintelligible preschoolers, many of whom demonstrated Childhood Apraxia of Speech and related disorders. She continues to provide similar services to private clients through a camp program in the summer months. She also sees clients privately and particularly enjoys working with children who exhibit CAS. Her website is www.gotospeech.com, and she can be reached at rjb.slp@charter.net.

Lisa Circelli, M.Ed., received her B.S. in ELED with a specialization in Early Childhood from Western Illinois University in 1995 and her M.Ed. in Reading and Literacy from Benedictine University in 2006. Lisa has worked in the field of education for the past 16 years. Currently Lisa is employed with KCSEC/Oswego 308 School District, as an Early Childhood Teacher. Lisa has worked with children in many different capacities, including in regular education settings from kindergarten to second grade, and special education settings from Pre-K through eighth grade. Although Lisa has had a few students with CAS, she did not know a lot about CAS until she worked with the children in the classroom. Lisa also learned about CAS from her students' parents and from her reading, but she has found that children are the best teachers.

Morgan Holubetz, M.S., CCC-SLP/L, received her B.S. in Speech-Language Pathology at Illinois State University in 2003 and her M.S. in Speech-Language Pathology at Illinois State University in 2005. She has been working as a speech-language pathologist for 6 years. She is currently employed by Edward Hospital in Naperville, IL. She has worked with a handful of students with CAS throughout the years. Although she learned about CAS in school, most of her knowledge and training has been on the job. When she first started working with children with CAS, there weren't many resources for her to go to. She says, "I think this book is a tremendous resource for parents, speech-language pathologists, and educators of all types. I am honored to have been selected to review this book and I look forward to adding it to my collection."

Amy Moll is a stay-at-home mom of two daughters. She volunteers her time assisting at their school library, helping out in the classroom and lunchroom, leading a Girl Scout troop, and supporting various events around the campus. Her younger daughter was diagnosed with Childhood Apraxia of Speech at around age three, so she makes frequent trips to and from speech therapy as well. Amy has a bachelor's degree in Analytical Finance from Wake Forest University. Prior to starting a family, she worked in the consulting and IT fields for the healthcare, travel, and public relations industries.

Amy is a hobby-level photographer and enjoys spending time with friends and family. She, her husband, and daughters reside outside of St. Louis, MO.

Teri Kaminski Peterson, M.S., CCC-SLP, is a board-certified speech pathologist holding the Certificate of Clinical Competence. She is the author of *The Big Book of Exlamations!* Graduating with a master's degree from Minnesota State University Moorhead, formerly Moorhead State University, she remains active in private practice in Minnesota.

Index

About the Author

Leslie Lindsay was formerly a Child and Adolescent Psychiatric nurse at the Mayo Clinic. She attended the University of Missouri-Columbia and earned a B.S.N. from the Sinclair School of Nursing with a minor in psychology. She and her family, including a daughter with CAS, live in suburban Chicago, along with their Bassett hound Sally. An active school volunteer and CAS advocate, she writes about a range of parenting issues on her blog and website, www.leslie4kids.wordpress.com.